Arthritis

The Botanical Solution

Nature's Answer to
Rheumatoid Arthritis, Osteoarthritis, Gout
and Other Forms of Arthritis

By Casey Adams, Ph.D.

Arthritis—The Botanical Solution: Nature's Answer to Rheumatoid
    Arthritis, Osteoarthritis, Gout and Other Forms of Arthritis
Copyright © 2009 Casey Adams
SACRED EARTH PUBLISHING
Wilmington, Delaware
http://www.sacredearthpublishers.com
All rights reserved.
Printed in USA
Front cover art by Sebastian Kaulitzki
Back cover "Vitruvian Man" and notes by Leonardo da Vinci, est. 1487
Original illustrations by Virginia Callow

The information provided in this book is for educational and scientific research purposes only. The information is not medical advice and is not a substitute for medical care or professional health advice. A medical practitioner or other expert should be consulted prior to any significant change in diet, sun exposure, exercise or any other lifestyle change. There shall be neither liability nor responsibility should the information provided in this book be used in any manner other than for the purposes of education and scientific research.

Publishers Cataloging in Publication Data
Adams, Casey
Arthritis—The Botanical Solution: Nature's Answer to Rheumatoid
    Arthritis, Osteoarthritis, Gout and Other Forms of Arthritis
First Edition
1.   Health. 2. Medicine
    Bibliography and References; Index

Library of Congress Control Number: 2009936479

ISBN 978-0-9816045-9-6

For those dedicated to recognizing nature's healing forces—
now and in the past

Table of Contents

Introduction

Arthritis is probably one of the oldest remaining medical mysteries. For thousands of years, humans have dealt with the crippling joint disease called osteoarthritis, and to a lesser degree, rheumatic arthritis, gout and other forms of arthritis. Rheumatoid arthritis appears to be a more modern disease—one that seems to have gradually increased in incidence over the last thousand years with the rise of the industrial era. More recently, over the past century, osteoarthritis, rheumatoid arthritis, gout, lupus and other arthritis forms have been dramatically on the rise.

Billions of dollars have been invested into arthritis research to find safe treatments that work for more than a few hours, days or weeks. Although there have been some commendable efforts and discoveries over the last century in understanding the mechanisms of arthritis and inflammation, leading to pain-relieving, inflammation-reducing drugs, these efforts have yet to disclose the precise causes and solutions to arthritis—nor have they resulted in treatments that curtail and reverse the disease in a satisfactory manner.

This does not mean we *cannot* know the causes and solutions to this range of disorders. It may mean, however, that perhaps we are looking at them with the wrong perspective.

Consider the *stereogram*. The stereogram is an image that contains another, 'hidden' image inside of it. The 'hidden' image inside the more obvious image can certainly be seen. Yet it blends into the more obvious image in such a way that we have to change our perspective in order to perceive it. For some, this might mean squinting at the image. For others, it might mean changing the light or stepping away from the image. Still others will need to walk away and come back with a new 'fresh' approach to the image. Whatever the strategy, perceiving the 'hidden' image requires continually looking at the entire image with a new perspective.

I believe that the causes and solutions for arthritis are much like the stereogram. The data are right in front of us, available for anyone to see. However, in order to perceive the conclusion and truly understand the causes and solutions to arthritis, we have to clear out the noise and look at the evidence with a new perspective.

Hopefully this book will help provide this perspective.

—*Casey Adams*, September 28, 2009, cadams@realnaturalhealth.com.

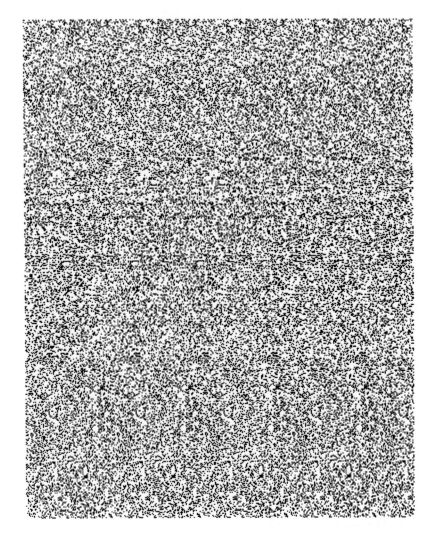

Stereogram: Can you see the 3-D teapot inside the image?

Chapter One

What is Arthritis?

Arthritis is a group of sometimes-debilitating diseases characterized by inflammation, stiffness, pain, restricted motion, nodules and tenderness within and around the joints.

The word 'arthritis' is derived from the Greek word *"anthron"* meaning "joint" and the Latin word *"itis"* meaning "inflammation." In other words, arthritis literally means "joint inflammation."

According to a review of research by the Arthritis Foundation (2008), about 46 million adults have been diagnosed by a doctor that they have some form of arthritis, lupus or fibromyalgia. Approximately 21% of adults—one in five—have been diagnosed with some form of arthritis. Two out of three of those diagnosed are under 65 years of age. About half of all adults over 65 years old have reported receiving an arthritis diagnosis.

Young people also get arthritis. About 300,000 youngsters (under the age of 18) are estimated to have juvenile arthritis in the U.S.

Arthritis is now the second-most diagnosed illness in the United States. Arthritis handicaps more people than cancer, cardiovascular disease or diabetes. About three quarters of a million people are hospitalized each year due to arthritis, and close to ten thousand die each year due to complications of arthritis.

About 19 million people have limited activity due to arthritis. It is estimated that about 40% of those with arthritis have activity limitations in the work place. This means that arthritis affects employer productivity as well. An activity limitation is considered present when there is a restriction of a particular range of physical movement. One sufferer might not be able to reach up and grab something from a shelf. Another might not be able to twist a screwdriver. Still another may not be able to bend down and pick up something off the floor.

About 80% of us know someone with debilitating arthritis.

More than one hundred different diseases are defined as forms of arthritis. While most involve inflammation of the joints, bones or associated ligaments and tendons, a few of them do not involve inflammation *per se.*

There are also several general characterizations of arthritis. Many forms of arthritis are considered *degenerative*—meaning they worsen with time and use. Generally speaking, just about any form of arthritis can be degenerative if it is chronic. Without corrective measures, whatever is causing the damage to the cartilage and joints will continue, and the resulting joint damage will worsen.

Several types of arthritis are also called rheumatoid. Because rheumatism in the strict sense refers to chronic, degenerating inflammation, we might also be able to call just about every form of arthritis rheumatoid. However, in modern medical pathology, rheumatoid arthritis is referred to as an infectious or spreading form of arthritis, where other tissues outside the joints are also infected. As we will discuss in greater detail, rheumatoid arthritis is often related to an infection or a toxin that has to be mitigated in order to curb the infiltration of the cartilage and synovial tissues.

General Symptoms

There are many symptoms of arthritis, depending of course on the type and cause. *(One's health professional should always be consulted before concluding any self-diagnosis.)* These include:

Pain: Around or within the joints. This can be anything from dull aching pain to acute, sharp pain. This pain is often disassociated with any particular event. For example, if we have just run ten miles, our joints may be painful for good reason. This may not necessarily mean we have arthritis. Different types of arthritic pain can worsen with movement or non-movement. If it will aches with no conceivable cause, arthritis might be the reason.

Stiffness: When rotating or otherwise moving a joint or joints. This can occur upon waking or after sitting for some time, although it is also normal to feel stiff after sitting or lying in the same position for an extended period (as this reduces local circulation). If the stiffness continues even after stretching and walking around, then arthritis may be the cause.

Redness: Pink or red color around our moving appendages. A noticeable red area without a discernable cause could indicate deepset inflammation. This means that the immune system has launched a mission intended to repair some kind of damage in the region. If we don't remember banging it, we might suspect arthritis.

Puffiness: Swelling on or around joints. This will usually accompany the redness, but sometimes not. A puffy non-red area is actually more serious than a red puffy area. Non-red puffiness indicates some damage to tissue or joints that is not being actively addressed by the blood and immune system. This scenario often results in a slower healing and repair process.

Tenderness: Touching can create the sensation of 'pins and needles' or it can throb with our heart beat—meaning a more active site of injury and inflammation.

Nodules: Appearing around or on top of joints or other body parts. These can be as small as a few millimeters, or larger than the joint itself. Usually the nodules are rubbery but semi-hard, as they are likely filled with fibrinoid necrosis—a mix of fibrin, protein and collagen. If the nodule is soft, spongy, painless and disassociates with (or "floats" over) the underlying tissues when massaged, then it may be a lipoma—a small deposit of fat surrounded by tissue. Nodules are often tender. Lipomas will have little or no feeling.

Warmth or heat: Arthritic joints may feel warm or even hot to the touch when compared to other body parts. Sometimes joints will be warm (or even ache) when we have an active flu or cold infection too. Unless we have a fever otherwise, the joint is inflamed.

Numbness: Part of the body is numb without apparent cause. Numbness after sitting on a limb for too long is normal: Numbness during movement or not. If the numbness occurs around our joints even after rubbing and movement, we should suspect arthritis.

Accompanying Signs

A number of other conditions can accompany arthritis. These might not indicate arthritis in themselves, but they can accompany other symptoms:

Cold hands or feet: If the feet or hands become colder than the rest of the body, this indicates a lack of circulation or a blockage of blood flow.

Chronic fatigue: Being tired upon waking, even after receiving a good night's sleep. Also feeling lethargic, purposeless, and exhausted for no good reason should be investigated.

Irritable bowels: The pain and inflammation associated with arthritis can also be accompanied by cramping, gas and indigestion.

Low-back pain: Back pain can come from a variety of issues related to vertebral discs, the pelvis, vertebral ligament weaknesses, and abdominal imbalances. However, arthritis can also cause low-back pain.

A Little Anatomy: The Joints

We should probably review some basic anatomy applicable to arthritis before we go any further. Surrounding and supporting our joints are various *muscles*. Connecting the muscles to the bones and joints are a series of *ligaments*. Depending upon the joint region and overall conditioning, the ligaments can range from flexible to thick and protective. Attached to the ligaments are *tendons*, which connect the joints with the ligaments and surrounding muscles. Within the ligaments lies a tissue structure called the *synovial membrane*. This protective membrane forms the outer layer of the *joint capsule*. The synovial membrane cells produce a clear, sticky substance called the *synovial fluid*—a substance that fills the inside of the joint capsule.

The synovial fluid has a runny gelatinous texture. It contains *hyaluronic acid*, fatty acids, enzymes (*collagenases* and *proteinases*), and *lubricin*. The combination of hyaluronic acid and lubricin—together with several lipids—reduce friction. The lubricin seems to create a thin barrier between moving surfaces. This barrier repels opposite chondral surfaces, while hyaluronic acid provides a protective layer between them.

Separating the synovial fluid, and lining the bone ends that meet in the joint—and providing their central pivot surface between bones—is the *articular cartilage*. This is also often called *hyaline cartilage* because it contains hyaline. This is not perfectly accurate, however, because articular cartilage is specific to joints, while other types of cartilage also contain hyaline. Articular cartilage is a slippery, smooth, white, glistening, and thin (usually not more than 6 millimeters) membrane covering the bony ends around the joints. The articular cartilage is made up of a complex of hyaline, collagen, elastin and proteoglycans such as chondroitin sulfate. Collagen is a fibrous protein that provides the strength, and tensility, while elastin provides elasticity. The cartilage absorbs shock and provides lubrication for the movement of the joint.

As hinted at, there are several other types of cartilage located throughout the body. Cartilage is critically important to the body and provides a number of purposes. Cartilage makes up the tissues of our nostrils, our ears, the discs in our vertebrae, epiglottis, larynx and trachea—and many other tissues in between. The main types of cartilage include *costal cartilage. temporary cartilage, articular cartilage* and *elastic cartilage.* Costal, temporary and articular cartilage are all hyaline cartilages. These are all noted for their smooth, elastic yet tough texture, allowing for bending and movement without breaking.

Articular cartilage cells are not directly vascularized. In other words, they do not receive direct blood flow. Rather, the cells are branched and structured to allow tiny canals—fed by the *canaliculi* emerging from the bone marrow—through which blood and nutrients can seep. However, this feeding requires pressurization from the cartilage space—created by the movement or compression onto the cartilage. This is why weight-bearing exercise is so important to the health of the joint.

With raw nutrients delivered by these canals, the cells of the cartilage—called *chondrocytes*—weave together a mixture of collagen, elastin and proteoglycans. This weave is like a netting of sorts. It provides strength yet tensility, and in the case of articular cartilage, the slipperiness to allow the joints to glide against each other. This does not mean that the cartilage on each joint actually touches, however. Between the two cartilage (or *chondral regions*) covering each bone within a joint lies a thin layer and cushion of synovial fluid. This adds additional viscosity and glide to joint motion.

A layer of fat cells may also accumulate around a joint. Joints also have other connective tissues. Surrounding the knee joint, for example, is a band of connective tissue called the *meniscus*. The two meniscus (or *semilunar fibrocartilage*) wrap around each side of the knee joint. The inside band is the *medial meniscus* and the band toward the outside is the *lateral meniscus*.

There are several types of joints:

Ball and socket	Shoulders, hips
Pivot	Neck, spinal column
Hinge	Elbows, knees, fingers, toes
Ellipsoidal	Wrists, ankles

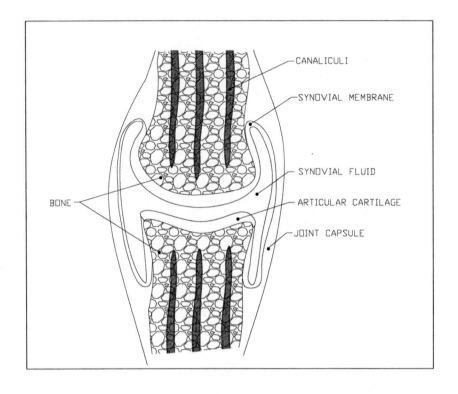

CANALICULI

SYNOVIAL MEMBRANE

SYNOVIAL FLUID

BONE

ARTICULAR CARTILAGE

JOINT CAPSULE

Osteoarthritis

This is by far the most common form of arthritis. This type of arthritis is considered degenerative, because there is a slow progression of destruction of the articular cartilage surrounding certain joints.

The fingers, wrists, elbows, shoulders, hips, knees, ankles, and the lumbar and cervical regions of the spine are most often the areas affected by osteoarthritis. These are also the parts of the body most used for weight-bearing work and tasks of precision.

Primary osteoarthritis

This is diagnosed when the cause is unknown and its occurrence is seemingly isolated. It often occurs either among weight-bearing joints or among the fingers. In other words, most health professionals do not understand why most people contract osteoarthritis. Some health professionals assume that osteoarthritis is caused by the wearing away of the cartilage over use and time. This is assumed because it is prevalent among the elderly and within joints bearing more of the body's weight and thus possibly subject to more trauma.

Even still, younger people also contract osteoarthritis. About 4% of young adults—from 18 to 24 years of age—contract obvious cases of primary osteoarthritis. In fact, in many of these cases, there are no symptoms of osteoarthritis—the diagnosis was made from an incidental x-ray or other diagnostic review. In other words, a lot more younger people may have osteoarthritis. With little or no obvious symptoms, it is hard to tell.

Meanwhile, about 85% of all adults in the U.S. between the ages of 75 and 79 are thought to have primary osteoarthritis. Between the genders, more men than women contract primary osteoarthritis before the age of 45. After the age of 55, more women than men contract primary osteoarthritis.

The wear-and-tear or incidental trauma hypothesis has been boosted by the skeletal findings of many archeological digs. Many remains thousands of years old have been found to have indications of osteoarthritis. Even many animals contract osteoarthritis. In fact, nearly every animal with a bony spine—including mammals, birds, amphibians, fish and even whales and dolphins can contract osteoarthritis—even though their contraction rates are far less than humans. A few animals that do not contract osteoarthritis include bats and sloths—both of which also spend a lot of time hanging upside down.

This does not mean that osteoarthritis is inevitable. As we will discuss, further investigations have determined that osteoarthritis is not necessarily caused by wear and tear. The cells that synthesize and put together the components of the cartilage develop some sort of abnormality that prevents them from continuing to build effective cartilage matrix.

We will discuss alternative cause theories in more depth later on.

Secondary osteoarthritis

This is generally considered to accompany another primary illness. Secondary osteoarthritis can follow Paget's disease, for example. In addition, secondary osteoarthritis is often diagnosed when it is preceded by repetitive motion injuries or other accidental traumas. Infections, stress, joint overload and other associated factors may also precede a diagnosis of secondary osteoarthritis.

The associations of acquired secondary osteoarthritis that have most been observed include: the contraction of another inflammatory disease; the deposit of crystals among the joints; a variety of metabolic disorders such as fibromyalgia; endocrine diseases related to the production of hormones; damage to osteocytes; blood leakage within a joint; or some type of bacterial or fungal infection. This form of arthritis is differentiated from rheumatoid arthritis most often because of the way it presents. In other words, the symptoms push the diagnosis. These become more obvious by comparing the identification charts shown with each arthritis type.

The pain and symptoms of osteoarthritis are usually within the region of the joints involved. There is little history of radiating or reflective pain. Osteoarthritis joint pain is often deep and achy. This often improves with rest. Movement will likely increase the deeper, aching pain. Stiffness can also bring about a 'pins and needles' pain, which can occur in the morning or after sitting for long periods. Because there are few if any nerve endings around the articular cartilage, when there is pain in osteoarthritis, some cartilage damage has already begun. While joint movement is recommended to keep circulation to the joint area, too much motion can also bring pain. Furthermore, too much weight-bearing movement while the joint is under duress may cause further damage.

Identifying Osteoarthritis

Osteoarthritis is not always recognizable or obvious in its early stages, as mentioned. Many people have it and continue to function normally—with few outward symptoms. However, early osteoarthritis will often be visible on x-rays as maligned joints. A few of the joints, such as fingers, thumbs, lower back, big toes, hips and knees may show the first symptoms of swelling. Pain usually begins in these areas, especially during and directly following exercise or work. Joint stiffness might follow sitting or waking, but the joints may also loosen up with 30 minutes of stretching, walking or other movement.

As the disease progresses, the joints may become unstable. The ligaments around the joints become weakened and stretched. This might cause the joint to crumble or falter. The hips may also become stiffer and more restricted. The affected joint will also become tender and painful to the touch.

Bony knobs or nodules can grow along the sides or otherwise near affected joints. These are called *Heberden's nodes*. They are usually hard, unmovable and often slightly red. They might grow to the size of a small marble.

Osteoarthritis frequently affects the lower spine, creating lower back pain. Usually this pain is fairly mild compared to disk problems or sacral problems. However, in more advanced stages, the abnormal growth of the vertebral joints may impinge upon nerves, cause numbness, and strange *referring pain* in different parts of the body. This may occur in the toes on one side, for example, and not the other.

Quick Chart for Identification of Osteoarthritis

Joints	Weight bearing: fingers, wrists, elbows, toes, hips, spine, knees, ankles
Regions	Asymmetrical and variable—joints on either side, often with joints that are more active or have greater weight bearing activity
First occurrence	Pain and swelling in one or several joints
Ongoing	Periodic worsening and resolving
Pain	Sharp, persistent, and piercing when moved
Movement	Joint stiffness in morning or after sitting, but usually loosens up within 30 minutes
Motion	Gradually more restrictive, frozen joints possible
Co-factors	Possible nerve compression, causing headaches, intestinal cramping and other problems
Appearance	Bony growths—Heberden's nodes may develop
Lab Tests	X-rays for abnormal joint formation

Progression of Osteoarthritis

A thinning of the articular cartilage is usually the first change to appear in osteoarthritis. This will narrow the joint and thicken the *subchondral bone*. Subchondral bones are bony plates that support the articular cartilage. Bony cysts may erupt as the plate thickens. Osteophytes may then grow out from the cartilage as a protective and inflammatory strategy. These create the bony protrusions we see in osteoarthritic patients.

As the articular cartilage thins, chondrocytes—the cells that make up the subchondral bone—begin to die and this opens up gaps within the cartilage. These gaps, or cracks in the cartilage may allow synovial fluid to leak through the cartilage and get into the joint tissue, creating a little sac or cyst within the bone—called *subchondral bone cysts*. As these cysts evolve, osteophytes can form around them, creating bone spurs. These spurs often appear as sharp, hard protrusions around the joint.

Around the cracks and the cysts, layers of fibrin will become implanted by the immune system. These will cause what is called *marrow fibrosis*, which is a narrowing of the bone marrow due to the build up of fibrin. This might be compared to atherosclerosis—the thickening of the artery wall caused by damage to artery walls. Unfortunately, marrow fibrosis will reduce the amount of circulation to the subchondral bone. This is part of the process for healing, as it reduces damage from toxins and infections and allows the site to be rebuilt. If this immune process is halted or encumbered, however, marrow fibrosis will eventually reduce the flow of nutrients and fluids to the chondrocytes, creating more damage.

The progressive degeneration of the articular cartilage generally leads subsequently to the thinning of the cartilage and the thickening of the subchondral bone. Once the subchondral bone is thickened and the cartilage thins, the joint becomes less mobile and more painful. This type of pain can be aching or sharp, depending upon the amount of weight bearing on the joint.

As the cartilage breaks down further, small pieces of the cartilage can be released into the synovial fluid within the joint capsule. This increases swelling and pain, as the inflammation process proceeds.

This thinning articular membrane causes a vicious cycle of damage. Unprotected subchondral bone begins to grind away within the joint. This can cause more subchondral bone surface to crack, allowing synovial fluid to leak into the subchondral bone tissue. This in turn causes more cysts, more fibrin and more thickening. This thickening in turn further thins and weakens the articular cartilage membrane.

Rheumatoid Arthritis

This type of arthritis is categorized as an autoimmune disease of chronic, recurring inflammation. The joints are inflamed symmetrically. In other words, the same joints on both sides of the body will be swollen and red, and quite possibly hot. The joints most affected include finger joints (metacarpophalangeals), elbows, ankles, shoulders and knees. The spinal column is sometimes affected by RA as well. Over time, RA can destroy the joints.

Typical occurrence takes place when a person reaches their 30s or 40s. RA has been occurring in about 1-2% of U.S. adults and is three times more likely to occur in women than men. Some reports indicate over two million people in the U.S. have been diagnosed with RA. This higher percentage among women is especially noticeable prior to menopause. Following the menopausal years, the occurrence for men and women roughly even out. While it will occur at any age, rheumatoid arthritis will often first appear between the ages of 25 and 50 years old.

While occurrence is often symmetrical, there is a great variance of where it will strike and how severe. Often the swelling and pain will increase dramatically for a while and then taper off significantly, only to re-emerge later. This periodic occurrence in RA outbreaks can be stimulated by a variety of factors. We will discuss some of the research around this later.

The cause of rheumatoid arthritis is officially considered unknown, but there have been a variety of relationships that have been observed by clinicians and researchers. These include possible genetic factors, immune system malfunction, various infectious agents, autoimmunity and others. About 70-80% of RA sufferers test positive for what is termed the *rheumatoid factor*. The rheumatoid factor is a unique immunoglobulin-antibody complex present in the blood and synovial membrane. The complex is often greater among IgM antibodies, but IgAs and IgGs are also usually present. The combination and placement of the antibodies is termed an *anti-idiotype*. It is interesting that RA factor is also found in many patients that do not have rheumatoid arthritis. RA factor has been found in significant numbers in diagnoses of lupus, systemic sclerosis, tuber-culosis, cirrhosis, pulmonary fibrosis, lepromatous leprosy, viral hepatitis and dermatomyositis. Some of these are significantly symptomatic of collagen-related vascular diseases.

Furthermore, as we will discuss more in detail, the likelihood of contracting RA is increased by the presence of certain genes. Still, by no means does having a particular allele (such as HLA-DR3 or HLA-DR1) guarantee one will contract RA.

While bacteria are not always found within the synovial fluid, there is reason to believe that many RA cases are connected with either a viral or a bacterial infection. Because the synovial mem-brane of an RA patient is often full of antimicrobial antibodies, cytokines and macrophages, the feasibility of microbial associations becomes more logical. In addition, RA patients often maintain high levels of virally infected B-cells in other locations around the body. Macrophages within the synovium also appear to be stimulated by the presence of some type of bacterial or toxic agent.

There are a variety of types of RA, depending upon the loca-tion of the body, the offending pathogen, and the progression of the disease. In about 10% of RA cases, nearly complete disability results.

How to Identify Rheumatoid Arthritis

There are a number of conditions that can cause joint inflam-mation. Therefore, establishing RA with certainty can be difficult. A physician will draw a synovial fluid sample to analyze for RA factor, and may also draw a tissue sample from a nodule to examine under a microscope. Erythrocyte sedimentation rate (ESR—a test of the red blood cell precipitation indicating inflammation) is increased in about 9 of 10 cases. Anemia is also often present.

RA will often begin suddenly in just one joint (on both sides) or several joints. Fingers, wrists, toes, hands, feet and elbows will likely become swollen first. The swelling will often be greatest after wak-ing or sitting for a long period.

Many RA patients also report increasing fatigue, dull, aching muscle pain, and even weight loss. A fever, especially during periods of inflammation, may be present.

The stiff joints will grow larger, and may show deformity after some time. They might also become frozen or stiff in the same position. Extending the joint may become difficult. Fingers can bend outward towards the pinky. Wrists can become swollen, and carpal tunnel syndrome may easily result from repetitive motion. Nodules may appear near the joints.

The inflammation can go up and down, creating periods of relief followed by periods of extreme pain and stiffness.

Worsening cases may result in inflammation of the blood vessels—called *vasculitis*. This can also damage nerves and cause sores on the legs. The lungs and heart may also be inflamed, creating breathing difficulty and chest pain.

Quick Chart for Identification of Rheumatoid Arthritis

Joints	Fingers, wrists, elbows, toes, others
Regions	Symmetrical—joints on both sides
First occurrence	Pain and swelling in one or several joints
Progression	Periodic resolution and then worsening
Pain	Dull, aching, worse after sleeping or resting
Movement	Joint stiffness in morning or after sitting, lasting more than one hour
Motion	Frozen joints
Co-factors	Fever during infection, nodules around joints
Appearance	Bending joints—fingers bent outward
Lab Tests	RA factor, nodule tissue, erythrocyte

Progression of Rheumatoid Arthritis

A thickening of the cells among the synovial membrane is often one of the first events in early RA. The membrane in a healthy person is usually about 2-3 cells thick. In an early RA patient, the membrane is often layered with 8-10 cells. This produces a thickening of the membrane—termed *hyperplasia*. The thickened membrane will often be filled with masT-cells and other immune system materials. The synovial membrane with hyperplasia is often termed a *pannus*.

With this thickening, the pannus will often creep into the articular cartilage. As this occurs, the cartilage will erode, and the bone adjacent to the cartilage will demineralize. Here the pannus may produce a substance called collagenase. This is considered the agent that erodes the articular cartilage.

Gradually the pannus also invades the joint capsule and sub-chondral bones. Fibrin collects within the spaces, and the joint begins to fuse. This thickening fusion is called *ankylosis*. Those bones around the joint also begin to be fused by the pannus invasion. As they fuse together, this is called *bony ankylosis*.

Alternatively and possibly concurrently, the T lymphocytes are stimulated within the cartilage tissue. This follows with the production of chondrocytes and lysomal enzymes, which eat away the cartilage further.

Rheumatoid arthritis produces a vastly modified synovial fluid. The fluid level will increase, become thicker, and full of protein and inflammatory cells.

RA also produces pronounced nodules, which are called rheumatoid nodules. These will often occur in on peripheral locations around the joint as well as over the joints. Often they are on regions that receive pressure, such as below the elbows, the shins and fingers. Sometimes they will appear internally, on areas such as around the heart, intestines, lungs, and neck. They are movable, rubbery and firm. They will often be tender as well. These nodules are made up of fibrin, proteins and broken down collagen, surrounded by lymphocytes, plasma and various immune cells.

Bone loss in RA will often occur adjacent and on each side of the joint, as the pannus invades the bone.

Spondyloarthropathy

This was considered a variant of rheumatoid arthritis, but now is considered an independent disease. Spondyloarthropathy includes a variety of diagnoses, including **ankylosing spondylitis, psoriatic arthritis, inflammatory bowel disease arthritis,** and **Reiter syndrome.**

In spondylarthropathy, there is rarely an RA factor present. Spondyloarthropathy often appears in the sacrum or vertebral (lower spine) region. There is also little of the symmetrical occurrence as evident in most RA cases. Here tendons and associated tissue systems will display inflammation and swelling. In addition, organs and other internal tissue systems may also become inflamed and painful.

Here is a summary of the main spondyloarthropathy diseases:

Psoriatic Spondylitis

About 7% of *psoriasis* sufferers will also develop this form of inflammatory arthritis. Psoriasis is a skin condition that results in rashes and reddened scales and patches. Psoriasis sufferers can also have thickened nails. Many psoriasis arthritis sufferers will usually have joint inflammation in the fingers and toes. Other joints may also become infected. Many cases are fairly mild and do not progress into the extreme symptoms RA sufferers can experience— where the joints can become mutilated and fused. This is also because there are often less joints involved in psoriasis arthritis.

Ankylosing spondylitis

This disease is primarily focused upon the lower vertebral column and the joints around the sacrum. About a third of ankylosing spondylitis patients will experience metabolic changes and systemic symptoms to various organs. About 40% experience an inflammatory eye disease called *iridocyclitis*. Peripheral effects can also result, producing numbing and painful affects in the legs and feet.

Ankylosing sponylitis will often begin in the sacrum and will spread up the spine through the vertebral bones and discs. The disease often begins during younger years, from ages 20 to 40 years old, and continues to develop with aging. Three times more men contract it than women do. Occurrence is frequent within families, indicating either a genetic relationship, or an association with diet or other lifestyle factors.

The bone destruction will often result in a fusing (joining) of multiple vertebrae. This restricts bending and twisting significantly. Vertebrae may also deform, causing nerves to set between them differently—causing pain as the nerves become irritated from rubbing up against these oddly shaped articulations.

Many spondylitis sufferers are able to live normal lives outside of a reduction of motion range. For a small percentage of cases, it can also be crippling, and even effect the heart and kidneys.

Enteropathic Arthritis

Crohn's disease, ulcerative colitis and *irritable bowel syndrome* will result in spondylitis about 10% of the time. IBS will result in peripheral arthritis about 20% of the time. Sometimes this follows intestinal bacteria infections. The link between colon infections and arthritis is made obvious when the resection (removal) of an infected part of the intestine often results in the relief of arthritic symptoms. This will occur in irritable bowel syndrome, but usually not in Crohn's disease. Joints affected may be the hips, sacrum, knees and the spinal column.

Quick Chart for Identification of Spondyloarthropathy

Joints	Principally in lower spinal region, but also hips, knees, fingers, sacrum, toes, neck, ankles
Regions	Lower back, buttocks, referred pain
First occurrence	Dull aching on one side of the buttocks, progressive lower back pain and leg pain
Progression	Gradual progression over many years.
Pain	Dull, aching, worse after sleeping or resting
Movement	Better with motion, stretching
Motion	Slowly restrictive spinal region
Co-factors	Psoriasis, colitis, spine restriction
Appearance	Posture adjustments
Lab Tests	X-rays, MRI

Juvenile Arthritis

When a child presents with practically any type of arthritis, the diagnosis given will often be juvenile arthritis. This type of arthritis may also be diagnosed as **Still's disease.** A variety of different types of arthritis will also be diagnosed as juvenile arthritis. Rheumatoid arthritis is one of them. Others include ankylosing arthritis, psoriatic arthritis and others. Only about 10% of juvenile arthritic children show positive for rheumatoid factor. About 80% of RA factor-positive juvenile arthritis cases are girls. More than 50% of children with positive RA factor will eventually develop extreme rheumatoid arthritis.

About 25% of juvenile arthritis cases do not have any systemic symptoms, and experience joint pain and inflammation on asymmetrical joints (no bilateral as most RA patients experience). These sufferers rarely develop severe cases — at about 15% of the total.

Systemic symptoms include rashes, fevers, pain in the spleen or lymph glands, chest infection, anemia, pericarditis, and high white blood cell count. About 60% of these children are boys.

About half of juvenile cases have what is called **pauciarticular arthritis.** This occurs when the arthritis inflammation only affects the larger weight-bearing joints, such as the hips, knees, and ankles. A third of these cases will contract ocular diseases such as iridocyclitis—an inflammation of the iris' and ciliary bodies. These cases are generally negative for rheumatoid factor.

Gout

Gout in itself is not arthritis, but it can create arthritis, or joint inflammation. Gouty arthritis includes several conditions in which uric acid content in the serum is increased. This will often result in the deposit of uric acid crystals in the kidneys and joints. This is also called **hyperuricemia.** About one third of gout cases appear to occur without the incidence of another disease—called **primary gout.** In **secondary gout,** there is an accompanying disease associated with the onset of gout.

Uric acid is a by-product of numerous metabolic processes in the body. As cells are broken down, uric acid is released. Uric acid is also a byproduct of animal products as well. If too much uric acid accumulates and body is unable to dispose of it, uric acid crystals will form and become deposited in the joint. These crystals can build up in the joints over a period of months or years. Some health professionals say it takes about ten years for uric acid crystals—also called *trophi*—to build up around the joints and cartilage enough to begin causing pain and reduced motion.

Metabolic errors in blood sugar processing and glycogen production have also been associated with secondary gout. As we will discuss, various dietary and issues related to water consumption are also involved in uric acid problems. Alcohol consumption is particularly associated.

Primary gout can also be related to an impairment of uric acid processing by the kidneys. This still may be connected to diet, however. Uric acid clearance from the kidneys involves glomerular cell filtration ability, tubular reabsorption and urate excretion by renal tubules. Should any of these processes fail or become overloaded, uric acid will build up among tissues and joints.

Associated diseases that can cause gout are primarily metabolic oriented diseases. If the kidneys are malfunctioning, for example, they may not excrete enough uric acid during urination. This can lead to what is called renal disease. Decreased uric acid elimination can also be associated with the increased production of uric acid in response to leukemia and lymphomas. About 80% of gout sufferers also have high cholesterol levels (*hyperlipidemia*). About half of gout patients also have *hypertension*—high blood pressure. Obesity is also a common factor in gout. About a third of high blood pressure patients also have hyperuricemia. Gout patients will have an average of 20% higher body weight than the general population. Currently about a third of the adult population in the U.S. is now obese.

How to Identify Gouty Arthritis

About 25% of gout sufferers also have kidney stones. These are urate stones, or uric acid crystals. Some also contain calcium. About one in ten people in the U.S. that have any kind of kidney stones also have gout. The number of gout sufferers among kidney stone patients goes up to 40% in Australia and Israel for some reason. This seems to indicate dietary links among these populations.

Increased uric acid content may exist for many years without symptoms. The body may also adjust to this through a number of periodic detoxification processes. However, at any point in time, especially following a trauma, a night of drinking, a large meal of animal proteins, or another overtoxification event, the joints may become suddenly painful and stiff. Often the first occurrence will be in one joint. In over half of gout cases, that first joint is the big toe—the metatarsophalangeal joint. This is called *podagra*. About 90% of all gout sufferers have a big toe attack at some point or another. This is because uric acid tends to crystallize in cooler temperatures, and among larger joints. Seemingly, because the toes are frequently colder and receive less circulation than other parts of the body, they begin to show symptoms first. Even as the condition worsens, rarely are the warmer shoulders, hips and spine joints affected.

Other joints may also have pain and swelling or be affected first. The instep of the foot is a frequent region. Ankles, elbows and wrists are also frequently painful. If there is no correction, the pain can become excruciating. Younger sufferers often experience more intense pain. The pain can worsen during the night.

Quick Chart for Identification of Gouty Arthritis

Joints	Big toe(s), foot instep, ankles, toes, wrists, elbows—rarely hips, spine or shoulders
Regions	Distal regions of arms and legs
First occurrence	Pain, swelling and redness within one or multiple joints
Progression	Worsens with trauma or stress, may then gradually resolve, returning again with another attack days, weeks, months or even years later
Pain	Sharp, throbbing, worse during sleep or rest
Movement	Painful to move joint most affected
Motion	Range of motion moderate
Co-factors	Fever, chills, nausea, rapid heartbeat.
Appearance	Swelling around joints with smooth, shiny skin with red or purple color
Lab Tests	Uric acid in blood, urate crystals in joints

Progression of Gouty Arthritis

The initial attack may occur even at a young age. After an initial attack, a sufferer may not have another attack for weeks, months or even years. Subsequent attacks will often be more painful than the initial one.

As the condition develops, the joints may become permanently maligned. Deformities are typical for long-standing, chronic cases. Lumps of urate crystals—accumulated trophi—may also build up under the skin near the joints. Trophi may also build up around the ears, wrists, elbows, kidneys and other areas. Sometimes these trophi will erupt and spread into neighboring tissues.

Pseudogout

The technical name for this disorder is **calcium pyrophosphate deposition disease** (CPDD). CPDD comes from the deposit of *calcium pyrophosphate dihydrate* (CPPD) within the joints. This disorder occurs primarily among the elderly. Often those over 85 years old will be symptomatic, although many live with CPPD for years without symptoms. Furthermore, about two-thirds of those diagnosed with CPPD have also had previous joint damage—from either injury or cartilage damage. For this reason, many doctors believe that CPPD manifests from joint damage. Weight-bearing joints such as the hips, wrists and knees are the most likely to be affected. Other joints can also be affected, however.

Following a surgery or other trauma, the pyrophosphate crystals can form within the synovial fluid. It is thought that nucleotides derived from nucleotide triphosphate pyrophosphohydrolase (NTP) increases pyrophosphate production. This is an enzyme involved in the processing of ATP—our energy production cycle. It is also involved in the conversion of collagen into cartilage.

About half of those over 85 show signs of CPPD. Women have about a 40% higher likelihood of contracting CPPD. Middle-aged people—often older than 50—may also contract CPPD. These cases are often the result of a specific metabolic disorder. There is also evidence of genetic disposition in some cases.

Quick Chart for Identification of Pseudogout

Joints	Knees, wrists, elbows, ankles, hips
Regions	Large joints
First occurrence	Pain within one or multiple joints
Progression	Trauma may spark attack, followed by chronic condition, worsening with time
Pain	Lingering, dull or sharper pain, worse with rest
Movement	Pain and stiffness to joint most affected
Motion	Range of motion restricted at affected joints
Co-factors	Fever, chills, nausea, rapid heartbeat
Appearance	Swelling around joints
Lab Tests	Calcium pyrophosphate crystals in joint fluid, also visible as white crystals on x-rays (urate crystals are dark)

Reactive and Septic Arthritis

Reactive arthritis occurs when there are infections occurring in other parts of the body that come to affect the joints. Infections that stimulate reactive arthritis include prostatitis (inflamed prostate), psoriasis (inflammation of the skin), *Salmonella, Shigella, Pseudomonas, Campylobacter,* or *Ureaplasma urealyticum* infections, and venereal diseases such as herpes, gonorrhea, *Chlamydia,* and others. We will discuss these later in more detail.

Septic arthritis or **acute infectious arthritis** is a form of reactive arthritis wherein bacteria invade the joints. These can be the same bacteria just mentioned or many others. Whether bacteria actually invade the joint capsule or simply stimulate inflammatory cytokines is not always clear in every case. A rheumatic arthritic joint will often be permeable to septic infection by microorganisms. Septic infections are also often accompanied by other symptoms such as fever and digestive difficulties. Symptoms of this form of arthritis include sharp, immediate and piercing pain within a few joints or even a single joint. This can occur at any age. Infective arthritis can affect young children as well, who may be infected by *H. influenzae* or *Streptococcus pneumoniae.*

A subset of septic arthritis is **disseminated gonococcal infection,** or DGI. This is often caused by a gonorrhea infection—a sexually transmitted disease. This can also cause fever, chills, random limb motion, and dermatitis. The skin can break out in pustules, vesicles and lesions. This can occur in different places on the skin, and can occur near the joint pain.

Nongonococcal septic arthritis is infective arthritis caused by bacteria other than gonorrhea. This form is actually a further descriptor for the same septic arthritis discussed above.

Lyme disease is another form of septic or reactive arthritis. Here the lyme bacterium, *Borrelia burgdorferi* in the U.S. and *Borrelia afzelii* in Europe, infect the body and sometimes the synovial fluid and cartilage. Lyme is officially thought to be caused by an infected tick bite, although other routes of infection have been identified in recent years. The bacterium has been shown to burrow and incubate into certain tissues, where it can emerge when the immune system is in a weakened state.

Quick Chart for Identification of Reactive/Septic Arthritis

Joints	Any movable joint
Regions	Dependent upon infection site and progression
First occurrence	Pain, swelling and redness in multiple joints
Progression	Moves with rate of infection and detoxification or treatment. Untreated, it may resolve by itself if infection is reduced by immune system. It may also worsen if infection is not purged
Pain	Throbbing and persistent. Worsening with time
Movement	Stiffness variable
Motion	Range of motion dependent upon swelling and type of infection
Co-factors	Fatigue, fever, chills, nausea
Appearance	Swelling, redness and heat around joints, pustules may appear, filled with fluid
Lab Tests	Blood, urine or joint fluid is tested for the presence of bacteria and/or specific types of antibodies

Other Forms of Arthritis

Calcium hydroxyapatite disposition disease (CHDD) is usually the result of the deposit of hydroxyapatite crystals within the synovial fluid, membranes and cartilage. Calcium hydroxyapatite is the central mineral that bones are made of. In many cases, *osteoporosis* may be involved, as the bones demineralize. Osteoarthritis or another form of arthritis may also be involved—but not necessarily. Joints crystallized with CHDD are often weight-bearing joints such as hips, knees, shoulders and fingers.

Ochronosis is a defect in the processing and breakdown of the enzyme *homogentisic acid oxidase*. This will result in the release of ochronotic pigment into the cartilage around the joints. This can affect any number of joints, including the intravertebral disks, and also cause *alkaptonuria*.

Hemochromatosis is caused by a toxic load of iron in the body. Half of hemochromatosis sufferers experience recurrent attacks of arthritis in the joints. Weight-bearing joints like knees, hips, and ankles are frequently involved. Other problems—including liver diseases such as cirrhosis and enlarged liver—can accompany hemochromatosis. In addition, cardiovascular problems and fatigue are common in hemochromatosis.

Hemoarthrosis is a form of arthritis where blood leaks into the joints. This can be caused by circulatory diseases, clots and organ breakdown. The symptoms of hemoarthrosis can mimic rheumatoid arthritis. Most any moving or weight-bearing joint can be affected.

Hepatitis is a liver infection that often causes arthritic symptoms. It can be caused by several types of viruses such as *Epstein-Barr, cytomegalovirus, mumps,* and of course *hepatitis A, B, C, D (with B),* E and G. Hepatitis often leads to cirrhosis—the mutilation of liver cells combined with the replacement of scar tissue. This can lead to a deficiency of a number of metabolic processes for which the liver is responsible. This in turn can then lead to damage to the cartilage or the deposit of crystals into the synovial fluid.

Sarcoidosis is a disease that is symptomatic of nodules of inflammation appearing around the body, principally around the lymph nodes or the lungs. Sarcoidosis can be fatal, and will accompany a severe loss of energy, appetite, difficulty breathing, blurred vision, weight loss and others. As it spreads, sarcosis can also damage the liver, thyroid, and joints. The bacteria species *Propionibacterium acnes* has been found in about 70% of patients with sarcoidosis. Still, physicians do not understand sarcoidosis well.

Lupus is an autoimmune disease that resembles rheumatoid arthritis in many ways. It affects many of the same joints in the same way. The difference is that lupus is a systemic disease—affecting many other parts of the body besides the joints. Unique symptoms of lupus include photosensitivity, nerve problems, inflammation of other organs, ulcers in the oral cavity, peeling sores on different parts of the skin, and the odd appearance of the *malar rash*. The malar rash sometimes resembles a butterfly—often appearing on the cheeks of the face.

Chapter Three

What Causes Arthritis?

The cause of most forms of arthritis puzzles modern medicine. Yet a lot of research has gone into arthritis over the past few years. Let's review what the research tells us about arthritis and inflammation, and see if we cannot arrive at some valid conclusions regarding the causes for arthritis.

We know that most forms of arthritis are accompanied by inflammation of the synovial membrane around the joints. What causes this inflammation? How far back should we go?

We could say an automobile accident was caused by the bumper of the car crashing into another car. Is this the real cause of the accident, however? Most of us would say the bumper was an incidental intermediary and not the cause. And we would be right.

Arthritis is also thought to be caused by inflammation. Furthermore, osteoarthritis is thought to be caused by joint cartilage eroding through wear and tear. In rheumatoid arthritis, a mysterious autoimmune disorder is the cause: The immune system is curiously attacking the body's own healthy cells.

This is not to say that medical researchers have not put considerable focus towards the mechanisms that drive the process of inflammation. The assumption they have made is that chronic inflammation in the joints is caused by a biochemical cascade towards inflammation. This leads to the assumed solution that halting the biochemical cascade towards inflammation will solve the problem.

This has been the strategy embarked upon by the pharmaceutical companies over the past fifty years. The concept is that pain and inflammation lay at the root of arthritis. Therefore, if we stop the pain and stop the inflammation, we stop the problem. Right?

The problem with this methodology is that again, it is treating the symptoms rather than the disease.

The actual causes for arthritis are different from its symptoms. We will show here that pain and inflammation are simply byproducts of our body's immune system repair process. They are not the problem. Without pain and inflammation—along with all the other parts of the immune system's healing process—our bodies cannot repair injuries and prevent disease.

The Immune System

When a heart is removed from a dead body and put into another body, the body's immune system immediately begins to reject it. This is because the body's immune system recognizes this heart as foreign. It came from another body. This means the immune system is smart.

The immune system is located throughout the body. We find immune cells on the skin, in the blood, in the lungs, in the bones and in every organ system.

The immune system has a number of intelligent abilities. The first is *recognition*. The immune system has the facility to recognize molecules that endanger the body's welfare. The immune system also maintains *memory*. The immune system can remember the identity of a toxin or pathogen by virtue of recognizing its *antigens* (byproducts or molecular structure). This is the rationale for vaccination. Vaccination exposes the body to a small amount of a particular pathogen so the immune system will develop the tools and the memory to recognize its antigens, so that the body can respond appropriately the next time it is exposed to it.

The immune system is incredible in its ability to maintain *specificity* and *diversity*. These characteristics allow the immune system to respond to literally millions, if not billions of different antigens. Moreover, each particular antigen requires a completely different response.

The immune system is an intelligent scanning and review system intended to gauge whether a particular molecule, cell or organism belongs in the body. This is determined through a complex biochemical identification system. We might compare this system to an iris scan, often used as a password entry system. Utilizing a database of information, the immune system checks molecular structures against this database. If the molecular structure matches a memorized molecule or cell that is considered foreign, the immune system launches an attack. This is often called an immune response or an inflammatory response.

Despite much research in the areas of vaccination, antibiotics, and inflammation, modern medical science is still perplexed with the *autoimmune syndrome*. A massive list of degenerative diseases are now considered autoimmune, including irritable bowel syndrome, Crohn's, asthma, allergies, fibromyalgia, lupus, urinary tract disorders and many, many others. Many physicians also classify most types of arthritis as autoimmune disorders. Some contend, however, that osteoarthritis is not an autoimmune disorder because it seems to be related to aging and wear and tear—"normal" processes. The problem, however, is that the cartilage damage observed in osteoarthritis is not being repaired by the immune system. Why can't the immune system repair the damage, as it does with most other types of injuries? Furthermore, why does inflammation continue to damage the joints in arthritis?

Most researchers agree that in arthritis, the inflammatory process has gotten out of control and is creating more damage than it is repairing. This might be referred to as a *derangement* of the immune system. Instead of bringing in the troops to halt the damage and heal the injury, the process has become deranged. Simply by this definition—that the immune system process is further damaging the tissues—most forms of arthritis can be classified as autoimmune. Most health professionals and researchers agree with this definition. Autoimmunity occurs when the immune system is somehow damaging the tissues instead of repairing them.

In order to understand autoimmunity, we must clearly understand how the immune system works.

Harmful microbes or chemical toxins invade the body via the digestive tract, the nose and sinuses, the genitals, the lungs, the skin, the ears and even the eyes. Bacterial or fungal infections can also be caused by normal residents of the body, should they grow beyond their typical populations. These include *H. pylori*, *E. coli* and *Candida albicans*. For the purposes of this discussion, we'll call both—microbial foreigners and toxic chemicals—*pathogens*, because they both can lead to disease or *pathology* if they are not removed. *Antigens* are sometimes used to describe these, but the definition of antigen must now include recent research showing that antigens can also be molecular combinations sitting atop cell membranes that stimulate an immune system response.

There are four processes the immune system uses:

The first is called the **non-specific immune response**. This utilizes a network of biochemical barriers that work synergistically to prevent infectious agents from getting into the body. The barrier structures include the ability of the body to shut down its orifices. We can close our eyes, mouths, noses and ears to prevent invaders or toxins from entering the body. Within these orifices lie further defensive barriers. Nose hairs, eyelashes, lips, tonsils, ear hair, pubic hair and hair in general are all designed to help screen out and filter invaders. Most of the body's passageways are also equipped with tiny cilia, which assist the body to halt invaders by snagging them. These cilia move rhythmically, sweeping back and forth, working the snagged invaders back out with their undulations. The layer of skin within most of the body's orifices, ducts and passageways is also covered with a mucous membrane. This thin liquid membrane film keeps many invaders from penetrating the body. The mucous membranes lining the passageways are also lined with immune cells and immunoglobulins that respond to pathogens.

The digestive tract is equipped with another type of sophisticated defense technology. Should any foreigners get through the lips, teeth, tongue, hairs, mucous membranes, and cilia and sneak down the esophagus, they then must contend with the digestive fire of the stomach. The gastrin, peptic acid and hydrochloric acid within a healthy stomach keep the pH around two. This is usually enough to kill or disrupt many bacteria. If a person mistakenly weakens this protective acid with antacids or acid-blockers, for example, the body's ability to neutralize invaders will be handicapped. In addition, a number of microorganisms are accustomed to acidic environments. A few can tuck away into clumps of food— especially food that has not been masticated (chewed) enough.

The next type of immune process takes place among the body's *probiotics*. The human body can house more than 32 billion beneficial and harmful bacteria and fungi at any particular time. Beneficial bacteria are in the majority in a healthy body. A healthy immune system works conjunctively with these probiotics. Probiotics can help identify harmful bacteria or fungal overgrowths and produce strategies to eradicate them. Most probiotics produce antimicrobial biochemicals that can damage or kill certain pathogenic bacteria. These form the body's own natural antibiotic system.

The body's third form of immune response involves a highly technical strategic attack that first identifies the invader's weaknesses, followed by a precise and immediate offensive attack to exploit those weaknesses. This is often called *humoral immunity.* There are more than a billion different types of antibodies, macrophages and other lymphocytes the immune system utilizes to mobilize and execute specific attack plans. As an immune cell scans a particular invader, it will analyze and recognize a particular biomolecular or behavioral weakness within the toxin or pathogen. Upon recognizing this weakness, the immune system will devise a unique plan to exploit this weakness. It may launch a variety of possible attacks, using a combination of proteins and lymphocytes of different varieties.

A humoral response utilizes specialized B-cells (or *B-lymphocytes*) in conjunction with specialized antibodies. Cruising through the blood and lymph systems, the antibodies and/or B-cells can quickly sense and size up viruses, toxins or bacteria. Often this will mean the antibody will lock onto or bind to the invader to extract critical genetic information. This process will electromagnetically scan the potential invader's genetic makeup, biomolecular makeup and potential vulnerabilities. Their specific vulnerability is often revealed by the nature of their antigens—specific molecular structure indicators. Each invader will have its own type of antigen, though similar invaders might have similar vulnerabilities. The B-cell then reproduces the specific *antibody* designed to record and communicate that specific vulnerability through the body's satellite transceivers. This antibody signals the precise information on the location and development of these invaders so the B-cells or *macrophages* can take them apart.

The fourth process the immune system utilizes is the *cell-mediated immune response.* This also incorporates a collection of smart proteins and specialized immune cells that wander the body looking for cells that have become infected. Infected cells are often discovered by their antenna molecules (antigens) that are positioned on the cell's membrane. Once recognized, the immune system will launch an attack against the cell, often utilizing a specialized type of immune cell called the T-cell.

Let's back up a bit and review the central immune players in more detail, and then discuss the role they play in arthritis:

White Blood Cells

The immune system produces at least five different types of white blood cells—also called leucocytes. Each is designed to identify and target specific types of pathogens. After identification, they will either initiate an attack with other components, or directly begin their attack. The main types are *lymphocytes, neutrophils, basophils, or monocytes.* Each plays an important role in the pathogen-identification and inflammatory process. All white blood cells are initially produced in the bone marrow.

Lymphocytes are the body's intelligent and specific immune response team. The primary lymphocytes are the T-cells (*thymus cells*) or B-cells (*bone marrow cells*). These cells and their specialized proteins work together to strategically damage and remove invaders. Then they memorize the strategy in preparation for a future invasion.

Both B-cells and T-cells are assembled by stem cells in the bone marrow. T-cells, however, undergo further differentiation and programming in the thymus gland. B-cells undergo a similar process of maturity before release from the spleen. Both T-cells and B-cells circulate via lymph nodes, blood stream and tissue fluids. Both also have a number of special types, including memory cells and helper cells to identify and memorize invaders.

B-cells are part of the humoral system, so they circulate through the blood stream and lymph looking for foreign or potentially harmful pathogens. These might include toxins, bacteria, viruses and others. Once identified, B-cells will stimulate the production of a particular type of antibody protein, which is designed to destroy or break apart the foreign object. There are several different types of B-cells. Most are monoclonal, which means they will adjust to the specific type of invader. Some B-cells are investigative and surveillance oriented. They are looking for roaming pathogens. Once activated, they can then damage these invading pathogens using a variety of biochemical secretions or physical activities. B-cells that circulate the bloodstream are often called *plasma* B-cells. Others—like *memory* B-cells—record previous invasions and remember how to remove them for future attacks.

T-cells, on the other hand, are oriented toward specific types of cells around the body. They are focused upon problems that occur within the body's cells, or those pathogens that have invaded cells.

There is a variety of different T-cells. Each is programmed in the thymus to look for a different type of invasion, and each has the capability of destroying different types of cells and pathogens. Many T-cells simply respond to a pathogen that has invaded the cell by destroying the cell itself—this is the *killer* T-cell. It does this by inserting special chemicals into the cell, or by simply submitting instructions for the cell to kill itself. Cell death—regardless of whether it is caused by a T-cell or not—is called *apoptosis*.

T-cells work through a communication system of *cytokines* to relay instructions and information to the various killer T-cells. The killer cells include *macrophages, natural killer cells* and *cytotoxic* T-cells.

The initial scanning of an infected cell by a *helper* T-cell utilizes electromagnetic scanning just as the B-cells do. The T-cell's support network also includes *delta-gamma* T-cells. Delta-gamma T-cells are stimulated by specific molecular receptors on cell membranes while helper T-cells communicate previous responses, memorize current ones, and provide other support. These cells exchange information and collaborate.

The helper T-cell scan surveys the molecular bonding patterns for indications of either bacterial infection or some sort of genetic mutation due to a virus or toxin. This 'antigen scan' might reveal invasions of chemical toxins, protozoa, worms, fungi, bacteria and viruses that have intruded or deranged the cell. The scanning helper T-cell immediately communicates the information by releasing cytokines—tiny coded proteins that disseminate the information needed to coordinate macrophage, NK cells and/or cytotoxic T-cells for attack.

Every particular toxin or pathogen has its own unique weakness for the healthy immune system to exploit. For some toxins, lymphocyte phagocytes or macrophages might simply engulf it and break it apart with specific chemicals. For others, a lymphocyte might secrete a particular chemical that poisons the antigen. When a cell is infected, an immune cell may just directly kill the entire cell. One specialized lymphocyte that does this is the natural killer T-cell or NK cell. Most T-cells contain tumor necrosis factor or TNF—a sort of self-destruct switch. When signaled from the outside or inside, TNF will initiate a self-destruct and the cell will die. Under some circumstances, entire groups of cells or tissue systems may be damaged. Macrophages may be called to cut off the blood supply to these deranged or infected cells to kill them off.

The healthy human immune system might be compared to a specialized hit squad, ready to reply with smart counteractive measures with precise coordination.

The two primary helper T-cell types are the Th1 and the Th2. The Th1 T-cell focuses on the elimination of bacteria, fungi, parasites, viruses, and similar types of invaders. The Th2 T-cells, on the other hand, are focused upon allergic and antibody responses. The Th2 is thus explicitly involved in the responses of inflammation and allergic reaction. This is important to note, because research has revealed that stress, chemical toxins, poor dietary habits and lack of sleep tend to suppress Th1 levels and increase Th2 levels. With an abundance of Th2 T-cells in the system, the body is prone to respond more strongly to allergens or toxins, causing problems like hay fever and allergies. This is why we sometimes see people who are under physical or emotional stress overreacting with hives, psoriasis and other allergic-type responses. High Th2 levels are also implicated in arthritis.

Neutrophils are white blood cells that circulate primarily within the blood stream, looking for abnormal behavior among various cells and tissues. Once they identify a problem, they will signal a mass assembly and begin the process of cleaning the area. This often involves inflammation, as they work to break down and remove debris. Neutrophils will also penetrate tissue structures, and will often accumulate within joints. In one study, neutrophils were shown migrating directly into arthritic joints (Gao *et al.* 1994).

Monocytes, on the other hand, are the precursors for the attack soldiers. They are produced in marrow, and can later be differentiated into either *macrophages* or *dendrite cells*. The macrophages are particularly good at engulfing and breaking apart pathogens. Dendritic cells are interactive cells that stimulate certain responses. They isolate and present pathogens to the T-cells, for example. Dendritic cells also stimulate the production of those special communication proteins called cytokines.

Cytokines

Cytokines are communication messengers that allow different types of cells to communicate. These come with complex names like *interleukin* (IL), *transforming growth factor* (TGF), *leukemia inhibitory factor* (LIF), and *tumor necrosis factor* (TNF). There are five basic types of cell communication: *intracrine, autocrine, endocrine, juxtacrine* and *paracrine.*

Autocrine communication takes place between two different types of cells. This message can be a biochemical message or an electromagnetic stimulus. The receiving cell in turn may respond automatically by producing a particular biochemical-electromagnetic message. We might compare this to leaving a voicemail on someone's message machine. Once we leave the message, the machine signals that the message has been received and will be delivered. Later the machine will replay the message. The immune system uses autocrine messaging to activate T-cells. Once stimulated, the T-cell will specifically respond with the necessary activity.

A paracrine communication takes place between neighboring cells of the same type, often passing on messages that originated from outside the tissue region. Tiny protein antennas will sit on cell membranes, allowing one cell to communicate with another. This allows cells within the same tissue system to respond together with coordination.

Juxtacrine communications take place via smart biomolecular structures. We might call these structures relay stations. They absorb messages and pass them on. An example of this is the passing of inflammatory messages via cytokines.

An intracrine communication takes place inside the cell. An externally generated message may be communicated into the cell through an antenna sitting on the cell's membrane. These communications stimulate specific metabolic processes within the cell.

The endocrine message takes place between endocrine glands and individual cells. The endocrine glands include the pineal gland, the pituitary gland, the pancreas, adrenals, thyroid, ovary and testes. These glands produce endocrines, which relay messages directly to cells. Their messages stimulate a variety of metabolic functions within the body. These include growth, temperature, sexual behavior, sleep, glucose utilization, stress response and so many others.

One of the functions of the endocrine glands relevant to arthritis is the production of inflammatory co-factors such as cortisol, adrenaline and norepinephrine. These glands coordinate and initiate instructions that stimulate inflammatory processes.

All of these communication systems are interactive, and they play a large role in the explanation of arthritis. For example, the *osteoclast* (cells responsible for breaking down bone tissue) increases seen in osteoarthritis appear to be stimulated by the cytokine autocrine IL-6. However, in the presence of estrogen domination, IL-6 production is decreased. This relationship is significant in the occurrence of osteoporosis among menopausal women.

Leukotrienes, Prostaglandins and Thromboxanes

These three biomolecules are an important part of the bio-chemical communication pathways that stimulate inflammation.

Leucotrienes are molecules that identify problems and stimulate immune responses. They pinpoint and isolate areas of the body that require repair. They both stimulate and moderate the process of inflammation. Once they pinpoint the site of repair, one type of leucotriene will initiate inflammation. Once the repair process proceeds to a point of maturity, another type of leucotriene will begin slowing down the process of inflammation.

This smart signalling process takes place through the bonding formations of the particular molecules. The type and number of leucotrienes on location tend to stimulate one response or another. Leucotrienes are paracrines and autocrines. They are paracrine in that they initiate messages that travel from one cell to another. They are autocrine in that they initiate messages that encourage an automatic and immediate response from cells—notably T-cells to engage them in the process of repair to an injury. They also help transmit messages that assist in the collection of blood, mucus, fibrin and other repair elements.

Leucotrienes are produced from the conversion of essential fatty acids (EFAs) by an enzyme produced by the body called *arachidonate-5-lipoxygenase* (sometimes called LOX). The central EFAs of the process are *arachidonic acid* (AA), *gamma-linolenic acid* (GLA), and *docosahexaenoic acid/eicosapentaenoic acid* (DHA/EPA). The lipoxygenase enzyme will produce a different type of leucotriene, depending upon the initial fatty acid. The important point of this is that the leucotrienes produced by arachidonic acid stimulate inflammation, while the leucotrienes produced by DHA/EPA inhibit inflammation. The leucotrienes produced by GLA, on the other hand, block the conversion process of polyunsaturated fatty acids to arachidonic acid.

Prostaglandins are also produced through an enzyme conversion from fatty acids. Like leucotrienes, prostaglandins are messengers that transmit particular messages to immune cells. Their messaging is either paracrine or autocrine as well. Prostaglandins are critical parts of the process of repairing injuries. They also initiate a number of other protective sequences in the body.

The central messages that prostaglandins transmit depend upon the type of prostaglandin produced. Prostaglandin I2 (also PGI2) stimulates the widening of blood vessels, the widening of bronchial passages, and stimulates a pain response within the nervous system. In other words, along with stimulating blood clotting, PGI2 signals a range of responses to assist the body's healing and protection processes at the site of injury.

Prostaglandin E2, or PGE2, is altogether different. PGE2 stimulates the secretion of mucus within the stomach, intestines, mouth and esophagus. It also decreases the production of gastric acid in the stomach. This combination of increasing mucus and lowering acid production keeps healthy stomach cells from being damaged by the content of our foods as well as the stomach acid itself during a trauma. As we will discuss later, this is one of the central reasons NSAIDs and COX inhibitor pharmaceuticals cause gastrointestinal problems.

Prostaglandins are produced by the oxidation of certain fatty acids by an enzyme produced in the body called *cyclooxygenase*—also called prostaglandin-endoperoxide synthase (PTGS) or COX. We know of three types of COX. Each converts fatty acids to different types of prostaglandins among different tissues. The central fatty acid implicated in inflammation is arachidonic acid. COX-1 converts AA to prostaglandin-2 (or PGE2) expressed in mucosal membranes including the digestive tract. COX-2, on the other hand, converts AA into PGE2, prostacyclin (PGI2) and thromboxane among injury sites and blood vessels. Prostacyclin stimulates blood vessel expansion and assists with clot formation, while thromboxane drives the clotting process. PGE2 stimulates bronchial expansion, fever, and the pain response at infected or allergic sites.

This means that the COX-1 enzyme instigates the process of protecting the stomach, while the COX-2 enzyme instigates the process of inflammation and repair within other parts of the body. In the case of arthritis, it is primarily the COX-2 process that lies at the root of joint pain and swelling.

Cyclooxygenase also converts EPA and GLA to prostaglandins. Just as lipoxygenase converts EPA and GLA to anti-inflammation leucotrienes, the conversion of EPA and GLA by cyclooxygenase produces prostaglandins that either block the inflammatory process or reverse it. This means that a healthy diet that supplies these two fatty acids will balance the joint inflammation response.

The arachidonic acid conversion process that produces prostaglandins also produces *thromboxanes*. Thromboxanes stimulate the platelets in the blood to aggregate. They work in concert with another substance called platelet-activating factor or PAF. These two biomolecules drive the process of clotting the blood and restricting blood flow. The restriction of blood flow is what maintains the swelling seen among arthritic joints.

Immunoglobulins

Immunoglobulins are proteins that are coded for a particular type of response and signaling. IgAs line the mouth and digestive tract, and try to prevent pathogens from infecting the body in the first place. IgDs sense infections and activate B-cells. IgEs attach to foreign substances and launch histamine responses—often associated with allergic responses. IgGs cross through membranes—responding to pathogens that have already intruded and are growing: expanding infections, in other words. IgMs are focused on brand new intrusions that have yet to grow enough to garner the attention of IgGs.

Each of these general immunoglobulin categories contain numerous specific types of immunoglobulins geared to specific pathogens and responses. Other immunoglobulin proteins also exist. Some of these will sit atop the membranes of macrophages and lymphocytes to better identify pathogens.

A subset of these is the *CD glycogen-protein complex*. CD stands for *cluster of differentiation*. CDs are molecules that sit on top of the membranes of the T-cells and macrophages to navigate and steer their behavior. In other words, the CDs provide the communication between the type of pathogen and the appropriate response the immune cell should take to remove the pathogen. They often negotiate, or 'bind to' pathogens, so the T-cell or macrophage can proceed to tear the pathogen apart, or insert the appropriate chemical to destroy the pathogen and the cell hosting it.

Many different types of immune cells have been assigned particular CD classifications by researchers. Each classification is based upon the molecular arrangement of the protein or its outer surface structure: This is called a *ligand*. The molecular arrangement (CD number) will also match to a specific type of *receptor* at the molecule, cell or pathogen. Each type of CD will produce a particular type of bonding relationship with the receptor on the cell to allow the accompanying immune cell its interactivity with the pathogen.

This relates to arthritis because certain types of CD cells are often found in the synovial membrane, telling health researchers that particular types of cells or pathogens are being hunted down by T-cells. In many cases, these CD numbers indicate that the cells and environment has suffered from toxins, bacterial or viral infection. They also often indicate the existence of deranged cells whose DNA has been damaged—consistent with the invasion of toxins, bacteria or viruses.

The Inflammatory Cascade

Let's review the inflammation process with these players in motion. First, know that inflammation is a healing response. It is the reaction by the immune system to an injury or invasion. The inflammation response blocks the site of an injury or infection while stimulating a process of repair and eradication of the offending pathogen and/or damaged cells. Without inflammation, our bodies simply will not heal correctly. Imagine for a moment cutting your finger pretty badly. First you would feel pain—letting you know the body is hurt and needs attention. Second, you will probably notice that the area has become swollen and red. Blood starts to clot around the spot. Soon the cut stops bleeding. The blood dries and a scab forms. It remains red, maybe a little hot, and hurts for a while. Soon the cut is closed up and a scab has been left in its place. The pain soon stops. The scab falls off and the finger returns to normal—almost like new and ready for reuse.

This is an absolute beautiful miracle of nature. Without this process, we might not even know we cut our finger in the first place. We might keep working, only to find out that we had bled out a quart of blood on the floor. Without clotting, it would be hard to stop the bleeding. We might get the bleeding to stop with a tunicate. But we'd probably lose the finger because it was receiving no blood flow whatsoever (clotting and inflammation slows down blood flow just enough to make repairs, but does not stop it). If we somehow got the bleeding to stop, the wound would remain open: We would have to sew it up manually! Were it not for our immune system and inflammatory process slowing blood flow, clotting the blood, scabbing and cleaning up the site, our bodies would be like our automobiles: Any little dent or scratch would remain until manually repaired.

Every injury or threat from a pathogen stimulates a particular strategy of response by the immune system. The type of strategic response is determined during an interactive investigation of the site by neutrophils, helper T-cells, helper B-cells, immunoglobulins, leukotrienes and prostaglandins. The cells themselves are also involved, as they will often signal the type of duress they are under with biomolecular signals given from their cell membranes. Once the intrusion and strategy is determined, the lymphocytes will directly attack the deranged or infected cells. Most T-cells and B-cells do not enter the cells themselves. They will usually secrete a chemical or signal to a chemical within the cell to conduct a particular process of detoxification or self-destruction. In arthritis, the later is often the case.

Leukotrienes immediately gather in the region of injury or infection, and signal to T-cells to coordinate efforts and begin the process of repair. Prostaglandins immediately initiate the widening of the blood vessels to the site to bring more T-cells and other repair factors (such as plasminogen and fibrin).

Prostaglandins also stimulate the substance P within the nerve cells, initiating the sensation of pain. At the same time, thromboxanes, along with fibrin, drive the process of clotting and coagulation in the blood, while constricting certain blood vessels to decrease the risk of bleeding.

In the case where the pathogen is an allergen, the inflammation response will also accompany and H1-histamine response. Histamine is primarily produced by the masT-cells and basophils after being stimulated by IgE antibodies. This parallel response serves to try to remove the pathogen using physiological responses, such as sneezing, watering of the eyes, coughing, and even a seizing of the throat (anaphylaxis). These measures, though sometimes considered dangerous, are all stimulated in an effort to remove the pathogen and prevent its re-entry into the body. As the H1 histamine binds with receptors, it also encourages alertness (also why antihistamines cause drowsiness). These are the body's natural responses to get away from the allergen, and remove it from the body. As the allergic process continues, *anaphylatoxins* are produced, which increase blood vessel wall permeability and smooth muscle contraction. This also promotes the process of detoxification.

As the T-cells arrive at the injury site, the process of repair begins. The bad guys are taken apart or destroyed. If they are bacteria, they are either engulfed by phagocytes and neutrophils or injected with poison. If the damage is within cells, the T-cells will stimulate a self-destruct switch within the cells or simply take them apart.

At the height of the repair process, swelling, redness and pain are at their peak. Here range of motion is also limited, and for good reason. The T-cells, macrophages, neutrophils, fibrin and plasmin all collect together to break apart pathogens and repair the damage. Motion is limited to allow the region to focus on repair. Blood circulation is stunted as coagulation sets up internal scabbing.

As the process proceeds, the pathogen should be arrested, and the mending of the area accelerates. Here macrophages continue the clean up and the other immune cells begin to retreat. Antioxidants like glutathione will attach to and transport the byproducts— the dead body parts—out of the body. As this proceeds, both prostaglandins and leucotrienes begin to signal a reversal of the inflammation and pain process.

One of the first events in the process is the production of *bradykinin*. Bradykinin slows the formation of clots and opens the blood vessels to allow the site of inflammation to clear. This happens as bradykinin connects with receptors, producing more *nitric oxide* (NO). NO slows inflammation by promoting the detachment of lymphocytes to the site, and reduces tissue swelling. NO also helps clear out debris with its interaction with the superoxide anion. NO was originally described as *endothelium-derived relaxing factor* (or EDRF)—because of its role in relaxing blood vessel walls.

Confirming the effects of bradykinin, a 2008 report (Meini and Maggi) from the Pharmacology Department of the Menarini Ricerche research facility found that injecting bradykinin into the synovial fluid within the osteoarthritic joint capsule significantly reduced pain and inflammation. A reduction in pro-inflammatory cytokines was also noted in the research.

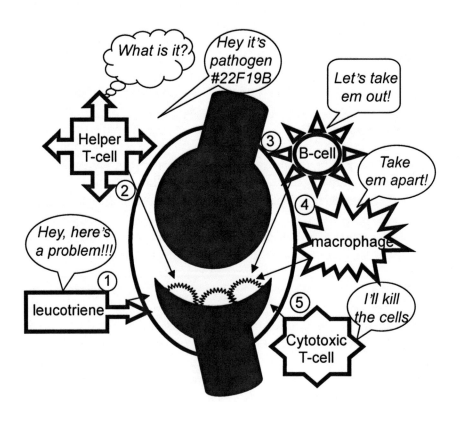

Note that the body produces nitric oxide in the presence of good nutrition and lower stress. Lower nitric oxide levels are associated with a plethora of diseases, including diabetes, heart failure, high cholesterol, premature aging, cancers and many others. Low or abnormal NO is also associated with smoking and obesity, and environmental factors like air pollution.

The Thymus Gland

One of the most important players in the immune system is the thymus gland. The thymus gland is located in the chest-region, in the center, behind the sternum. The thymus is a major component of the lymphatic system. Some even compare the thymus gland of the lymphatic system to the heart of the circulatory system of blood vessels.

The thymus gland activates T-cells and a number of hormones that modulate and stimulate the immune and autoimmune processes. The thymus converts a type of lymphocyte called the thymocyte into either a T-cell or a natural killer cell. These activated T-cells are released into the lymph and bloodstream ready to protect and serve. Within the thymus, they are infused with surface markers of CDs—which identify particular types of problematic cells or invading organisms.

In other words, the thymus codes the T-cells with receptors that will bind to particular cells or toxins. The type of cells or toxins they bind to are determined by the *major histocompatibility complex,* or MHC determinant. During the process of converting thymocytes to T-cells, their receptors are programmed with MHC combinations. This allows them to tolerate particular frailties within the body while attacking what the body considers to be true invaders (Kazansky 2008).

Therefore, it is the MHC that gives the T-cell the ability to identify the difference between *self* and *non-self* parts of the body. A *non-self* identification will produce an *immunogen,* or a factor that stimulates an immune response. Once the immunogen is stimulated, the inflammatory process proceeds, with a cascade of COX enzymes, prostaglandins, inflammation and pain.

The thymus gland grows and develops from birth. It is most productive and at its largest during puberty. From that point forward, depending upon the diet, stress and general health of the person, the thymus gland may begin to shrink. By forty, an immunosuppressed person will often have a tiny thymus gland. In elderly persons, the thymus gland is often barely recognizable, and for many, completely non-functional.

Throughout its productive life, the thymus gland produces T-cells that are given the appropriate MHC programming. If the thymus gland is functioning, it will continue to produce T-cells with revised MHC programming coding. The revised coding accommodates the various genetic changes that can happen to different cells around the body as we age and adapt to our changing environment. With a shrunken and non-functioning thymus, however, its ability to re-program T-cells with new MHC—enabling them to identify the body's cells that have adapted—is damaged. The T-cells will have to keep working off the old MHC programming. This in turn leads those T-cells to identify cells that have adapted—including intestinal cells, bone cells, synovial cells, and cartilage cells—as genetically deranged cells. This lies at the heart of the autoimmune puzzle.

Joint Inflammation

Now let's translate this information specifically to joint inflammation. Joint inflammation differs from typical inflammation only slightly, because the joints are surrounded by a capsule that has less blood supply than many other tissue systems. This can significantly slow both the processes of damage discovery and inflammation response, as well as injury site repair and clean up.

In order to initiate the process of inflammation, there must be some sort of invasion, damage or derangement among the subchondral bone, the synovial fluid, the synovial membrane, or the cartilage. This invasion, damage or derangement of the cells or tissue environment of the joints can be caused by a variety of factors. Preliminary research over the past few decades has concluded that arthritis is associated with a narrow range of factors. The chart on page 47 summarizes those associations given the most attention by conventional western medicine.

The fact that T-cells and B-cells are found within the synovial fluid of arthritis sufferers indicates that there is an infection or toxic invasion of the joint. T-cells indicate damage to cells.

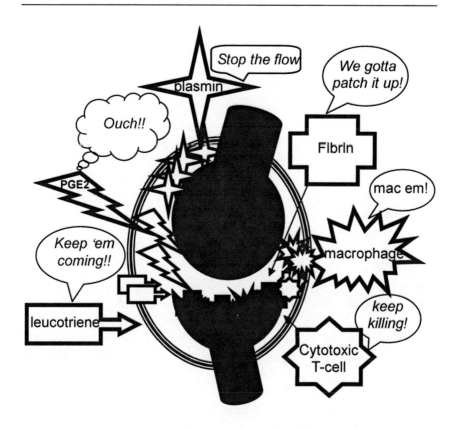

Chronic inflammation associated with T-cells and B-cells within the synovial fluid indicates that the joint invasion is not being adequately addressed by the immune system. The continuing damage to subchondral bone and cartilage indicates ineffective inflammation.

In research comparing the synovial fluid of osteoarthritis patients to synovial fluid of rheumatoid arthritis patients, OA synovial fluid was found to contain more masT-cells than RA synovial fluid (Renoux *et al.* 1996). MasT-cells are associated with the release of histamine. OA synovial fluid has also been found to contain more nitrite content than RA synovial fluid. Synovial fluid of both RA and OA patients contains abnormal levels of substance P as well—indicating the common presence of pain (Menkes *et al.* 1993). Curiously, RA synovial fluid often contains more cholesterol and fats than normal synovial fluid (Prete *et al.* 1993).

Different types of cytokines and antibodies have also been found in arthritic synovial fluid. Synovial fluid of both OA and RA patients often contain significantly more T-cells than B-cells as well. This indicates that the joint invasion has penetrated and damaged not only the fluid and cartilage, but also chondrocytes.

The T-cell system's memory protocol utilizes cytokines to help translate and store the information inside helper T-helper cells. This allows the immune system to catalog and later access the specific genetic, molecular and physiological makeup of an invader scanned even decades earlier. When the helper T-cell sees this pathogen again, it can immediately mount the same defense and healing strategy used against the previous pathogen.

What has gone wrong in the case of chronic arthritis, then? The immune system has indeed launched a healing strategy, yet with no real results—only more damage. This indicates a problem: A problem with the process or perhaps the damage has become unrepairable. For one reason or another, the immune system is not doing its job. It is possibly overworked. It is possibly overstimulated. Perhaps the pathogen is simply too strong for the immune system to fix, or the damage is too great. We can narrow this down to the pathogen being too strong, the damage being too great, or the immune system being too weak.

Many health professionals breeze over this and decide to narrow it down to one possibility: They say the immune system is attacking the *wrong thing* (healthy cells). Because there are lots of healthy cells available to attack, the inflammation continues. They say the immune system is confusing *self* with *non-self*, and the body is essentially attacking itself. They say the immune system has gone on some sort of crazy binge and it has begun self-annihilation. They generalize that autoimmunity is caused by a *good immune system gone bad*. This kind of explanation is quite easy because there is an unknown, mysterious bad guy we can blame. We might compare this explanation with the concept of the *bogeyman*. Yes, the *autoimmune bogeyman* is doing this to our joints.

This kind of explanation also allows us to avoid the possibility that we could be doing anything wrong with regard to our diets, lifestyles or our environment. No one is to blame. It is easy.

A more logical explanation is that the immune system is still doing the right thing, but it is overpowered by the problem. Either the immune system is too weak for the problem or the problem is too strong for the immune system. Therefore, the immune system cannot adequately fix the problem.

As for the idea that the immune system is attacking the body's own healthy cells   why are we so sure that those cells are healthy? If we see T-cells and cytokines in the neighborhood, this should indicate that the cells are not healthy.

If the cells were somehow damaged by microorganisms or oxidative radicals from toxins, then they should be considered unfit by the body's immune system. In the case of arthritis, we are talking about a group of cartilage or synovial cells that have been damaged. Just because the cells are still functioning does not mean they are healthy. The immune system must be attacking them for a reason. They are damaged or infected. There is no mystery.

There is also the possibility that a few or combination of all of these circumstances are taking place in arthritis. As we delve further into the science, we will find a few common denominators.

Without question, our bodies are under constant attack. For most of us, the immune system works pretty dog gone well. Most invading toxins and organisms are broken up and disposed of within seconds of contact with the body. If they grow within the body, the immune system launches full-scale war—an illness—to knock them out. Unless, of course, the body is burdened with too many toxins and organisms to remove at once—stressing the immune system to its breaking point. This is called *immunosuppression.* In this state, the immune system is exhausted. Immune cells and their supporting players—the liver, the adrenals, the kidneys, and the thyroid—are creeping along. To what degree does immunosuppression have to do with arthritis?

Conventional Arthritis Causes

Physical damage	Wear and tear, age, trauma or injury.
Infection	Systemic infection of bacteria, fungi, or virus, possibly exacerbated by trauma
Genetics	DNA sequencing handed down through families
Autoimmunity	Immune system misidentifies the body's own cells

Let's review these various associations critically, and open the discussion to other potential factors.

Wear and Tear, Damage or Trauma

Physical injury or wear and tear is thought to be a possible cause of some arthritis—especially osteoarthritis. While this is certainly a consideration, the body has countermeasures for both. In the case of physical injury, the body has a method of replacing the chondrocytes and the cartilage matrix. With rest, plenty of water, good nutrition and measures to increase circulation—heat and cold—the body's immune system should be able to remove the damaged tissue and regain full operational effectiveness. In this case, inflammation would be a temporary occurrence as the body heals itself.

In chronic wear and tear, this becomes more complex because the injury may be repetitive. In other words, the shearing and physical shock to the region may recur before the wound gets a chance to heal. This is often the case for carpal tunnel syndrome, which can be caused by the repetitive motion of typing on a keyboard or other device.

These issues are often simply resolved by changing habits. Once the pain signals us to make adjustments, we can make postural changes, or change the way we move in other ways. This should give our cartilage the opportunity to be repaired. As new chondrocytes are generated, new cartilage will be woven together. Assuming the body has the right raw materials (nutrients) for the job.

Crtilage can become damaged when it loses some of its key ingredients and protective agents such as collagen and lubricin. This in turn can accellerate the loss in the protective synovial fluid between and around the cartilage.

This brings us to the situation of recurring inflammation and destruction within the synovial membrane and synovial fluid. As we noted before, because the inflammation is not shut off and the area is not cleaned up, autoimmune syndrome is assumed.

We know that osteoarthritis and rheumatoid arthritis—and most other types of arthritic inflammation—often accompany an avalanche of immune cells and their co-factors into the synovial membrane and synovial fluid. These include T-cells, monocytes, and dendritic cells. Leucotreines and prostaglandins also proliferate. As these inflammation agents encroach, there is a breakdown of the cartilage cells and a growing number of damaged synovial cells called *fibroblast-like synoviocytes* (or FLS). These synoviocytes are unique in that they resist the process of cell death. In other words, these abnormal synovial cells become very difficult to knock off.

This poses a problem for T-cells programmed to remove abnormal or damaged cells. These proliferating FLS cells are very difficult for the T-cells to remove: Unless, of course, the T-cells can be reprogrammed and retrained with new MHC from the thymus to kill off the FLS. In the absence of this, the inflammation continues, as the T-cells keep working on removing the abnormal synovial cells. Here the problem appears to relate to a handicapped, burdened or deficient immune system.

Bacterial Infections

The role of microorganisms in arthritis has been controversial over the past few decades, because assaying live plate counts from synovial fluid has proved difficult. Over the past decade, however, assay methods have improved, and antibody profiles and DNA analysis has provided the smoking gun indicating prior or existing infections within arthritic joints. A growing number of studies are now associating numerous types of bacterial infections with a range of arthritis types.

In one review of multiple studies from the rheumatology department of a Turkish hospital (Ogrendik 2009), it was found that people with chronic infections of oral anaerobic bacteria—the kind that infects the gums, such as *Porphyromonas gingivalis, Tannerella forsynthensis,* and *Prevotella intermedia*—were more likely to have RA. Furthermore, antibodies from these bacteria were found in greater levels within the synovial fluid of RA patients.

Severe, life-threatening cases of arthritic joints infected with bacteria are often diagnosed as *septic arthritis.* For this reason, septic arthritis diagnoses are far less prevalent than diagnoses for rheumatoid arthritis. However, the number of RA cases that are actually septic in nature is unknown. Indeed, septic arthritis diagnoses are from 14 times to 35 times more likely in previously diagnosed RA patients (Favero *et al.* 2008). Whether this means that the original RA cases were actually septic and had not yet progressed to that point is unknown. Quite often, the link between bacterial or viral infection and a particular case of arthritis is difficult to make by a doctor without significant testing of the synovial fluid and membrane.

It also appears that the diagnosis of septic arthritis is growing. This may be related to more awareness among physicians, increased synovial fluid testing, or the growth of these infections. Some physicians simply consider the septic arthritis diagnosis *severely infected arthritis*, while rheumatoid arthritis is milder, albeit possibly still infective. In other words, an RA case may actually be septic or infective arthritis in its preliminary stages. Septic diagnosis is also often referred to as *polyarticular septic arthritis*. Truly, this diagnosis is severe, with a mortality rate of about 50% (Dubost *et al.* 1993). There is also an association between corticosteroids and septic arthritis. Septic arthritis rates increase among RA patients who have been prescribed corticosteroids (Goldenberg 1989). For this reason and others, which we will discuss, corticosteroids are losing their shine in conventional treatment for RA.

There also appears to be a link between septic arthritis and surgery. In a recent study of 4,068 arthroscopic surgery patients at the Peking University Institute of Sports Medicine (Wang *et al.* 2009) revealed that 21 had septic arthritis following the surgery.

Infective arthritis that arises after a worsening of an infection elsewhere is often called *reactive arthritis*. While these words may implicate arthritis as some kind of bystander to the real disease, the infection has often simply expanded into the joints.

Illustrating this effect, in a 2009 study of arthritis in horses (Dumoulin *et al.* 2009), synovial fluid was drawn from 220 severely inflamed joints. Out of 149 horses that had other symptoms of infection, 72% of those joints actually contained microorganisms.

Pseudomonas aeruginosa has provided a clear link between bacterial infection and arthritis. Pseudomonas can infect hot tubs and other moist, warm environments. A *Pseudomonas* attack can almost immediately severely infect and inflame the joints. Often the infection will subside within a couple of weeks, assuming the body's immune system can clear out the invasion. Occasionally, the infection continues. In one case study (Keynes *et al.* 2009), an elderly person was treated for a urinary tract infection of *Pseudomonas*. The joints of the patient were soon infected as well. Synovial fluid aspirate culturing confirmed the bacteria had invaded the joint capsule. The patient soon died of the infection.

Tuberculosis has been found also invading the joints, in a septic form of arthritis created by the *Mycobacterium tuberculosis* bacteria. The tuberculosis infection and inflammation tends to move slowly, often gradually involving the spine and larger joints.

Chlamydia trachomatis has been found at an alarming rate in the synovial membranes of arthritic patients. In one test from Tunisia (Siala *et al.* 2009), synovial samples were drawn from 34 arthritic patients. Nine had reactive arthritis, seven had undifferentiated oligoarthritis, two had rheumatoid arthritis and two had osteoarthritis. Out of the 34 patients, a total of 20 patients—59%—were positive for *C. trachomatis* within synovial tissue and/or fluid using PCR testing—a process where polymerase is used to isolate and identify DNA sequences.

Fungi have also been found to infect joints. *Candida albicans* has been known to infect joints, causing arthritic inflammation. A joint infected with fungi is officially called *fungal prosthetic joint disease*—assuming that the fungal infection is found.

Osteomyelitis of the vertebrae—spondylodiscitis—is a condition that mostly affects adults. Its occurrence has been rising over the past few years. *Staphylococcus aureus* is the most common cause of osteomyelitis (Pintado-Garcia 2008). *Staphylococcus aureus* and its new superbug version, MRSA—Methicillin-resistant *Staphylococcus aureus*—has been increasingly found among RA cases as well. RA is also sometimes associated with *Staphylococcus polymyositis*.

Here is a list of microorganisms that have been associated with either rheumatoid, septic or reactive forms of arthritis:

Bacteroides fragilis	*Gardnerella vaginalis*
Borrelia burgdorferi	*Kingella kingae*
Brucella melitensis	*Listeria monocytogenes*
Brucellae spp.	*Moraxella canis*
Campylobacter jejuni	*Mycobacterium lepromatosis*
Chlamydia trachomatis	*Mycobacterium marinum*
Clostridium difficile	*Mycobacterium terrae*
Corynebacterium striatum	*Mycoplasma arthritidis*
Cryptococcal pyarthrosis	*Mycoplasma hominis*

Mycoplasma leachii sp.	*Serratia fonticola*
Neisseria gonorrhoeae	*Sphingomonas paucimobilis*
Ochrobactrum anthropi	*Staphylococcus aureus*
Pasteurella multocida	*Staphylococcus lugdunensis*
Pneumocystis jiroveci	*Streptococcus agalactiae*
Prevotella bivia	*Streptococcus equisimilis*
Prevotella loescheii	*Streptococcus pneumoniae*
Pseudomonas aeruginosa	*Streptococcus pyogenes*
Pyoderma gangrenosum	*Streptococcus uberis*
Roseomonas gilardii	*Treponema pallidum*
Salmonella entertidis	*Vibrio vulnificus*
Scedosporium prolificans	*Yersinia enterocoolitica*

There are a number of different types of microorganisms. Here are the basic categories:

Types of Microorganisms

Fungi	Yeasts, molds and others; over 100,000 species; live in earth, air, water and damp, moist environments; can infect the body via food, water, air, touch
Bacteria	Single-celled organisms; live in water, earth, air, on and inside other living organisms; can infect via food, water, air, touch
Mycoplasmas	Ancient slow-moving bacteria; live primarily on earth and water; infect mostly via food, water and touch
Parasites	Tiny organisms that infect and live within another living organism. Includes worms, protozoa, amoeba
Thermophiles	Opportunistic bacteria that can live in very hot environments, such as boiling water or an oven
Psychophiles	Opportunistic bacteria that can live in the very cold, such as artic or freezers
Nanobacteria	Extremely small bacteria that often have hard calcium shells. Are now thought to cause some diseases once considered autoimmune-related.

Over the past few decades, bacteria have gotten stronger, thanks to the prolific use of antibiotics.

Indeed, the rise of superbugs such as MRSA has been specifically related to the amount of unnecessary antibiotics being given to people and animals. This is because bacteria are living organisms, and they tend to *adapt* to their surroundings. If they are attacked enough times with a certain challenge, they are likely to figure out how to work around that challenge, and possibly even thrive in spite of it.

Many other forms of antibiotic-resistant strains of bacteria have also evolved over the past few decades. Over a few generations, they have simply become stronger and more able to counteract these antibiotic measures. Worse, as one species of bacteria figures out how to counteract a particular antibiotic, it will store that knowledge within a genetic compartment called a *plasmid*. This plasmid can then be passed on to other species, enabling the antibiotic resistance to spread to other strains and species.

So many different species of bacteria reside within and around us. They reside within our bodies, houses, on our doorknobs, and within our foods. *Campylobacter* species is one of the most common food borne bacteria—often prevalent in meat. It causes diarrhea, fever and cramping, but rarely death. The *E. coli* O157:H7 bacteria can sometimes be lethal (verocytosis) in immune-suppressed people. Mostly *E. coli* infections result in nausea and diarrhea, however. *Salmonella* is prevalent in the intestines of some wildlife, including birds, reptiles and other animals (including humans) and can sicken humans. *Clostrium botulinum* can grow in food or juice containers, especially cans—producing a sometimes-deadly disease called botulism. *Giardia, Shigella, Staphylococcus aureus, Mycobacterium tuberculosis, Yersinia enterocolitica, Campylobacter jejuni, Cryptosporidia* and *Listeria monocytogenes* can also infect food, especially if they are prepared from infected water sources or from infected food handlers' hands. *Trichinosis*, quite common in pork, can also seriously sicken. Testing has also shown that 1 out of 20,000 commercial eggs are contaminated by *Salmonella enteritidis*.

While warm, moist environments are favored, bacteria can survive extreme environments. They can survive in the fridge, the freezer and even in low-oxygen vacuum containers. In colder temperatures, bacteria can hibernate and incubate. A little warmth and moisture will revive them. Many food-borne bacteria colonize via the release of spores, which can survive harsh conditions—including pasteurization. A single spore can quickly grow into an entire colony of bacteria.

Bacteria surround us. *Staphylococcus* species can live in any warm or moist environment. *Tuberculosis* can live within moisture droplets. It can be passed on from person to person through coughing, sneezing or physical contact (hand-to-mucosal membrane). *Borrelia burgdorferi* is also known as lyme disease. While lyme is commonly considered passed on through tick bites, new information has surfaced that other insects can also carry lyme. *Pseudomonas aeruginosa* can live among hot tubs and bathrooms, and can enter the body through the skin. *Streptococcus pneumoniae* proliferates in indoor environments. It can be passed on through breathing air droplets or physical contact with mucosal membranes.

Intestinal permeability may also allow entry to opportunistic bacteria that normally dwell in the intestines. Intestinal permeability is caused by gaps in the brush barrier that exists between the villi of the small intestine cells. When the brush barrier is eroded from a lack of probiotics, tobacco, alcohol, pharmaceuticals and other chemical toxins, bacteria can "leak" into the bloodstream. For example, *Blastocystis hominis*, a bacterial pathogen often found in the intestines, has been found in synovial membranes of infectious arthritic patients (Kruger *et al.* 1994).

Viral Joint Invasion

Unlike bacteria and fungi, viruses are not living organisms. Rather they are spores that derange DNA. Yes, viruses too have been associated with arthritis in research. In a 2009 study from the Harvard Medical School (Rosenau and Schur), synovial fluid was drawn from fifty RA patients who were RF-negative positive. The fluid was taken prior to knee replacement, and frozen until being analyzed. After full analysis of the cell lines, the IgM antibodies were examined for potential links to prior viruses. Eleven of the fifty patients—22%—had IgM antibodies to the measles virus. The presence of antibodies among the synovial fluid cells indicates that there was at some point, an active viral infection among the synovial fluid and membrane, indicating a clear viral link with the arthritis.

A number of other viruses have also been linked to arthritis. Epstein-Barr virus has also been connected with numerous cases of rheumatoid arthritis (Pohl 2009). Lupus has also been linked with Epstein-Barr (James *et al.* 1994). HIV (Human Immunosuppressive Virus) has presented with arthritis (Zaki 2009). Influenza has also presented with arthritis. This type of flu infection is often called *invasive influenza*. The infection sometimes causes what is considered either rheumatoid arthritis or osteomyelitis. The most often seen invasive version is *Haemophilus influenzae A*. Other viral infections known to cause arthritic conditions include hepatitis B virus and hepatitis C virus, HIV, the parvovirus B19, Epstein-Barr, the human T-cell lymphotropic virus-I, and the alphaviruses.

Viruses like Epstein-Barr will infect B-cells, deranging their immune response activities. Once infected, these B-cells can travel throughout various tissue systems, infecting other tissue cells and other B-cells. In this case, we can see that the immune system itself can become deranged by an infection. Such a derangement is seen also in a number of other afflictions, such as multiple sclerosis.

Viruses can gain access to the body's cells through a number of means. These include airborne droplets; contact exchange through hands or other parts of the body; touching door handles or any other common object; sexual contact; and saliva or blood contact.

There are two basic kinds of viruses: DNA viruses and RNA viruses. DNA viruses damage the cell's DNA, changing the master instructions for that cell. An RNA virus will damage the cell's ability to replicate its DNA instructions, sometimes even replacing those instructions with new instructions.

Once the virus has changed the cell's DNA or RNA, that cell begins to function differently. Some super-viruses are incredibly resilient, using damaged cells to pass the virus on to other organisms. Some viruses, despite an immune response from the body to attempt to eradicate them, can remain dormant inside some cells or tissue systems. These viruses may become active when triggered, often when the body is stressed, traumatized and/or the immune system is compromised. The *herpes simplex* virus is such a latent virus. It often becomes dormant within cells of the nervous system, intermittently becoming active. Once active, it will cause herpes' characteristic open wounds outside the mouth or in the case of

HSV2, around the genitals (although HSV2 can also invade facial tissues as well).

Viruses are genetic spores. They infect other cells by coercing infected cells to pass along the altered genetic sequencing. This often takes place by altering the transcription process. Once a virus has deranged the infected cell's DNA sequencing, the DNA's transcription to RNA becomes altered. Because RNA drives enzyme-protein synthesis, this mutation translates to altered enzyme activity. This alteration of proteins and enzymes secure the virus' ability to spread. Many feel this survival indicates a virus is alive. However, a virus is actually a messaging system—similar to a juxtacrine. It delivers a particular and often destructive message.

We might compare a virus to a computer email worm virus. The typical computer worm virus first invades certain files inside the computer, and uses the computer's own software to replicate itself. The initial virus program might have been originally written by a devious computer programmer. Once the programmer's emails are sent out, however, the coding within the worm's file does the damage automatically. The original programmer may be long gone by then—perhaps on vacation—while the worm could still be destroying software all over the world.

Other viruses can also become latent. Even common viruses such as rhinoviruses (including the common cold), various types of influenza, shingles, mononucleosis, cytomegalovirus, and a host of other viruses can hibernate. If a weakened immune system does not completely eradicate viral spores and infected cells immediately following an infection, the virus may gain entry and remain dormant and unnoticed in some less-traveled space in the body, awaiting the opportune time to re-emerge. This opportune time is usually when the immune system is weakened, or body is hit with a trauma (which will also burden the immune system).

Once these viruses begin infecting cells, the infection may grow from the more easily penetrable tissues of the organs and skin to the tissue systems with more barriers. This can include the bones, the cartilage and the synovial membrane. Once such a virus penetrates these tissues, the repair process can get complex.

In most tissue systems, the repair process of a virally infected cell is to surround the tissue area, destroy the infected cells, and guard the uninfected cells. This often requires a tremendous amount of focus by the immune system. Inflammation, fever, nausea and other processes to recycle and detoxify the system prevail. In the joints, the process will also include swelling, pain, restricted motion, and the need for rest and recovery.

A virus that infects the joints is often one the immune system has not successfully eradicated from more easily accessible tissue systems—where there are fewer barriers and more blood circulation. In general, those who have stronger immune systems also happen to have shorter durations of viral infections. Studies have shown that these people also tend to take better care of their bodies, and have better diets. Anyone can contract the flu—healthy or not. A weakened immune system will more likely contract it and become ill longer, according to epidemiological research of larger populations (Avery 1999).

Any sort of crisis, whether stress-related, diet-related, or environment-related, will weaken the immune system. This *immunosuppressive* state opens the door to optimistic viruses.

Germ or Field?

The depth and range of viral and bacterial infection risk is humbling. How can we expect to avoid and counteract all of these microorganism threats? Better yet, for those who currently have arthritis, which microorganism(s) could have caused it and how could we possibly have avoided contracting them?

This is a perplexing question for researchers and scientists who study pandemics and epidemics. They want to know, firstly, how do viruses and bacteria get to a point where they become a threat to society? Then, of course, they want to know how to stop infections from overwhelming society. In fact, there is a growing list of diseases that are now being connected to microorganisms—diseases that physicians thought previously were unrelated to pathogenic microorganisms. A shining example of this is the ulcer. It has only been over the last couple of decades that researchers have confirmed that *Helicobacter pylori* bacteria—or their overgrowth—is implicated in most ulcers. About 70-90% of all peptic ulcers (and 95-100% of all duodenal ulcers) are associated with an infection of the *H. pylori* bacteria. For many decades, medical science had concluded that peptic ulcers were caused by a combination of stress and diet. Gastric cancer is also associated with *H. pylori*.

Further on this example, it is now estimated that *H. pylori* infections occur among about 70% of the population of developing countries and 5-15% of developed countries (Pellicano 2009). The mode of transmission is currently unknown, but water and general sanitation are receiving the most research attention. In poor and developing countries, most children become infected with *H. pylori*. In developed countries, where sanitation is higher, usually infections occur among adults—but at levels far less than developing countries. The interesting factoid is that *gastric ulcers are rare among developed countries* (Everhart 1994)

In addition, very few people who are infected with *H. pylori* get ulcers and gastric cancer. For developing countries, the percentage is even less. So we can conclude from these facts that while *H. pylori* is associated with gastric ulcers and gastric cancer, having *H. pylori* does not mean that one will contract an ulcer or stomach cancer.

Why? If *H. pylori* cause ulcers, why doesn't everyone who is infected have an ulcer?

This question of infection by microorganism versus disease pathology is not limited to *H. pylori*, either. Every year hundreds of thousands—if not millions—of people eat some packaged food that is contaminated with *Salmonella*, *E. coli*, or some other pathogenic organism. Out of the millions that eat contaminated food, only a tiny proportion might get sick, and only a few die. According to the CDC, between 1996 and 1998, out of an estimated 76 million foodborne illnesses in the U.S., only 325,000 were hospitalized and only about 5,000 died. How is it that so few actually got sick enough to go to the hospital? How come so few died?

Some interesting population statistics come out of a comparison for this same period of foodborne illness outbreaks in other countries. Americans had 26,000 cases of foodborne illness for every 100,000 persons in the U.S. during this period. The UK had 3,400 cases per 100,000 of people (population). France had 1,210 cases per 100,000 people. Why are more Americans getting sick from foodborne illnesses than are people from the UK or France?

We might consider solving this problem by trying to determine how environmental conditions differ between the United States and

France. The environment *outside the body* would be the typical consideration. But what about the *environment inside the body?*

Over the past century, our society has increasingly been focused on bacteria as the cause for so many other ailments. And for good reason. Our current bacteria focus in the medical community began in the 1860s with Louis Pasteur's insistence upon the *germ theory*—a proposal made earlier that all disease was caused by microorganisms. To prove his point, Pasteur cruelly infected various animals with bacteria and studied their demise against uninfected controls. Yes, he proved that bacteria *can* cause certain diseases, assuming inoculation beyond the point of immunity.

However, he missed a central component of the equation. The fact is, our planet is covered with infectious bacteria in numbers far beyond calculation. Each human body contains trillions of bacteria of many species—both probiotic and pathogenic. So if the outside and inside worlds are covered with pathogenic bacteria, why are we not all sick and infected all the time? Why aren't we all dead—killed by this onslaught of bacteria? How could some of us be healthy with all this pathogenic bacteria around?

Microbiologists Antoine Bechamp and Claude Bernard—peers of Pasteur—took issue with Pasteur's germ theory. They proposed the important issue in disease is not the bacteria, but the *field,* or environment within the body. In other words, a healthy body with a strong immune system [and probiotic populations] can effectively counter infectious bacteria. Those who get sick, they proposed, were those with weakened, compromised immune systems.

We can confirm the field theory quite simply. A simple review of the statistics mentioned earlier regarding food-borne outbreaks, and an investigation of the specific cases of those who died or became seriously ill will tell us. The more immunosuppressed a person is, the more likely they will not be able to counteract the infection.

In fact, many of our foods contain *E. coli, Salmonella* and many other bacteria species. These do not make people sick. Why not? Because they do not have the colony strength to prevail against a healthy body's various immune systems.

Unfortunately, the germ theory prevailed within western conventional medicine. This unfortunate turn of events caused the unleashing of the genie of antibiotic drugs and so many other pharmaceutical panaceas over the last century. While many of these medicines have helped millions recover from crippling infection—preventing many deaths—the over-prescription of antibiotics has also created an epidemic of immunosuppression and destroyed internal probiotic populations. And those bacteria the antibiotics were working against are now coming back to haunt us. New superbugs like MRSA and other strains are more powerful than the previous bacteria. Now they are also killing more people, and many of our antibiotics are not working. Many of these superbugs are also causing debilitating arthritis and sepsis, causing illness and death—camouflaged by different disease names.

In fact, it now is becoming increasingly difficult to determine whether antibiotics have saved more people than the superbugs they created have killed. Epidemiological research shows that superbug infections can result in a variety of disease pathologies. They act in subterfuge. A superbug might result in pneumonia, flu, diarrhea, liver disorder or gastrointestinal disease—even arthritis. So it is hard to compare these statistics fairly. While it is easy to show that so many people have taken antibiotics, and that many bacterial infections have been averted, it is difficult to measure how many illnesses the new antibiotic superbugs have created: At least using today's diagnostic measurement systems.

As we pan to the future, we are faced with the reality that the germ theory solution will likely create new epidemics that fare worse than the ones antibiotics previously prevented.

All the evidence we have on foodborne illness, epidemics and pandemics indicate that immunosuppressed people fare the worst. It is the often among the elderly—who are dealing with immune systems weakened by age and stress. Or among babies—whose immune systems have yet to fully develop. Or among people who have had repeated illnesses or are fighting one particular illness. Or among those who are challenged by stressful environments.

A new definition of immunosuppression is arising out of the thousands of studies that have been done with probiotics and infection over the past decade. Increasingly we are seeing that the quantity and species of probiotics we have in our bodies relate to how we respond to bacterial infections.

This may be a new idea to some. You see, like animals in the forest, bacteria colonies tend to control each other's populations. In a healthy body and natural environment, our bodies harbor enough probiotics with 'smart' antibacterial strategies to keep most pathogenic bacteria colonies from growing too large.

Our body's probiotics make up about 70% of our immune system. How so? Because the trillions of probiotics that inhabit our mouth, sinuses, intestines and many other parts of the body are skilled at producing a number of their own antibiotics. Furthermore, the difference between probiotic antibiotics and static manufactured versions is that like infectious bacteria, probiotics are living organisms. So their arsenal tends to change and adapt to the pathogenic bacteria. We might compare this to the old *Mad Comics* "Spy versus Spy" cartoon. Every time one spy tried something different, the other spy changed strategies and countered him—frustrating the first spy. In the same way, the antibiotics that probiotics produce are responsive and *smart,* while the static versions that man has produced can easily be outsmarted.

Beyond this of course, the body's immune system also produces a number of smart weapons—antibodies and lymphocytes that identify and break down other microbial and viral infections. In addition, probiotics (and botanicals) will work conjunctively with the immune system to stimulate certain immune responses.

Keeping the immune system and probiotic colonies strong and healthy is vital to retarding bacterial infection. Those with healthy immune systems and probiotic populations will have less chance of getting sick from eating a limited amount of contaminated foods.

Virtually every body contains *E. coli* and *Salmonella,* as mentioned previously. *E. coli* is a common bacterium residing in the intestinal tract. Depending upon our environment, anywhere from three-quarters to a seventh of us host the *H. pylori* bacteria, yet show no sign of any infective response. Why do we not get sick from these "dangerous" bacteria? Because our probiotic bacteria populations and immune systems keep these populations in check. Like the many other bacteria in our bodies, including *Candida* and *Staphylococcus* species, *E. coli* in controlled populations actually perform a number of tasks useful to the body.

This does not mean that we should not be careful with our foods and surroundings. Nor should we not take antibiotics in the case of life-threatening emergencies. Our minds are also part of our immune system. We should carefully wash our hands and wash our foods to limit our exposure.

While *H. pylori* itself has little to do with arthritis, it is notable because the situation is analogous to arthritis. Like ulcers, arthritis has traditionally been disconnected with bacterial infection. It is much easier to culture the stomach and determine *H. pylori* presence than it is to culture synovial membrane and fluid. And because *H. pylori* and ulcers are fairly easy to connect, they have been more thoroughly researched among various populations. We can thus draw various conclusions and comparisons with infective arthritis. At the very least, we can conclude that infective arthritis research is in its infancy in modern medicine.

Chemical Toxins

We have always been surrounded by bacterial and viral pathogens. This is not true of many of today's chemical toxins. Only over the past century have our bodies and cells been bombarded by the toxic chemicals that pervade our homes, waters, air and now bodies.

As this grand synthetic experiment has unfolded, we have discovered many of these chemicals are quite lethal. Many also threaten humankind's future existence. After only a few decades of massive synthetic chemical manufacturing, we are beginning to suffer the horrific price synthetic chemicals come with: We are faced with increasing epidemics of asthma, lung cancer, COPD, and other bronchial diseases. The water we drink has become toxic. Much of our drinking supplies are laced with DDT, PCB, nitrates, and hundreds of other dangerous toxins. Much of the non-organic food we eat is now to full of various synthetic residues. We are gradually discovering that agribusiness' use of chemical fertilizers and pesticides is slowly poisoning our bodies. The toxins are building up in our cells—mutating our DNA and suffocating our immune systems.

Most of the furnishings we purchase now are filled with formaldehydes, synthetic materials and other synthetic preservatives. Most office buildings and many houses still contain hazards like asbestos and other components that cause toxicity. Our entire environment is laced with synthetic chemistry. If the human race stopped chemical production today, we still would have done so much damage over the past fifty years that it would take centuries for the earth's detoxification systems to purify herself.

The core issue with synthetic chemicals is that they run contrary to the fragile balance existing among nature's biochemical recycling systems. As a result, they clog the arteries of our ecosystem. Today there are mountains of synthetic chemistry loading up our dumps, landfills, lakes, rivers, and oceans. These mountains are decomposing very slowly—outgassing and breaking down into potent toxins released into the environment. *Time Magazine* reported on June 25, 2007 that Americans generated 1,643 pounds of trash per person in 2005. A mere 32% of it was recycled.

Much of this waste is plastic. The problem with plastic is reflective of its benefit—it lasts far longer than do natural materials. While a plastic bag might not tear and rip as fast as a paper bag as we walk from the grocery store, a plastic bag will have as much as a 500-year half-life—depending upon its material. That is a long time. What happens to the bag while nature works to biodegrade it? It clogs our soils and waters. For this reason our lands, waters, and bodies, are steadily becoming laced with polymers and plasticizers.

Plastics are made through reactions between monomers (small molecules) and plasticizers to create longer-chain molecules. Examples of monomers include hydrocarbons such as petroleum. Combining ethane monomers and plasticizers forms polyethylene. Combining styrene monomers and plasticizers renders polystyrene. Combining vinyl chloride monomers and plasticizers results in polyvinyl chloride, or PVC. Combining propylene monomers and plasticizers gives us polypropylene.

Nature produces its own types of natural polymers such as rubber. In an attempt to improve upon nature, in 1855 the lab of Alexander Parkes mixed pyroxylin from cellulose with alcohol and camphor to form what is thought to be the first type of plastic. This clear, hard plastic was 'improved' by Dr. Leo Baekeland decades later with a polymer process using phenol and formaldehyde in the first decade of the twentieth century. "Bakelite" became a wildly successful product as it effectively replaced shellac and rubber as a general sheathing material. Because it was heat-resistant and moisture-proof, it quickly became the insulator of choice for engines, appliances, and electronics. Dr. Baekeland eventually sold his General Bakelite Company to Union Carbide in 1939 and retired a very wealthy man to Florida. His life was made easy through the 'miracle' of chemistry.

Nylon was an invention of DuPont researchers in the late 1930s. It was made initially with benzene from coal. The introduction of polypropylene as a synthetic rubber followed shortly thereafter. Polypropylene was an accidental discovery by a couple of researchers who were trying to convert natural gas for Phillips Petroleum. The American industrial complex gearing up for World War II focused its attention on this synthetic version due to a shortage of natural rubber. Thanks to synthetic rubber, each military person was estimated to have 32 pounds of rubber in clothing and equipment. A tank needed about a ton. We might consider that America's military might is at least partially due to its synthetic rubber making. Again, chemistry has seemingly made our lives easier.

The synthetic polymer revolution surged after the Second World War. The plastic revolution emerged, and both consumers and manufacturers rushed to replace naturally derived goods with synthetic polymers.

One might argue that combining earth-borne commodities like hydrocarbons cannot be so unnatural. After all, hydrocarbons are produced by the earth as part of her recycling process. However, the process of converting these hydrocarbon monomers into polymers requires various catalysts and *plasticizers* to complete. Plasticizers are used in plastic production to give the long polymer chain its flexibility. Without plasticizers inserted between the polymer chains, there could be no flexibility among the plastics. Without plasticizers, polymers are clear, hard substances: rock-like. The various gradations of flex added to polymer chains give the resulting plastic its particular usefulness and characteristic. A plasticizer will provide strength along with this flexibility, making the material difficult to tear or break.

Most plasticizers are *phthalates*. Phthalates are derived from phthalic acid, an aromatic ringed carbon molecule also referred to as dicarboxylic acid. Originally synthesized in 1836 through the oxidation of naphthalene tetrachloride, phthalic acid can also be synthesized from hydrocarbons and sulfuric acid with a mercury catalyst. Most aromatic carbon rings like the phenyl ring or the benzyl ring made using this process have proven to be hazardous to our environment and physical well-being. Note there are a number of aromatic carbon rings that are produced in nature as well. These do not come with the same hazards for some reason.

There are hundreds of different plasticizers now in use in humankind's production of different plastics. Most are either aromatic carbons or similarly hazardous compounds. While bound within hydrocarbon polymer chains they appear innocuous. However, as plastic polymers break down in the environment, these plasticizers are released. Our backyards, landfills and oceans—our entire environment—are quickly becoming inundated with the release of these plasticizers.

While the cumulative effect of these compounds entering our bodies for many years has yet to be determined, there is some evidence that most plasticizers are estrogenic. They can attach to estrogen receptors, and thus confuse the body's stimulation of different mechanisms such as growth and inflammation. Estrogen ligand and receptor balance is also critical to our flow of various other hormones and neurotransmitters such as serotonin, dopamine, progesterone and many others. We should also note that rates of menopausal and chronic fatigue disorders and breast cancers, which are all directly related to the balance of hormones, neurotransmitters and estrogen balance, have been rising dramatically over the past 20 years. Estrogen balance has also been associated with arthritis—in both rheumatoid arthritis and osteoarthritis (Gerosa *et al.* 2008; Mundy 2007).

Benzene for example, is the typical source of the phenyl plasticizer. Benzene has been classified as a volatile organic compound and a carcinogen by the Natural Institutes of Health National Toxicology Program. Benzene is also among the top twenty most used industrial chemicals. It is used to make adhesives, paint, pharmaceuticals, printed materials, photographic chemicals, synthetic rubber, dyes, detergents, paint and shockingly, even food processing equipment to name a few. Today benzene is found throughout our environment—in our air and water—and has been implicated in numerous cancers.

A study released in 2005 by the *Environmental Working Group* found 260 contaminants in drinking water supplies around the country. Of these 260 chemicals, the U.S. *Environmental Protection Agency* regulates 114 to some extent; and another five have been assigned secondary standards—non-enforceable minimum contamination goals. That leaves an astonishing 141 chemicals with no standards in the drinking supplies of over 195 million people. Not all 141 chemicals are being served to all 195 million people at once. The report specified that at least 40 of these 141 chemical toxins were being serviced to at least one million people, while another 19 were being supplied to at least 10,000 people. In some cases, single water supplies had up to an additional twenty unregulated contaminants. In other words, some water supplies are much worse than others. Depending upon their proximity to industrial waste, commercial farm waste, chemical fertilizer use, pesticide use, herbicide use, sewage dumping, and the existence of underground storage tanks, there can be a range of toxins in our water.

The report also broke down the unregulated contaminants into several categories; including methyl tertiary butyl ether or MTBE from gasoline, perchlorate from rocket fuel, fifteen water disinfection byproducts, four plasticizers, seventy-eight consumer and industrial production chemicals, and twenty gas, coal and other fuel combustion chemicals. Fifty-two of these unregulated chemicals have been linked to cancer. Seventy-seven have been linked to reproductive or growth problems. Sixteen more have been connected with compromising the immune system. By far the biggest source of both regulated and unregulated chemicals in this study was industrial waste with 166 chemicals, followed by agricultural pollutants with eighty-three chemicals. Household and urban pollution came in third with twenty-nine chemicals and water treatment plants contributed a jaw-dropping forty-four pollutants to tap water systems.

Agriculture spreads 110 billion pounds of chemical fertilizer over almost 250 million acres according to a 2002 USDA report. This accounts for about one-eighth of the entire United States. Meanwhile about one-tenth of the U.S. is being drenched with herbicides and pesticides. Meat production is another dramatic contributor. There are about 248,000 feedlots in the U.S., primarily housing cattle or pigs. These feedlots produce about 500 million tons of manure annually, laden with hormones and antibiotics. This means our thirst for commercially farmed meat is limiting our future ability to consume our body's most precious requirement: water. As Fawell and Nieuwenhuijsen (2003) document in their review of various water contaminants throughout the world, water contamination has been linked to a variety of disease pathologies, especially in areas with increased industrial and commercial agricultural economies.

The problems of synthetic chemicals are pervasive. Estimates suggest some 80,000 chemicals have been approved for commercialization over the past fifty years. The *Toxic Substances Control Act of 1976* was set up to evaluate chemicals being introduced. Only about 65,000 have been reviewed. However only a small percentage of these chemicals have been carefully analyzed and reviewed as to their environmental and health effects. Hundreds of thousands of people die each year—and some say the number approaches one million just in the U.S.—from chemical pharmaceuticals, despite the 'watchful' eyes of governmental agencies. Several hundred thousand die in the U.S. from cancer each year. Millions die worldwide from cancer, a disease suspected to be caused primarily by cellular mutation due to environmental stressors like chemical toxicity.

The Environmental Working Group's Human Toxome Project has revealed some frightening statistics on the poisoning of our bodies by chemicals. In one study of nine adult participants, blood and urine contained 171 of the 214 toxic chemicals for which they were analyzed. These included industrial compounds and pollutants like alkylphenols, inorganic arsenic, organophosphates, phthalates, polychlorinated biphenyls (PCBs), volatile and semi-volatile organic compounds and chlorinated dioxins and furans. In another study, the EWG found 287 of the 413 tested chemicals in the umbilical cord blood of ten mothers after giving birth. These included the chemical types mentioned above and more, including fifty different polychlorinated naphthalene compounds (EWC 2007).

A polychlorinated biphenyl is a grouping of chlorine atoms bonded together with biphenyl. Biphenyl is a molecule composed of two phenyl rings. It is an aromatic hydrocarbon occurring naturally in coal and petroleum. When synthetically combined with chlorine—another naturally occurring element—the result is highly toxic. PCB was banned in the early 1970s when biologists studied a population of dead seabirds and found they died of a toxic dose of PCBs. For more than forty years, PCBs have been used in paints, pesticides, paper, adhesives, flame-retardants, surgical implants, lubricating oil and electrical equipment. Referred innocently as "phenols" for many years, the PCB ban followed suspicion by a number of years. Massive PCB contamination in the Hudson River was found caused by local electrical manufacturing plants. Some two hundred miles was eventually designated a toxic *superfund site.* This woke us up to PCB toxicity. PCBs break down slowly and bioaccumulate in living organisms. When PCBs get into our waterways they build up in the smallest organisms and work their way up the food chain, eventually reaching humans. Today the ban on PCBs does not include many applications considered "closed," such as capacitors and vacuum pump fluids. This means there are still considerable PCBs in our buildings and electrical equipment. PCB poisoning can cause immediate liver damage. Symptoms can include fever, rashes, nausea, and more.

Biphenyl A is another sort of biphenyl, used in many types of containers, including baby bottles. BPA can easily leach into food or formula when the bottle is exposed to heat or sunlight. A 2000 Centers of Disease Control study found 75% of those tested had phthalates in their urine, and subsequent studies have found some 95% of the U.S. population has detectable levels of biphenyl A within body fluids. Biphenyls are considered endocrine system disruptors. Long-term effects as their residues build up in our cells, organs and tissue systems are largely unknown.

By some accounts there are nearly nine hundred different pesticides being used in the United States. Of those, at least thirty-seven contain organophosphates—one of our more toxic chemical combinations. Organophosphates kill insects through nervous system disruption. These neurotoxins are also toxic to humans' nervous systems. The nerve gases serin and VX are organophosphates, for example. Organophosphates block cholinesterase—a key neuroenzyme—from working properly within the body. With cholinesterase blocked, acetylcholine is not regulated. Unregulated acetylcholine causes an over-stimulation of nerve activity, resulting in nerve damage, joint damage, paralysis, and muscle weakness.

Organophosphates are spreading through ground water, air and through dermal contact. They are exposing us through our breathing, touching, swimming, and drinking. Initial symptoms can include nausea, vomiting, shortness of breath, confusion, and muscle spasms. Some of the more common organophosphates include malathion, parathion, diazinon, phosmet, clorpyrifos, dursban and others. The Environmental Protection Agency actually banned diazinon and dursban in a phase-out beginning in March of 2001, to last through December 2003. Curiously, both diazinon and dursban are still in use today. Phased bans like this can take several years to allow companies to run out their inventories. Since these bans were aimed at consumer products, organophosphates are also still used profusely in commercial agriculture—our food production.

In a 2003 study done by the Centers for Disease Control and Prevention, thousands of people were tested for 116 chemicals. Thirty-four of these were pesticides such as organophosphates, organochlorines, and carbamates. Nineteen of the thirty-four were found in either the blood or urine.

The use of pesticides on agricultural land, playgrounds, parks, home lawns, and gardens throughout the United States is growing by a staggering amount. In 1964, approximately 233 million pounds of pesticide active ingredients were used. By 1982, this amount tripled to 612 million pounds. In 1999, the U.S. Environmental Protection Agency reported that some five *billion* pounds of these chemicals were used per year throughout America's crops, forests, parks, and lawns.

One of the fastest growing of these pesticides has been imidacloprid, a neonicotinoid. Introduced by Bayer in 1994, imidacloprid is used against aphids and similar insects on over 140 different crops. Touted as a chemical with a fairly short half-life of thirty days in water and twenty-seven days in anaerobic soil, imidacloprid's half-life is about 997 days in aerobic soil. While it has a lower immediate toxicity compared with hazards like DDT, imidacloprid's use is now widespread. It is rated by the Environmental Protection Agency and the World Health Organization as *"moderately toxic"* in small doses. Larger doses can disrupt liver and thyroid function.

While this pesticide does well at killing off increasingly resistant pests, it also can decimate bee populations.

A world without bees, as described in Rachel Carson's classic *Silent Spring,* would insure a destiny of hunger and destitution in human society. In France for example, some 500,000 registered hives were lost in the mid-1990s. Imidacloprid was implicated, and was subsequently banned for many crops in that country. Massive bee destruction has occurred in other regions of Europe also appear connected to imidacloprid use. A 2006-2007 loss of hives throughout Europe and the U.S.—referred to as *colony collapse disorder*—is now increasingly being connected to imidacloprid and possibly other chemicals as well. At first, a virus was suspected. Now several viruses have been seen. In other words, these chemicals *weaken the bees' immunity* to bacteria, viruses and other pathogens. Imidacloprid and other chemicals can weaken the bee's immune system just as they can weaken the human immune system—depending of course on the level of exposure.

Chlorinated dioxins are also pervasive in today's environment. Significant sources include cigarettes, pesticides, coal-burning factories, diesel exhaust, and sewage sludge. Dioxins are also byproducts of the manufacturing of a number of products, including many resins, glues, plastics, and chlorine-treated products. Dioxins also bio-accumulate in fatty tissues and can take years to fully degrade. Dioxins are known endocrine disruptors. They have also been linked to liver toxicity and birth defects.

Thanks to our massive industrial complex, there are now thousands of *volatile organic compounds* in our environment. A VOC is classified as such if it has a relatively high vapor pressure, allowing it to vaporize quickly and enter the atmosphere. Gasoline, paint thinners, cleaning solvents, ketones, and aldehydes are a few of the chemicals considered sources of VOCs. Methane-forming VOCs like benzene and toluene are also carcinogens. VOCs are often used as preservatives for pressed wood and other building materials. As a result, many buildings contain VOCs locked within its building materials. Once soaked in or inborn with the fabrication, VOCs are trapped within the material, causing them to outgas over time. This outgassing process is speeded up when the building is demolished or taken apart. As the building materials are broken up, VOCs can be released at toxic exposure levels.

VOCs will form ozone as they interact with sunlight and heat. VOC poisoning symptoms include nausea; headaches; eye irritation; inflammation of the nose and throat; liver damage; brain fog; and neurotoxic brain damage. Using cleaning or painting solvents indoors is a common cause of VOC poisoning.

In a study by Janssen *et al.* (2004) and *The Collaborative on Health and the Environment,* some two hundred diseases were found to be attributable to exposure to industrial chemicals. The diseases documented are some of the most prevalent diseases of our society—cancers, cardiovascular disease, and a variety of autoimmune diseases—including several forms of arthritis. They are also known to cause hormone disruption, which can indirectly instigate bone and cartilage damage. The researchers found that over 120 diseases have been specifically linked by research to exposure to specific industrial chemicals—again including arthritis (Lean 2004).

This and other research has indicated associations between arthritis and specific chemicals. A significant link between rheumatoid arthritis and industrial silicon dioxide has been made. Silicon dioxide is a byproduct of sand blasting, asphalt pavement manufacturing, cement manufacturing, brick cutting and jackhammer work. Silica dust can be inhaled at these sites and cause a pathology called *silicosis.* A significant association with silica and silicone has also been made to lupus. Tobacco smoke and a number of pesticides and solvents has also been significantly associated with rheumatoid arthritis. These have included polyvinyl chloride, epoxy resins, formaldehyde and organic solvents (Holladay 1999; Mayes 1999; Cooper *et al.* 2002; Dooley and Hogan 2003, Petri and Allbritton 1992, Hardy *et al.* 1999).

What are the possible mechanisms for chemical toxins causing arthritis? Exposure from inhalation can travel through the bloodstream into joints. Skin absorption can expose joint tissues through the epidermal and interstitial fluid. Toxins in food can be absorbed into the bloodstream either directly through the intestines or via the colon's uptake (especially when there is a deficiency of fiber, which can bind toxins).

Included in this discussion of toxins should be pharmaceuticals. Most pharmaceutical drugs are treated by the body as toxins. They must be broken down by the immune system just as any other chemical toxin must. Some pharmaceuticals even specifically interfere with the immune system. The level of toxicity of a pharmaceutical is fairly simple to measure: Liver enzymes. Liver enzymes increase as a result of higher toxicity levels, because the liver is working harder to clear the toxicity. It is for this reason that many drug manufacturers recommend that physicians periodically perform liver enzyme testing for patients taking their drugs.

Some drugs also have effects particularly concerning for arthritis. Oral contraceptives have been linked with a higher risk of lupus, for example (Sanchez-Guerrero *et al.* 1997). The mechanism is thought to be because synovial health is related to a balanced flow of estrogen and other hormones—as we have mentioned. Contraceptives work by significantly altering a woman's hormonal cycles.

Besides some of these specific effects, many synthetic chemicals create or become free radicals once they enter the body. As these circulate, they will damage cells throughout the body. Damage to artery cells, muscle cells, immune cells, or synovial membrane cells is likely—especially at exposure levels beyond what the immune system can neutralize. They will damage whatever cells, tissues and environment they come into contact with, because free radicals are molecularly unstable and need to complete their deficiency by deranging molecules. This means they will also derange the tissues and cells those molecules make up around the body.

Chemical toxins will also significantly burden the immune system. As they enter the body, the body will launch immune cells like lymphocytes to try to neutralize the toxins before they destroy cells. Should they enter or otherwise destroy cells, the immune system must launch a cytotoxic attack against the cells. This is the link between environmental toxins and autoimmune diseases such as arthritis. The immune system must destroy cells that have been damaged by toxins. A cell's cytoplasm or organelles like mitochondria may be saturated with toxic radicals. The cell's DNA may also be deranged by radical molecules formed from toxins. Either of these conditions can cause the immune system to identify a cell as being damaged—and decide the cell needs to be destroyed.

Genetic Factors

By comparing the gene sequences of arthritic patients with un-affected people, researchers now estimate that genetic factors may influence about 50-60% of all rheumatoid arthritis cases (Kobayashi *et al.* 2008).

However, our understanding of genetics is still in its infancy. This is indicated by the progress of our genome research. Over the last two decades, geneticists have focused on assembling the combined gene combinations that together would make up the genome of particular organisms. Genome research has expanded into a worldwide focus on establishing the genome of humans and other species. The assumption in the beginning of this research project—which involved hundreds of scientists from different specialties over two decades—was that we would find within the genome the answers to all the mysteries of nature, the body and disease pathologies.

Many of these assumptions were found to be erroneous. One assumption, for example, was that they would find an increasingly complex assembly of genes up the hierarchy of species. This research revealed that humans only have about 25,000 gene combinations—about the same amount that a small fish or a mouse has. Plants contain more genes than do humans, it turns out. In other words, gene combinations are no more complex in humans than they are in many other creatures.

Furthermore, the initial assumption was that the combination of genes in humans would unlock the keys to all disease pathologies. Preliminary research connected certain gene combinations or gene expressions to particular diseases. It was assumed that every disease had a particular genetic trait to match. This worked out pretty well in the beginning until researchers began discovering that many people with gene sequences associated with a disease never contracted that disease. And sometimes two or three diseases were connected to the same genetic trait. For example, Angelman syndrome and Prader-willy syndrome both relate to the same chromosome 15 deletion. These and other problems revealed that perhaps our understanding of genes and disease etiology was not as advanced as we'd like to think.

The other mystery for geneticists is that zygotic identical twins—which have the same DNA at conception—do not necessarily develop the same diseases later in life. Identical twins often have very different pathological outcomes.

This is supported by the research. Many twins have dramatically unique and individual lifestyles from each other. Depending upon how much time they spend together, they will often make distinctly different choices in life. In general, they display significantly unique and often diverse behavior. Hur and Rushton (2007) studied 514 pairs of two to nine year old South Korean monozygotic and dizygotic twins. Their results indicated that 55% of the children's prosocial behavior related to genetic factors and 45% was attributed to non-shared environmental factors. It should also be noted that shared environmental factors could not be eliminated from the 55%. The environmental versus genetic association could well be higher if the twin's early shared environments had been removed. In another recent study from Quebec, Canada (Forget-Dubois *et al.* 2007), an analysis of 292 mothers demonstrated that maternal behavior only accounted for a 29% genetic influence at 18 months, and 25% at 30 months. In a study done at the Virginia Commonwealth University's Institute for Psychiatric and Behavioral Genetics (Maes *et al.* 2007), a large sampling revealed that individual behavior was only about 38-40% attributable to genetics, while shared environment was 18-23% attributable and unshared environmental influences were attributable in 39-42%. In a study (Whitfield *et al.* 2004) of genetically identical twins and lung capacity from Pennsylvania State University, lung expiration capacity was only 14% attributable to genetic factors. 30% was due to shared environments and 56% was due to non-shared environmental effects. These and other studies confirm that our environment (including what we eat) has a much greater affect upon our health than our genetic factors.

Among autoimmune diseases, genetic dispositions among twins and families are illustrated, but the evidence is stronger that environmental issues are more important. For example, a study from the University of Western Ontario's Clinical Neurological Science Department (Ebers *et al.* 1996) reviewed the research on twins and autoimmune complexes such as multiple sclerosis, and also performed a genome search of 100 sibling pairs, looking for MS gene markers. Their research on multiple sclerosis concluded that while monozygotic twins showed higher concordance levels (matching pathologies) than dizygotic twins and siblings (25-30% versus 4%), they concluded that "environmental factors strongly influenced observed geographical differences." They also concluded that, "Studies of candidate genes have been largely unrewarding."

Studies more specific to arthritis have revealed a range of only 12-15% in concordance between monozygotic twins for rheumatoid arthritis (Silman *et al.* 1993, Jones *et al.* 1996; Aho *et al.* 1986). This indicates an even weaker connection between genetics and RA exists—as has been proposed. In other words, if RA were significantly genetic, then we would see that among twins with the RA genetic traits, both twins would contract the disease somewhere between 33% and 100% of the time—and preferably more than 50% of the time.

To further close the door on the genetic association with RA, the *British Medical Journal* (Swendsen *et al.* 2002) published a nation-wide study from Denmark on RA among monozygotic twins and dizygotic twins. This concluded no significant difference between monozygotic twins and dizygotic twins with regard to 1) onset of RA; 2) presence of RA factor; or 3) any other RA association. In other words, RA occurrence was no more shared between genetically identical twins than non-genetic identical twins—the opposite of what should happen if RA was genetic.

This does not mean that every disease labeled as autoimmune has no significant genetic association. Multiple sclerosis is the example mentioned above. The risk of multiple sclerosis among children of MS parents is 20 times higher than the general population. Yet there is still no certainty that an MS parent will have offspring that will contract MS. MS is still very rare, even among children of MS parents.

Certainly, in either case—both RA and MS—there may be genetic associations, but the evidence leans towards environmental influences being more important. If we look at the above research more closely, 25-30% concordance on MS and the 12-15% rate on RA between genetically identical twins are lower than the accepted placebo rate of 33%, not to speak about the Denmark study showing no concordance. In other words, common MS and RA incidence among genetically identical twins could also be subject to environmental or empathetic influences common to both twins. This could include common environmental toxins, common diets, common water intake, common breast milk and so on. They could also relate to the potential for empathy between the siblings.

Distinct disease pathologies despite genetic sameness is further evidenced by the fact that identical twins will have distinctly different fingerprints, irises and other physical traits, despite their identical genetics. Many twins also differ in handedness and specific talents. Researchers have found that twins will make significantly different lifestyle choices later in life such as sexual preference, drug abuse, and alcoholism.

We might compare this to automobile ownership. Say two people purchase the exact same make, model and year automobile at the same time. Comparing the two cars in the future will reveal the cars had vastly different engine lives and mileages. They each had different types of breakdowns, and different problems. This is because each car was driven differently. One was likely driven harder than the other was. One was likely better taken care of than the other was. They may have been the same make and model, but each had different owners with different driving habits. While the model might have a particular weakness in its design, this weakness may only affect performance if the car is driven a certain way.

Because twins have the same genetics—just as the cars shared the same make, model and manufacturer—their unique disease factors stem from the fact that each body is operated differently by a different individual under different conditions.

This distinction between inherited genes and continued environmental inputs is a realm that scientists are just beginning to explore. Realizing that even the same genes or the same genetic abnormalities will not render the same pathologies, researchers want to better understand the full matrix of causation in differentiated gene expression. Even twins who shared the same diet and environment will still have vastly different disease pathologies. This means there are missing elements the research still must consider.

These missing elements have forced a re-calibration of the genetic theory, and the rise of the concept of *epigenetics*. In general, epigenetics is the acceptance of additional factors that affect the switching off and on of gene expression and non-expression. It has been hypothesized—and confirmed by the research—that ones DNA is not as important as how gene expressions—or *phenotypes*—are switched on or off. If the genes are expressed, particular metabolism consequences result. If they are not expressed, there are different consequences.

The original concept of epigenetics was penned by geneticist Conrad Waddington in the early 1940s to explain in general how environmental circumstances could affect ones genetic instructions. The concept, however, was given increasing focus in the 1990s and early 2000s as geneticists discovered the various many holes genome assumptions contained.

The biochemical relationships of gene expression have focused upon the action of DNA methylation or histone regulation. These biochemical messengers have been observed switching alleles on or off. For example, mice experiments at McGill University's Douglas Hospital Research Center (Szyf *et al.* 2008) found that phenotype switching could be turned on and off with increased nurturing from the mother. Those baby mice receiving affectionate nurturing from mama would switch on genes differently than those mice that received less nurturing.

Biochemical mechanisms like phosphorylation, sumoylation, acetylation, methylation, and ubiquitylation also appear to be mechanically responsible for phenotype expression—which connects them to the availability of nutrients like oxygen, water, vitamin B, Co-Q-10 and so on.

As we review this research, it becomes evident that even if a parent has had an autoimmune disease such as arthritis, the child's environmental factors play a stronger role. The component missing from inclusion in the genetic assumption has been the common diet and common living environment between parents and their children. With rare exception, children consume the foods and recipes chosen by their parents. Dinners and cooking methods, for the most part, are passed down from generation to generation. As a result, the diet the children have may be practically identical, with the exception of brand names and packaging, to the diet the grandparents had.

Furthermore, the house and those environmental toxins present in its furniture and building materials are often presented equally to the parents and the children. The outside environment—automobile pollution, pesticides on the lawn and park, etc.—is also mutually presented to parents and children to a large degree. Because parents pass certain diet and lifestyle proclivities to their children at an early age, those children are more likely to not only assume those diets and lifestyles. They are also likely to pass those habits on to their children. Even if the child does not assume the lifestyle choice of the parent as an adult, the environmental exposure has already been done. In other words, we can prevent further exposures to our bodies and to the next generation. But we will still have to deal with our own childhood exposures.

This "passing" of lifestyle habits is undoubtedly more important than the genes parents pass on to their children. Why? Because even if the children received the genes predisposing some weakness towards a particular issue—take arthritis—then those genes still have to be switched on in order for the arthritic pathology to take place. And how do we switch on the genes? By our choice of environment and lifestyle choices such as diet, air, water consumption and exercise.

Both foodborne and environmental chemical toxins can become potent free radicals once inside the body. These can damage cell membranes, organelles and nuclei. A damaged cell membrane may cause the cell and its DNA to adjust as the cell adapts to the damage. Worse, a damaged or weak cell membrane may allow oxidative radicals from toxins to enter the cell and damage the cells organelles and even the nucleus. Should the nucleus be damaged, the DNA molecule itself may be damaged, resulting directly in genetic damage. Studies have demonstrated that many "autoimmune" responses are simply caused by the immune system removing a group of cells that are genetically damaged. Sometimes toxins or viruses may even genetically damage immune system cells. Once genetic damage takes place, the cell's activities become altered. As these specialized are altered, their genetic instructions may allow toxins to roam free and bad cells to continue to grow and divide.

These adaptive genetic changes will be seen by immune cells when they scan the body's cells. Genetically altered cells stimulate an immune response to remove those cells. This is precisely the mechanism observed among autoimmune-related diseases.

Those altered gene sequences that remain, unscathed by the immune system, will then be passed on to the children—giving the children an increased likelihood of the same autoimmune response. However, in order to *turn on those altered autoimmune-sensitive genes,* the child will have to be exposed to the same type of environmental conditions or toxins that stimulated the parent's autoimmune response. In some cases, this means toxins in the diet and environment, or other immune suppressors like stress or trauma. Oftentimes, especially for autoimmune disorders like arthritis, this switching process does not take place for many decades. Why? Because the immune system may be strong enough to neutralize most of the toxins before they have a chance to switch on the autoimmune genes. In any case, the body's welfare is the genetic intent.

A 2003 report from University of North Carolina's Department of Rheumatology and Immunology (Dooley and Hogan) discussed these factors in more detail, concluding that, "Rather than disease-specific genes for individual auto autoimmune disorders, there may be "autoimmunity genes" that increase the risk for development of autoimmune disorders in families. Autoimmune disorders may result from multiple interactions of genes and environmental factors."

In other words, for those of us who may have had parents with rheumatoid or other forms of arthritis, we may have inherited certain gene sequences that may turn on the disorder—as a matter of defense against lethal toxicity. This means that we will have to pay closer attention to our level of toxins, and the burdens we put on our immune systems. If we keep our immune systems strong and active, and prevent the mass derangement of cells from toxic radicals, we will likely prevent those genes from turning on in the first place. Epigenetic research and the research on twins appear to confirm this progression.

Autoimmunity

About 3% of the U.S. population suffers from systemic or tissue-specific autoimmune disorders (Jacobson *et al.* 1995), with women making up about 85% (Walsh and Rau, 2000). A significant amount of research data confirms the conclusion that environmental exposures contribute significantly to autoimmune disease in general (Cooper *et al.* 2002; Hess 1997).

As we investigate autoimmunity in more detail, we unfold a number of relationships between autoimmunity and environmental factors. We also discover a strong link between autoimmunity and the viability of the immune system itself. This relationship becomes apparent as most autoimmune diseases occur during the middle age years or elderly years. The relationship between our environment and autoimmune disorders is also highlighted by the rise in auto-immune disease as our environment becomes increasingly contaminated with chemical toxins.

In 2008, the Immunosciences Lab in California released a study (Vojdani) that tested the fluids of 420 patients with a variety of autoimmune-type disorders. These were screened with 96 different antibodies for a variety of different infectious and protein-type antibodies. A significant number of the autoimmune-patients tested positive to one or multiple *autoantibodies*. This leads to a thesis that some autoimmunity is related to a derangement of the immune system from previous infections, and/or the immune system has been overloaded with too many toxins.

We have discussed how the thymus can weaken with age, stress and toxic overload. The thymus is where T-cells are programmed with the antigen-antenna called T-cell receptors or TCRs. These direct the T-cells to identify particular types of infected cells or toxins. The thymus accomplishes this through a molecular assembly process called the MHC—major histocompatibility complex. This ability of the thymus gland is corrupted by stress and toxins. Over the years of toxic load and bombardment, the thymus will begin to collapse and become increasingly unproductive. As this happens, the immune system's T-cells are not programmed with the most up to date instructions. Should the thymus not be productive, T-cells will not be appropriately programmed with the updated MHC and TCR information.

This lack of updated programming could well be the missing link that causes T-cells to begin attacking the body's own cartilage and synovial membrane cells: Especially if those cartilage cells have become altered as a result of adapting to new toxin exposures.

We thus have a combination of events going on here. The synovial and cartilage cells (among others) begin to become deranged after so many years of exposure to toxicity and/or lack of nourishment. Plus, the immune system's programming features become worn down due to the same overexposure to toxins.

This is only logical, since over time the body's cells must adapt to all the stressors that we throw at them in order for our body to keep living in a toxic world. How else could we survive so many lethal toxic threats? As the cells begin to adapt and change, they become increasingly unrecognizable by the immune system's older programming.

How do we know the cells will change so much as to become unrecognizable by a weakened immune system?

The human cell is quite adaptive, but only to a point. Like most things, the cell becomes weakened when it is pushed too far for too long. We might compare this to a rubber band. It can be stretched to accommodate a range of stretches over a period of time. At some point and after so many stretches too far, the rubber band starts to fray and become overstretched. At some point it will break. Just before and after being stretched to the breaking point, it pretty much becomes useless.

Practically every environmental change or toxin that differs from what our body is naturally designed for or used to forces the body and immune system to adapt. Even our probiotics must adapt to environmental changes. Furthermore, chronic changes that recur can push a cell to adapt permanently. This means it must make slight changes to its DNA sequencing and RNA processing.

Over time, most stressors can force an adaptation of genetic structure to accommodate the disturbance. This happens increasingly in the modern world, as our cells adapt to new stresses, new foods and new toxins our environment presents to us. Our cells learn to adapt to the chemicals in our foods: preservatives, food dyes and overly processed and isolated ingredients. Our cells learn to adapt to the chemicals in our immediate environment: formaldehyde, PCBs, plasticizers and petrochemicals. Our cells learn to adapt to the stresses of our modern culture: not getting enough sleep, rushing for time, and dealing with money. For some of us, our cells must learn to adapt to deficient water. For some of us, our cells must learn to adapt to a lack of good nutrition. Any environmental condition that is constant will force the cells to adapt. Over time, all these adaptations are reflected in our cells' gene sequences.

In the case of the intrusion of a toxic chemical, for example, the immune system stimulates a detoxification event to clear the toxin. This might be to dispatch macrophages to take apart the toxin. Should the toxin not be cleared, the free radicals produced by the toxin may enter and/or damage cells within the body. Once cells are invaded, the cell may have to adapt to the toxin in order to accommodate it.

Viruses are more specifically tuned to forcing genetic changes. In either case, the immune system will often initiate an inflammatory response and detoxification event to rid the damage to the cell. This might include swelling, sneezing, coughing, watery eyes or otherwise. In the later case—the adaptive process—the cell must begin to operate under duress and its DNA and RNA functions must develop procedures for these altered mechanisms. This adaptation is often reflected in the DNA sequencing.

We might compare this to how we adapt to weather. When there is hot weather, we will wear different clothes and move more slowly. During cold weather, we put on many more clothes and shiver more to create heat. During the wintertime, we adapt to the cold weather with many changes to our house and habits.

As the cell adapts, it may also produce a reflective molecular signal on the cell membrane. This ligand can signal the TCR of the appropriate T-cell that it is deranged or genetically different.

This might be compared to a ship raising a flag that it is under duress for other boats to see from far away. This signal can be read by T-cells that are searching for cells that have been invaded. Once the T-cell 'reads' such a signal on the surface, it dispatches the appropriate immune response. If there is a large group of 'flagged' cells, the immune system will likely launch a full-scale inflammatory attack against the region.

In the case of a lack of nutrients or water for extended periods, the DNA and RNA within the cell may be forced to adapt to a condition where the cell operates with less fuel. We could compare this to taking a long walk through the desert with no water.

The first nutrient deficiency to damage the cell is oxygen. Without oxygen, our cells will starve for energy and will not be able to function. This can take place within minutes. The second most dangerous nutrient deficiency is water. Should the cell not have enough water, it will begin to deteriorate. We'll discuss this shortly.

Our DNA will undergo direct damage from interfering electromagnetic waveforms from unnatural EMF waveforms as well. This has been illustrated in the research on nuclear bomb victims. Electromagnetic waveforms originating from alternating currents, including those arising from electronic appliances, cell phones, high transmission power lines and so on will subtly stress the cell's ability to communicate within itself and with other cells. The cell must then adapt to these new environmental waveforms by making genetic accommodations. The need for chronic adjustment can result in the mutation of DNA. This mutation may also turn the cell into a cancerous cell.

The accommodation of the cell and genetic information is evidence that the waveform bonding sequencing of DNA can be altered to accommodate external influences. We have seen this evidenced through genetic analysis of various family trees. Should an ancestor have a particular environmental exposure, their adaptation will be passed on to the next generation. This is why we find that the people in cultures that have lived in sunnier regions have higher levels of melanin in their skin cells—giving them darker skin. For those who moved north and lived primarily indoors during long winters, melanin content is greatly decreased. This leads to whiter skin color. In both cases, our skin color today is reflected by genetic accommodations to our ancestors' environments.

In the same way, we find our bodies can accommodate many environmental toxins: Despite these toxins' ability to damage our cells and burden upon our immune system. Why have our bodies seemingly adapted to the avalanche of plastics and the plasticizers that come with them over the past three decades? The plethora of plastics have certainly increased our immune system burden, disrupted our hormones and damaged our livers. Yet many of us have little in the way outward allergies, sensitivities or other obvious symptoms of plastic use. The problem is that we cannot readily recognize the results of genetic accommodation to plasticizer toxicity. These may include hormone imbalances, chronic fatigue, reduced immunity, allergic reactions to natural elements like pollen and grass, and of course autoimmune diseases such as arthritis.

Our cells are adjusting to new environments all the time. For example if we were to move to a warmer location—with greater solar radiation through contact with infrared radiation—our cells will begin to operate with slower metabolism, allowing the body's core temperature to remain balanced. Though this might stress the cells somewhat, this sort of adapting mechanism is not considered harmful primarily because the sun's rays (except perhaps mid-day UV rays) are considered healthy to the body. However, should our body move into a building where it is exposed to toxic chemicals, our cells might react more violently, with allergies and physical stress, as those cells attempt to adapt to this new environment.

As this process continues, the body's immune cells may recognize that the cells are under duress as they attempt to adapt to our environmental or dietary toxins. This may in turn stimulate the inflammatory immune response. Should some of those cells be synovial membrane cells or subchondral bone cells, the response may well result in arthritic inflammation.

As we will discuss further, conventional western medicine's solution to autoimmune disorders is to try to stop the symptoms by interrupting the pathways of inflammation and immune response. While it may temporarily slow the inflammatory response, this solution also can weaken the entire immune system by blocking the body's healing mechanisms. This puts more burdens on the body because the body cannot efficiently detoxify and heal itself from the offending toxins or pathogens. This 'solution' ends up increases the burden upon the body's already-overloaded immune system.

This strategy would be analogous to punishing our dog because he barked at a thief who was invading our home.

Nutritional Factors

Modern medicine has has focused upon the immune factors for arthritis because laboratory assays of the synovial fluid of arthritis sufferers is often chock full of T-cells, B-cells, cytokines, leucotrienes, prostaglandins and macrophages. This of course indicates an immune system launch—the veritable smoking gun.

Over the past decade, however, several studies have brought nutrition into the equation. The relationship between arthritis and nutrition arose as the inflammatory cascade and the COX and LOX enzymes were examined more closely. It turns out that nutrition is more than just a contributing factor to arthritis.

Every cell in the body utilizes nutrients such as vitamins, amino acids, fatty acids and minerals to produce cells, proteins, enzymes and tissue systems. Cartilage is a critical tissue system that requires a combination of minerals, polysaccharides, amino acids and lipids to build. If these raw materials are absent or deficient in our diet, the resulting cartilage will also be deficient in structure, tensility and longevity. Nutrients play protective factors too. Many nutrients are antioxidants, preventing damage to cartilage and synovial tissues from free radicals.

Calcium, magnesium, vitamin D and boron have all been shown to improve arthritis in animal studies (Devirian and Volpe 2003). In one study (Newnham 1994), 50% of arthritic rats given boron each day had a significantly favorable joint response, in comparison with 10% in the group receiving the placebo.

As we discussed in depth, a critical part of the arthritis inflammatory cascade involves the conversion of fatty acids to prostaglandins, thromboxanes and leucotrienes. These three molecules stimulate the process of inflammation, as they signal specific pathogens. These are not the bad guys, remember. These are a critical part of the body's healing response.

As long as there aren't too many hanging around. Too many of these compounds can transmit too many messages, making it more difficult for the body's inflammation *shunting* (or reversing) process to take hold. Too many prostaglandins can stimulate too much substance P and thromboxanes, which stimulate clotting—attracting fibrin and plasmin to the location. Too many leucotrienes will stimulate T-cells into attack mode. Too many prostaglandins and thromboxanes without shunting (stimulated by the adrenal's production of cortisol) can put pain and inflammation into overdrive.

This trio of inflammatory messengers are created by two conversion processes of arachidonic acid—a fatty acid. The critical enzymes used for this conversion to prostaglandins, thromboxanes, and leucotrienes are cyclooxygenase (COX) and lipoxygenase

(LOX). A significant amount of research over the past decade has confirmed that a disproportionate amount of arachidonic acid in the diet will produce increased levels of inflammation (Calder 2008 and many others) due to an oversupply of these messengers.

In fact, research headed up by Dr. Darshan Kelley from the Western Human Research Center in California illustrated that diets high in arachidonic acid stimulated four times more inflammatory cells than diets low in arachidonic acid content. And this problem actually increases with age. In other words, the same amount of arachidonic acid-forming foods will cause higher levels of arachidonic acid the older we get (Chilton 2005).

This also relates to many other health-related problems as people age. For example, higher arachidonic acid levels in the bloodstream correlate with greater platelet aggregation. This creates a higher risk of blood clots. Higher levels of arachidonic acid can also cause difficulties with glucose utilization, lung efficiency, intestinal health and so many other disorders related to inflammation.

So how do we lower our arachidonic acid levels?

By lowering our intake of foods with high arachidonic acid levels, and lowering our intake of oils that convert easily to arachidonic acid. And by rebalancing our diet to include fats that do not convert so easily to arachidonic acid.

This simply means that when we eat an over-abundance of too much of the wrong fats, our body tends to be on a 'hair-trigger' when it comes to inflammation, whereas if we balance our fat intake with good fats, we help mediate inflammation. An abundance of arachadonic acid or oils that easily convert to arachadonic acid encourages our inflammatory mechanisms into overdrive. So what foods produce or convert more easily to arachadonic acid?

According to the USDA's Standard 13 and 16 databases (Chilton, 2006), animal meats and fish produce the highest amounts of arachidonic acid in the body. Diary, fruits and vegetables produce little or no arachidonic acid. Grains, beans and nuts produce none or very small amounts. Processed bakery goods produce a moderate amount of AA.

Hundreds of studies have now confirmed that an increase in long-chain fatty acids such as DHA, EPA, ALA and GLA in the diet slows down inflammation in the body. How do they do that?

Because these fats convert to other compounds—such as phospholipids used for cell membranes—leaving less fat available to convert to prostaglandins, leucotrienes and thromboxanes.

In a study from Germany published in Rheumatology International (Adam *et al.* 2003), sixty-eight patients with diagnoses of rheumatoid arthritis were divided into two groups. For eight months, one group maintained a typical western diet (meat diet high in arachidonic acid) diet, while the other group ate a diet low in arachidonic acid for eight months. Parts of each group also supplemented DHA/EPA oil or a placebo. The western diet had no reduction in pain and swelling. The placebo (no DHA oil) group in the low arachidonic acid group had a 14% reduction in pain and swelling. The DHA supplemented-western diet group had 11% reduction in joint pain and 22% reduction in joint swelling. The DHA supplementation, low-arachidonic acid group had a reduction in joint pain of 28%, and a reduction in joint swelling of 34%. Therefore, while taking a DHA oil supplement can reduce pain and inflammation, the western diet—high in arachidonic acid—will continue to contribute to chronic inflammation: Like taking a few steps forward while taking a few steps back.

We will discuss later further research indicating that between the two—DHA and EPA—DHA is the primary agent in reducing inflammation.

Saturated fats have also been connected specifically to arthritis. In a study at the Loma Linda University School of Medicine, 23 people with rheumatoid arthritis ate a low fat diet of 10% calories from fat. They were compared to a control group eating an unregulated diet high in saturated fats. The low-fat group experienced a 20-40% reduction in joint inflammation as a group. Dr. Edwin Krick, the study leader and professor at the medical school, recommended a diet low in saturated fats for arthritic sufferers.

We will discuss the science of fats in more detail later.

Outside of fat content, the association between arthritis and diet has not been subject to repeated clinical study. Still there has been a good amount of indirect evidence and supporting clinical research indicating that a diet rich in mineral-rich, antioxidant foods can significantly reduce the occurrence and risk of inflammatory diseases such as arthritis.

There are several reasons for this. The first is that inflammation is reduced if free radicals and other toxins are neutralized by circulating antioxidants. Antioxidants have been shown to significantly reduce the severity of a number of disorders, including atherosclerosis, heart disease, liver disease, diabetes and others. This is because they support the immune system's process of removing toxins before they do any further damage. This was illustrated in a study (McAlindon *et al.* 1996) at the Boston University School of Medicine. The study revealed that people consuming more than 200 milligrams a day of vitamin C were one-third less likely to experience a worsening of their osteoarthritis. Dr. Timothy McAlidon, a professor at the University suggested that the reduction in free radicals by the antioxidant vitamin C was the likely mechanism. He also commented that, "Vitamin C may also help generate collagen, which enhances the body's ability to repair damage to the cartilage."

Vitamin D has also been shown to slow down the progression and pain associated with osteoarthritis (McAlindon and Biggee 2006).

Research on the role foods rich in minerals and phytonutrients play in the inflammatory cascade is in its infancy. Still, the antioxidant and immune-stimulating abilities of phytonutrients have been shown to help prevent cancer and inflammation—and reduce the risk of a variety of diseases. We have no reason to believe that arthritis is any exception.

Joint and Cartilage Hydration

There is significant reason to believe that dehydration at least contributes to nearly every form of arthritis. This conclusion was famously drawn by F. Batmanghelidj, M.D., one of western medicine's foremost experts on dehydration.

Dr. Batmanghelidj points out that the cartilage surfaces maintain a significant percentage of water—just as bone cells maintain calcium. Water is held within the cartilage's molecular matrix, rendering increased lubrication. This lubrication allows the two opposing cartilage surfaces to glide over one another in joint movement. These two cartilage surfaces glide over one another easily when the surface cells and synovial fluid are properly hydrated. When they become dehydrated, there is more friction. This increased friction damages cartilage faster than can be replaced. Dr. Batmanghelidj calls this region of abraded cells the "abrasive peel."

According to Dr. Batmanghelidj, the cartilage is hydrated from the serum of the blood delivered through tiny capillaries within the bone marrow (canaliculi) that lead to the bone's base attachment to the subchondral bone and cartilage. Because red blood cell production in the bone marrow hold a higher priority than joint lubrication, in an environment of reduced hydration, the bone marrow will take up the available water first—leaving the joint dehydrated (Batmanghelidj 1991; 1997).

A lack of adequate hydration for any duration in a tissue region will also stimulate the release of histamine to help regulate water usage. This will stimulate further inflammation as the immune system seeks to rid the body of cells that are now dysfunctional due to dehydration.

In addition, the body will respond to dehydration with a number of stop-loss measures. Histamine will stimulate antidiuretic hormones to control water loss as well as stimulate vasopressin, which controls artery wall pressure and renal water regulation systems. Histamine (H1) stimulates arachidonic acid pathways, which encourages greater inflammatory response. The sum total effect of dehydration is thus one of depressing immune function while stimulating hyperinflammatory response.

Dr. Batmanghelidj goes on to describe how, in a dehydrated state, the injured cartilage will stimulate "local remodeling hormones" that restructure joint surfaces along lines of force and pressure. This causes the deformation of joints that is seen among severe arthritic patients, according to Dr. Batmanghelidj.

Earlier we discussed how arthritis has been found among a variety of ancient bones—indicating to scientists that arthritis is not exclusively a modern ailment. A dramatic discovery of this was the "Iceman," whose remains were found in 1991 and analyzed by an international group of scientists. The "Iceman" was carbon-dated to have lived 5,300 years ago. His bones indicated that he had an advanced case of osteoarthritis. Through analysis of bone minerals and content, his remains also indicated that he also suffered from a significant case of long-term dehydration (Murphy et al. 2003).

Alkaline Diet

This discussion of nutrients should also include the reflective effects of a healthy diet: A balance of pH among the blood, urine and intercellular tissue regions. The reference to an acidic environment has been made by numerous natural health experts.

It is essential that the pH of the body's fluids be properly balanced. A balanced pH creates a state of homeostasis within the blood, lymph, and intracellular/extracellular fluids. Many nutritionists loosely term this as a *state of alkalinity*. Strictly speaking, however, an alkaline environment is also not healthy. The blood, interstitial fluids, lymph and urine should be *slightly acidic* to maintain a proper balance in metabolism (Beddoe 2002).

A measurement of the level of acidity or alkalinity using a logarithmic scale is called pH. The term pH is derived from the French word for hydrogen power, *pouvoir hydrogene,* which has been abbreviated as simply pH. pH is measured in an inverse log base-10 scale, measuring the proton-donor level by comparing it to a theoretical quantity of hydrogen ions (H+) in a solution. Thus, a pH of five would be equivalent to 10^5 H+ *moles* worth of cations in the solution. (A *mole* is a quantity of substance compared to 12 grams of the six-neutron carbon isotope.) Put another way, a pCl (chlorine) concentration would be the negative log of chlorine ion concentration in a solution, and pK would be the negative log of potassium ions in a solution.

The pH scale is 0 to 14, for 10^{-1} (1) to 10^{-14} (.00000000000001) range. The scale has been set up around the fact that water's (with mineral content) pH is log-7 or simply pH 7. Because pure water forms the basis for so many of life's activities, and because water neutralizes and dilutes so many reactions, water was established as the standard reference point and considered the neutral point between acid and base solutions. In other words, a substance having greater hydrogen ion concentration characteristics than water will be considered a base (alkaline), while a substance containing less H+ concentration characteristics than water is considered an acid.

Of course, a solution concentration may well be lower than log-14 or higher than log-1, but this is the scale set up based upon the typical ranges observed in nature. Using this scale, any substance measuring a pH of 7 would be considered a neutral substance, though it still has a significant number of H+ ions. In humans, a pH level in the range of 6.4 is considered a healthy state because this state is slightly more acidic than water, enabling alkaline ionic (mineral) currents to flow through the body. Better put, a 6.4 pH offers the appropriate *currency* of energy flow because there are enough negatively oriented ionic molecules present to match the number of positive ions. The earthly minerals like potassium, calcium, magnesium and others are usually positively oriented—or alkaline (cationic) in nature. These minerals bond with lipids and proteins to form the structures of our cell membranes, and tissue structures—including bones, cartilage and synovial tissues.

Natural health experts over the past century have observed that an overly acidic environment created by a diet abundant in processed foods, chemical toxins and purine-heavy animal meats lend towards diseased states. More recently, research has confirmed that these inputs increase free radical levels. Most microorganisms also flourish among acidic environments. Combined, these can damage tissues, including joint cartilage and synovial membranes.

A number of nutritionists and physicians have shown that a diet high in purines—which are highly prevalent in red meats, fish, asparagus, mushrooms and beans—also contribute to higher levels of uric acid crystals. In a study from Russia (Vopr Pitan 1985), for example, gout patients were given a specialized diet with daily levels of 70 grams of protein (typical protein levels in the US and Europe are well over 100 grams) made up of 85% plant protein, 85 grams of fat and 350 grams of carbohydrates. The diet resulted in a dramatic reduction of uric acid concentration in the blood, a normalized pH in the urine, an increase in kidney filtration, and improvements in general well-being among the diet group.

In another study by the Department of Rheumatology at the Vancouver General Hospital (Choi *et al.* 2008), 11,351 men were studied over a six year period. Men with gouty arthritis were significantly more likely to have adult-onset diabetes and metabolic disorder—both often related to diet. In another study at the Johns Hopkins University Medical School (Yeager 1998), 1200 medical students were followed for more than 30 years. Those with greater weight gains during early adulthood were most likely to develop gouty arthritis later in life.

An overly acidic environmental is also consistent with high arachidonic acid levels. Most of the same foods traditional nutritionists called "acid-forming" many years ago also happen to produce an abundance of arachidonic acid in the body. Perhaps they knew something science is only beginning to recognize.

Illustrating this was a study at the University of Oslo in Norway (Kjeldsen-Kragh 1999). Fifty-five people with rheumatoid arthritis followed either a vegetarian diet or an omnivorous diet for one year. After both three months and one year, the 27 people in the vegetarian group improved significantly in "all clinical variables and most laboratory variables" when compared to the 26 people in the omnivore group. This same effect was found in a previous study at the University of Oslo with 53 RA patients (Kjeldsen-Krash *et al.* 1994). This later group was studied for two years, and it was found that the vegetarian group sustained their improvements over the entire two-year period. The clinical results included the Stanford Health Assessment Questionnaire Index with such variables as pain score, duration of morning stiffness, Ritchie's articular index, number of swollen joints, ESR and platelet counts.

Dr. Jethro Kloss, a leading American naturopathic physician nearly a century ago, took this position with his arthritis treatments. In treating both consulting patients and inpatients to his treatment center, he advised arthritis or rheumatism sufferers to avoid tea, coffee, liquor, white flour products, refined sugar products, fried potatoes, meat, pork and bacon (Kloss 1946).

As we will discuss in more detail, a healthy plant-based diet creates a better balance between alkalinity and acidity in the blood, lymph and urine. This enhances kidney filtration, detoxification systems, microorganism control, nutrient delivery, and immune system function.

Conclusion

Here we have discussed a number of factors that have been associated with arthritis. We have also boiled down these factors to a few essential mechanisms relating directly to inflammatory arthritis. We have found that practically every single association is related to a weakening of the immune system associated with increased exposure to toxins, a poor diet and/or infectious microorganisms. Let's quickly review the associations and conclusions:

Physical damage to the joints from either wear and tear or injury trauma has been weakly associated with osteoarthritis, although there is no explanation of why there is no healing with rest. The immune system's primary job is to heal injury. The pathway for healing involves an inflammatory response through the production of prostaglandins, thromboxanes and leucotrienes, followed by the delivery of T-cells and B-cells to take apart damaged cells and begin the process of repair. A scabbing of the site allows for the replacement of healthy cells and cartilage. If the immune system is overburdened with too much toxicity, deficient due to an inactive thymus, or over-reactionary because of poor diet choices, the immune system's process of repair will be deranged. This will result in the inflammation process continuing without resolution or healing of the damage.

Infection to the joints by way of bacteria or viruses should be prevented by a healthy immune system and adequate probiotic colonies. Assuming they are available and properly programmed, the combination of immunoglobulins, cytokines, B-cells and T-cells should be able to identify and remove pathogens before they damage synovial membrane cells or cartilage tissue. Any bacterial overgrowth should also be controlled by probiotic populations. Should infectious pathogens gain entry to these cells, the immune system's T-cell network should still be able to remove the bad cells and allow the healing process to move forward. A depressed immune system and/or inadequate probiotic colonies will be hampered in these activities.

Chemical toxins absorbed into the body via consumption or exposure will burden the immune system. They require the immune system to break them down and escort them out of the body. This is especially the case for those with a diet low in antioxidants and other nutrients. The bombardment and constant overload of toxins over time will tax the immune system to the point where the adrenal glands and the thymus become stressed—slowing their function. This in turn creates an immune system not as efficient or effective at removing infection or toxins.

Genetic defects have been associated with some types of arthritis, but there is little indication that these genetic defects are unrelated to the common diets and environments held between the parents and children. Furthermore, *epigenics* research indicates that even if a particular genetic trait toward a disease is present, that trait will still need to be *switched on* in order to become active. This means there still must be some environmental or dietary trigger that switches the gene on. Here again, a reduction in toxin exposure combined with an effective immune system will play a significant role. It is not as if we have no control over our arthritic destiny.

Autoimmunity is not the mysterious mechanism western medicine makes it out to be. Autoimmunity relates specifically to the immune system's identification of a cell or network of cells (tissues) as infected or deranged. Quite simply, this means that either the immune system is working right and those cells have been corrupted, or the immune system is operating ineffectively and cannot complete the job. A factor of an ineffective or burdened immune system might be a depleted thymus gland. A defective thymus gland will be unable to attach new coding instructions to T-cells. After years of repeated toxin exposure for synovial and subchondral cells, and/or oxidative radical damage to cartilage tissue, the cells adapt and alter their DNA makeup. Once this alteration is observed by T-cells not programmed with recent MHC coding, the immune system begins attacking to remove those altered cells. In any event, the autoimmune paradigm still requires initiation from cell damage by toxins or microorganisms. Without these events, the immune system would not have cause to launch an immune response—unless of course the immune system cells themselves have been damaged, again by toxins and/or microorganisms.

Nutritional defects created by an undersupply of water and other nutrients, and an oversupply of arachidonic acid appear to be more than a coincidence for arthritis. An increasing number of researchers and health experts have observed that these are over-riding factors for inflammation. These factors relate to back to the immune system, because nutrient or water deficiencies and arachidonic acid overload contribute to the immune system's inability to clean up an injury site. In AA fatty acid overload, the immune system's inflammation triggers like prostaglandins, thromboxanes, and leucotrienes are overstimulated. In nutrient deficiency, the immune system is over-burdened because it must remove under-nourished and over-stressed cells. The immune system must also work overtime to clear out the toxic load that good nutrition would have neutralized and helped detoxify.

In *Ayurveda*—the oldest medical system in continuous practice—this build-up of toxins, inflammatory factors and poor nutrient choices is collectively called *ama*. Arthritis is thus called *amavata* in Ayurveda—inflammation and pain caused by the build up of too much *ama*.

Chapter Four

The Pharmaceutical Option

Note: While this discussion of pharmaceuticals draws from references written by medical researchers, physicians and drug manufacturers; any conclusions, action steps or treatment plans associated with these or other pharmaceuticals should be done in consultation with an attending medical doctor licensed to prescribe such treatments.

We may become amazed at the number of different medications being prescribed or sold over the counter for arthritis. Yes, it is truly astonishing how hard the pharmaceutical industry has worked over the past few decades to develop new pharmaceuticals that reduce pain and inflammation.

The studies do illustrate, as do many testimonials, that many of these medications temporarily reduce pain and inflammation associated with arthritis. However, in many cases this accomplishment has come with a cost. Some might say the cost is worth it, while others might say the cost has been too great. Let's examine the evidence.

As for costs, we are speaking, of course, about the side effects of these and other pharmaceuticals. Cost in dollars is another subject altogether. Before we review the pharmaceuticals themselves, let's examine some of the statistics regarding the application of pharmaceuticals and associated conventional medical treatments:

The *Journal of the American Medical Association* (Lazarou *et al.* 1998) reported that in 1994, 2,216,000 Americans were hospitalized, permanently disabled, or died as a result of pharmaceutical use. This is over 2.2 million Americans annually with *reported* injury from pharmaceuticals. The study, done at the University of Toronto, also showed that approximately 106,000 people die each year from taking *correctly prescribed* FDA-approved pharmaceuticals. This does not include the number of deaths resulting by misuse, overdose or addiction to these same drugs.

Furthermore, the U.S. FDA was sent 258,000 adverse drug events in 1999. Harvard researcher and associate professor of medicine Dr. David Bates told the *Los Angeles Times* in 2001 *"...these numbers translate to 36 million adverse drug events per year"* (Rappoport 2006). The plausibility of this number is confirmed in another study published in the *Journal of the American Medical Association* in 1995

97

(Bates *et al.*). This revealed that over a six month period, 12% of 4031 adult hospital admissions had either a confirmed adverse drug event or a potentially adverse drug event.

In addition to these facts, estimates from several sources have confirmed that about 16,000 deaths occur and about 100,000 people are hospitalized from NSAID use alone. This computes to 50 NSAID-related deaths and 300 hospitalizations every day as a result from NSAID use. About 100 million prescriptions of NSAIDs are written in addition to millions of over the counter purchases.

The infliction upon Americans by incorrectly applied medicine does not stop there. *The Nutrition Institute of America* reports that over 20 million unnecessary antibiotic prescriptions are prescribed per year. Over seven million medical and surgical procedures a year are unnecessary. Over eight million people are hospitalized without need. Our medical institution is quite simply suffocating in its own mismanagement.

According to a nationwide poll conducted by Louis Harris and Associates released in 1997 by the *National Patient Safety Foundation* and the *American Medical Association,* an estimated 100 million Americans experienced a medical mistake: 42% of those randomly surveyed. Misdiagnosis and wrong treatments accounted for 40% of those mistakes. Medical medication errors accounted for 28%, while medical procedure errors accounted for 22% of these medical mistakes (NPSF 1997).

In a study of four Boston adult primary care practices involving 1202 outpatients, 27% of responders experienced adverse drug events (Gandhi *et al.* 2003).

In a 2004 interview with Dr. Lucian Leape, a physician, medicine professor, expert in patient safety, and author of numerous studies, reported that over the past ten years since the 1997 NPSF studies were performed, improvements in our medical system have been inadequate. Barriers to improvement cited physician denial, hospital environment, lack of leadership and little system review (Leape 2004).

Indeed, over the past few decades, our medical industry has become the leading cause of death and injury in the United States. Carolyn Dean, M.D., N.D., in her book *Death By Medicine* (2005), compiled the following medical statistics for 2005:

Adverse Reactions	106,000 Deaths
Medical Errors	98,000 Deaths
Bedsores	115,000 Deaths
Hospital Infections	88,000 Deaths
Outpatient Adverse Reactions	199,000 Deaths
Unnecessary Procedures	37,136 Deaths
Surgery-Related	32,000 Deaths
Total Deaths	**783,936 Deaths**

This accounting of deaths out-numbers both U.S. heart disease death rates and cancer death rates. In 2002 for example, 450,637 people died of heart disease and 476,009 died of cancer.

Noting these facts, we present a review of pharmaceuticals prescribed or sold over the counter for arthritis, together with their adverse side effects. The FDA requires pharmaceutical companies to state the more pronounced adverse side effects of a medication along with advertising or dispensing. This is not just for fun and games. This is to alert people that taking pharmaceuticals is a risky scenario.

Admittedly, in manufacturer-sponsored research, some of these adverse side effects are only found in a small percentage of the study group. This percentage may be anywhere from .1-10% of those taking the drug. However, we must remember that these studies are closely monitored by physicians and the manufacturers to minimize adverse side effects. They carefully review the patient for contraindications, or medications that may interact with the drug. This means the likelihood of the drug being given to the wrong person is probably much less than if prescribed by a physician who just heard about the drug from their pharmaceutical sales representative, and/or does not closely monitor the patient during the medication's use. Outside of the confines of a carefully monitored study to be turned in to the FDA, there is a stronger likelihood of the dosage being incorrectly prescribed, the dosage being increased by the patient without the knowledge of the doctor, or the medication being taken along with alcohol or illicit drugs. Perhaps even the drug might be taken during a hot, sunny day. If the drug is contraindicated with sunlight—which many are—this could also increase its risk of serious side effects. The likelihood of the medication being taken on an empty stomach when the medication is supposed to be taken with food, or other medications being prescribed before or after the drug that interact with the drug all can make the side effects more pronounced, or even cause new adverse side effects. With the increase of medical specialists in modern medicine, this becomes a greater issue, as multiple physicians are prescribing medications that may interact. There are all sorts of other adverse reactions that can occur when medications are taken at home or otherwise away from the close scrutiny of study medical doctors and drug trial managers.

Sadly, multiple drug prescribing is becoming increasingly commonplace among the elderly—those who also suffer the highest rates of arthritis. In America, a growing number of elderly persons (especially those who regularly see a doctor) are taking multiple medications. A 2004 Duke University study showed that 21%—7 million Americans—over the age of 65 take drugs classified as "dangerous." The over-65 population is 15% of the overall population, and this group is taking one-third of all drug prescriptions. Study researchers added that the research actually understated the problem, as elderly persons commonly take at least ten to twelve prescription drugs concurrently.

This puts quite a heavy chemical load upon an already overburdened liver and immune system. No wonder there are so many adverse effects from pharmaceutical use.

Arthritis Medications

Many of the medications prescribed or sold over the counter are irrespective of the type of arthritis. This is because their aim is to block the inflammatory process. The goal is to reduce pain and inflammation in general. Because pain and inflammation result from a number of pathologies, many arthritis medications are considered *broad-spectrum*.

As we've discussed, the cause of most forms of arthritis is still considered a mystery to researchers and physicians. Thus, the focus of most arthritis medication is to provide temporary pain relief and reduced inflammation rather than provide a cure. While developing a cure can be done without knowing the cause, it certainly helps. The bottom line is that most arthritis pharmaceuticals are aimed towards treating the symptoms (pain and inflammation) but not dealing with the cause of the disease. For this reason, the initial arthritis drugs of choice tend to focus upon nonsteroidal anti-inflammatory drugs (NSAIDs) or selective COX-2 inhibitors.

The pharmaceutical path therefore presents a process that aims to interfere with the body's inflammatory process—a process the body uses to repair injury and prevent further disease. This is certainly a good strategy for the short-term solution of stopping the pain for a while or shutting down the inflammatory process. The major dilemma this presents, however, is that when the body's natural immune process is blocked, it is not just blocked for joint inflammation—it is also blocked for any other healing process required around the body. This leaves the body unable to properly heal other injuries while using these types of medications. This is one of reasons we find that people die during the use of some of these medications. They may not die from the medication or the disease itself, but from a disease that spun out of control because the body's immune system was hampered.

To be fair, medications that reduce uric acid levels, or antibiotics used in response to a bacterial infection can get at the foundation of joint inflammation related to gout or septic arthritis, respectively. In some cases, these may become absolutely critical for the survival of the patient. And in some cases, reducing pain and inflammation may be critical to keeping a patient alive. Certainly many medications may have their appropriate time and circumstance in critical care. Unfortunately, this is not how most pharmaceuticals are being used, and the statistics related to their over-use and inappropriate use mentioned above reflects this. Our intention here is not to make judgments, however. We merely present the facts.

That said, rheumatoid arthritis pharmaceutical treatment has been evolving over the past few years. A number of drugs that modulate the immune system in one form or another have emerged. Certainly, these advancements in cytokine management and other strategies may offer better results in many cases. Here again, we need to remember that modulating the immune response will likely hamper immune activities elsewhere in the body. Certainly, we also need to closely review the adverse side effects and consider their risks.

As for osteoarthritis, pharmaceutical treatment still focuses primarily on pain relief and inflammation reduction. Generally, pharmaceutical treatments for osteoarthritis include NSAIDs, analgesics, and selective or non-selective COX inhibitors. There are also a few new pharmaceuticals that are now on the market for osteoarthritis, which we will discuss.

COX Inhibitors

NSAIDs provide pain relief and reduced inflammation by interrupting the enzyme cyclooxygenase. Cyclooxygenase or COX oxidizes certain fatty acids to initiate a chain reaction that produces prostaglandins and thromboxane. These are key components involved in the process of healing wound sites and removing pathogens. Prostaglandins initiate the pathway resulting in pain response. They also collaborate with thromboxane to stimulate the process of clotting, scabbing and wound repair. This involves the delivery of fibrin, nutrients, plasminogen and other regenerative agents to the site of injury.

When an arthritis patient shows up in a doctor's office, they usually have a lot of pain, swelling, and lack of movement. The first inclination of most doctors is to suggest medications that provide immediate pain relief along with a reduction of the swelling. NSAIDs are often prescribed first.

However, over time, NSAID analgesic dosage must be increased to get the same relief. This can be due to the inevitable tolerance to the drug as well as a worsening of the pain, or a combination thereof. This can present a real problem as larger doses produce more side effects.

The primary NSAID recommended is the COX (cyclooxygenase) inhibitor. These drugs will bind to the COX enzyme, reducing thromboxane and prostaglandin production. This of course slows process of swelling, heat and tissue repair. This also blocks the process of healing our cuts, bruises, and internal damage to cells around the body. In other words, NSAIDs do not just reduce the COX enzymes related to our joints. The reduction is system-wide. This means our bodies can have difficulty healing from internal injuries. Then there is COX-1.

The three main COX enzymes are COX-1, COX-2 and COX-3. NSAIDs will inhibit the activity of both COX-1 and COX-2. The problem with inhibiting the COX-1 enzyme is that this blocks the metabolic process that produces protective secretions among the mucosal membranes of our esophagus, stomach and duodenum. Without this protective lining, the stomach can suffer damage from food and the gastric acids the stomach wall cells produce. This blocking of protective mucus is what causes the characteristic ulcer and GI pain seen in NSAID use.

Meanwhile, we also must accept that limiting the COX-2 enzyme will also restrict other healing responses around the body. For this reason, we have seen a number of adverse side effects emerge from both nonselective COX inhibitors and selective COX-2 inhibitors. Pharmaceutical COX inhibition reduces the body's ability to remove toxins and orchestrate a healing response.

Following are the most popular prescription and over the counter pharmaceuticals being sold and recommended by physicians. The drug data and adverse side effects are taken from pharmaceutical manufacturer published reports, studies, medical references, and the *Physician's Desk Reference:*

Acetylsalicylic acid or aspirin (Aspirin, Ecotrin®, many others, over the counter) is a synthetic molecule designed to mimic the effects of willow bark and meadowsweet herb. For thousands of years, herbalists and ancient healers used both willow bark and meadowsweet for the relief of pain. In 1828, salicin was isolated from the bark of the willow tree by Joseph Buchner. Two years later, salicin was isolated from the flower of the meadowsweet plant by Johann Pagenstecher. In 1838, a method of isolating salicylic acid from willow extract was discovered by the Italian Raffaele Piria. Meanwhile, German chemist Karl Jacob Lowig extracted the same salicylic acid from meadowsweet extract. In 1874, salicylic acid began to be produced for commercial use. Twenty-three years later, in 1897, Charles Garhardt, a chemist at the Friedrich Bayer & Company, synthesized a similar derivitive by adding an acetyl group

(OCOOH), to produce the more stable acetylsalicylic acid. The Bayer company proceeded to call it *aspirin* and began large-scale production.

Aspirin's mechanism of action in the body continued to be mysterious, however. Finally, in 1971, Sir John Vane determined that aspirin's active constituent, acetylsalicylic acid, inhibited prostaglandin synthetase (later identified as cyclooxygenase) causing its anti-inflammatory and anti-thrombosis effects. Sir John Vane received the Nobel Prize for Medicine in 1982 for this hypothesis.

Like willow and meadowsweet, aspirin has an immediate effect to reduce pain. Aspirin binds to cylooxygenase-2 within the cells. This allows it to block the pain and inflammatory process. Cylooxygenase-2 produces prostaglandins that in turn send messages to the brain that a particular part of the body is injured. When cylooxygenase-2 is blocked, the process of converting arachidonic acid to prostaglandins is halted.

Cylooxygenase-2 also stimulates the production of thromboxanes. These stimulate the process of blood clotting within the platelets—called platelet aggregation. This is again part of the healing process, because if a blood vessel were to be pierced, our blood would leak out, causing immediate death unless the vessel was sealed somehow. In other words, thromboxanes stimulate clotting, preventing our bodies from bleeding to death.

Adverse Side Effects: This also produces the side effect that aspirin is also known for—as a blood thinner. Because many heart attacks, strokes and other cardiovascular problems are caused by blood clots, low-dose aspirin is used to keep the blood thinner than normal. This also creates another problem, however: The tendency to bleed slows down wound healing. And because it takes increasing amounts of aspirin to provide the same pain relief when used continuously, this adverse effect can become more dangerous.

The problem with ASA, like other isolated chemicals, is that its positive effects come with a price of several adverse effects. Aspirin is notorious for damaging the lining of the stomach, and causing a variety of digestive issues, including acid reflux, ulcers, nausea and gastritis. Aspirin has also been known to cause liver toxicity, Reye's Syndrome (especially in children), and tinnitus—ringing of the ears. Aspirin's blood-thinning effects can create internal bleeding from a variety of internal injuries. The dangerous part of this is that the person may be bleeding internally without knowing it.

Acetaminophen or paracetamol, (many brands, over the counter) on the other hand, has been shown to be significantly more dangerous than aspirin. A number of studies have confirmed that acetaminophen causes acute liver damage and kidney failure. Some research has indicated that more than a third of Americans take acetaminophen at least once per month. The ubiquitous advertising by the many drug manufacturers that include acetaminophen as an active ingredient have removed much if not all consumer concern for the dangers of acetaminophen. Instead of seeing it as a potentially harmful drug, consumers have grown accustomed to acetaminophen on the bathroom shelf ready to take at the first sign of a headache or body ache.

Current theory holds that acetaminophen works by blocking the oxidized COX enzyme, thereby blocking prostaglandin production but not thromboxane synthesis. Apparently, for this reason, acetaminophen does not produce the same level of blood thinning. Some believe the COX-3 enzyme is also blocked, but COX-3 is not connected to inflammation, so this theory is disputed.

In addition to acetaminophen, there are several other ingredients in many of the popular NSAID brands. These can include chlorpheniramine, dextromethophan, diphenhydramine, guaifenesin, pamabrom, pseudoephedrine and doxylamine. These provide antihistamine (blocking histamine production), anticholinergic (blocking the neurotransmitter acetylcholine), and decongestant diuretic properties.

Adverse Side Effects: One of the basic problems with acetaminophen is that it will cause acute liver failure. In a 2009 study done at the University of Maryland's School of Medicine (Mindikoglu *et al.* 2009), 661 acute liver failure patients that were forced to undergo a liver transplant to survive were analyzed. The study concluded that 40% of all the liver failures were as a result of acetaminophen use. As for the other larger drug categories, 8% of the liver failures resulted from antituberculosis drugs, 7% from antiepileptic drugs, and 6% from antibiotics. In comparison with the other drugs, the acetaminophen-caused liver failure patients also required more dialysis.

Outside of this, stomach bleeding and gastric upset has been seen, and a disputed study showed an increase in asthma, eczema and conjunctivitis among young children (Beasley *et al.* 2008).

The adverse effects of some of the ancillary drug ingredients included in many acetaminophen-containing OTC drugs include liver damage, nausea, vomiting, fluid loss, hypertension, anxiety and tachycardia.

Ibuprofen (prescription and over the counter) is a fast-acting drug that provides anti-inflammatory effects and pain relief for a few hours. Brand names Advil®, Nuprin® and Motrin® use ibuprofen as the central active agent. Ibuprofen is an NSAID that inhibits both COX-1 and COX-2. This has the combined effect of reducing inflammation, reducing fever associated with inflammation, and relaxing tense muscles. Because the inflammatory process is inhibited by the blocking of the COX-2 conversion process, there is also a reduction of pain associated with the inflammation.

Adverse Side Effects: As mentioned, one of the most concerning side effects of ibuprofen is its blocking of critical COX-1 enzymes, robbing the digestive tract of healthy mucosal lining. Problems that result from constant ibuprophen use include GI bleeding, ulcers, acid reflux and indigestion. These can in turn cause nausea, vomiting, diarrhea and ulcers in the esophagus.

Side effects from ibuprofen also include a thinning of the blood, which increases the risk of bleeding. Liver enzymes are often significantly raised during ibuprofen use. This indicates possible liver damage over time. Other side effects have included dizziness, headaches, high blood pressure and loss of sexual potency. Other side effects that have been seen include heart problems, kidney damage, and lung damage. Some heart attacks have occurred with higher dosages. Ibuprofen also sometimes causes photosensitivity.

Naproxen (prescription and over the counter) and naproxen sodium are also anti-inflammatory, pain-relieving agents. Naproxen is the active constituent in Anaprox®, Midol Extended Relief® and others. The U.S. is one of the few countries in the world that allows the sale of naproxen over the counter. Canada and Australia are one of the few others that do.

Adverse Side Effects: Naproxen has many of the same side effects that other NSAIDs have. It has a history of causing GI bleeding, ulcers, and complete perforations of the stomach. Naproxen has also caused circulation problems, breathing problems, liver damage, problems with blood clotting and others. Naproxen has also been implicated in heart attacks and strokes.

A 2006 study (ADAPT) of 2528 human subjects showed that naproxen has a significant risk of cardiovascular-related deaths, heart attacks and strokes. Out of 713 patients on naproxen, 8.25% suffered a heart attack, a stroke, or heart failure, while only 5.68% of the placebo group suffered any of these events.

Meloxicam: (Prescription only, Mobic®) This is a COX inhibitor, but this drug requires less dosing per day because it takes longer for the body to break down. This however, is also a possible cause for concern, as it may further burden the liver and/or kidneys.

Adverse Side Effects: As with other COX-1 and COX-2 inhibitors, meloxicam causes gastrointestinal bleeding, ulcers, perforation and other intestinal difficulties. Headaches and tinnitus have also been reported.

Etodolac: (Prescription only, Lodine®) This is another COX enzyme conversion inhibitor, with medium dosing required.

Adverse Side Effects: The research has shown that etodolac can cause headaches, nausea, diarrhea, constipation, dizziness, drowsiness, kidney impairment, rashes, constipation, abdominal pain and ringing in the ears. Like the other COX inhibitors, etodolac also causes GI bleeding and ulcer issues. Anyone with a history of heart disease or asthma is warned against the product by the manufacturer.

Nabumetone: (Prescription only, Relafen®) is another NSAID that is prescribed to relieve pain associated with rheumatoid arthritis and osteoarthritis.

Adverse Side Effects: Like the other COX inhibitors, nabumentone causes GI bleeding, ulcers and other intestinal issues. Studies have also shown that nabumentone also can cause nausea, liver toxicity, dizziness, abdominal pain, and the inability for the blood to clot effectively.

Research has shown that etodolac can cause headaches, nausea, diarrhea, constipation, dizziness, drowsiness, kidney impairment, rashes, constipation, abdominal pain, lightheadedness, and ringing in the ears. Anyone with a history of heart disease or asthma is warned against the product by the manufacturer.

Sulindac: (Prescription only, Clinoril®) Another nonspecific COX inhibitor.

Adverse Side Effects: Like other COX inhibitors, GI bleeding and ulcerous effects in the stomach and small intestines are common side effects. Also, rashes, kidney impairment, lightheadedness, ringing in the ears, weakness, internal bleeding, liver toxicity and an exacerbating of asthma and hives have been seen.

Choline magnesium salicylate: (by prescription only, Trilasate®) is a salicylate, like aspirin. It thus acts the same, by blocking COX enzyme conversion. However, the potential for Reye's Syndrome is apparently slightly reduced with this drug.

Adverse Side Effects: Gastrointestinal bleeding and ulcers in the stomach and small intestines are side effects of all isolated salicylates. Liver toxicity, internal bleeding, and tinnitus have also been seen among users of this form of salicylate.

Ketoprofen: (by prescription only, Orudis®, Oruvail®) is another NSAID that blocks the COX enzyme conversion process. This reduces the pain and inflammation associated with arthritis.

Adverse Side Effects: Ketoprofen has similar side effects as many of the other NSAIDs in that it can cause GI bleeding, intestinal cramping, ulcerations, nausea, vomiting, and diarrhea. In addition, there are a number of other side effects with ketoprofen. These include headaches, fainting, persistent sore throats, stiff necks, rashes, itching, yellowing eyes and dark urine—indicating liver issues.

Diclofenac (prescription only, Cataflam®, Voltaren®, Arthrotec®); **oxaprozin** (Daypro®); **diflusinal** (Dolobid®); **piroxicam** (Feldene®); and **indomethicin** (Indocin®) are all COX inhibitor NSAIDs. Thus, they all block the inflammatory cascade that helps the body protect and heal itself and the production of mucosal membrane lining of the stomach and other mucosal surfaces.

Adverse side effects: Very similar to the other NSAIDs. They all can cause gastrointestinal problems. They can all cause ulcers because they block the body's secretion of protective mucosal lining in the stomach and small intestine. They also potentially can cause cardiovascular problems and potentially bleeding issues, and to varying degrees, headaches and nausea.

This is not a complete list, either. One must wonder why there are so many different NSAIDs out on the market today that basically work the same, by blocking the COX enzyme process. Most also cause many of the same side effects. This fact has been confirmed in numerous studies many times over, as each drug manufacturer has had to run human clinical trials in order to get clearance from the FDA to distribute the drug.

In the end, patients and doctors have had to go through one COX-inhibitor after another looking for a solution to pain and inflammation without the associated GI problems and other adverse side effects. Because the COX-1 enzyme stimulates the release of the mucosal lining along with other processes in the body, we find similar side effects for nonselective COX inhibitors.

We can only conjecture there are so many different NSAID drugs because while nearly all of them reduce pain and inflammation, they all produce similar adverse effects. This means that doctors and patients are continually looking for better alternatives. Undoubtedly, for each new drug, there was the hope that *this* drug would not have the same adverse effects as the others. Yet again, those drugs also have similar side effects, simply because the body is a complex arrangement of a myriad of mechanisms. To change one mechansim is likely to imbalance another. As we'll discuss, this is precisely the reason nature created botanicals with a variety of constituents that alter several mechanisms in a balanced manner.

Selective COX-inhibitor NSAIDs

One of the pharmaceutical industry's responses was the invention and formulation of *selective* COX inhibitors. These theoretically halt the conversion and cascading process towards pain and inflammation through the blocking of the COX-2 enzyme. Because these drugs attach to a molecular component of the COX-2 enzyme not present in the COX-1 enzyme, the drugs theoretically do not interfere with the important pathways of the COX-1 enzyme. Or so they thought.

Initial research by the drug manufacturers of Celebrex® and Vioxx®—by far the most financially successful selective COX inhibitors—did indeed show a reduction of gastrointestinal problems in comparison to conventional COX inhibitors. These drugs became wildly popular, and the drug manufacturers made billions.

Then they hit a snag. In 2000, Merck, who manufactured Vioxx, submitted a study (Bombardier *et al.* 2000) to the FDA that those taking rofecoxib (Vioxx®) experienced increased cardiovascular events (like heart attacks and strokes) at significantly greater levels than experienced in patients taking naproxen. As this information filtered through the ranks of the FDA and the medical community, a slow concern arose over selective COX-2 inhibitors. In 2002, the FDA responded by requiring Merck to print label statements on Vioxx® warning about these effects. Follow-up studies confirmed that rofecoxib doubled the risk of heart attacks and strokes (later evidence revealed levels possibly over four times). By 2004, the uproar forced Merck to withdraw Vioxx® from the market. The media has since exposed a number of irregularities between study authors and publications that indicated that critical evidence may have been either delayed or eliminated from the published data. In 2005, following urging from the FDA, Pfizer withdrew a similar coxib, valdecoxib (Bextra®) from the market.

However, celecoxib (Celebrex®) remains on the market. Subsequent studies have focused upon other selective COX-2 inhibitors—coxibs. Controversy has also arisen here. In the spring of 2009, Dr. Scott Reuben announced that he published fake and inaccurate data for twenty-one studies of coxibs, including celecoxib and rofecoxib. The story, reported in the *Wall Street Journal* on March 11, 2009, indicated that Dr. Reuben had been a paid speaker for Pfizer who traveled the country promoting the use of combined NSAID and coxib prescriptions for arthritis patients. The article indicated that study information was given to the FDA, but apparently the data was not part of the FDA's original clinical package from the manufacturers. While medical publications retracted many of the articles associated with these studies, there was no effect upon the marketability of the drugs.

In follow-up studies on the gastrointestinal effects (Laine *et al.* 2003; Chen, *et al.* 2008) of coxibs compared to NSAIDs, it has become apparent that while selective COX-2 inhibitors do cause less GI difficulties among patients, there are still more gastrointestinal problems when compared to placebo. This leaves the physician and patient in a conundrum: Pain, ulcer or heart attack?

That said, here is a short review of the one of the remaining selective COX-2 inhibitors still on the market:

Celecoxib: (Celebrex®, prescription only) About one million prescriptions are filled for Celebrex each and every month. This is still one of the most popular prescription non-steroid anti-inflammatory drugs on the market.

Adverse Side Effects: According to the manufacturer's own research, celecoxib may increase the chances of heart attack or stroke, possibly leading to death. It is not advised before or after certain heart surgeries. Skin reactions may occur. Stomach and intestinal problems have been found. These include bleeding and ulcers. These may occur without notice and may cause death—again this is according to the manufacturer's information. They also inform people that the elderly are at an increased risk of ulcer and gastrointestinal bleeding. Celecoxib is not advised for anyone who has responded negatively to aspirin, especially with any asthma or allergy symptoms. They also warn against use if the person is pregnant, has a history of ulcer or intestinal problems, has high blood pressure, has had any heart problems, or has had liver or kidney problems.

This last issue about the liver is important to note, because as we discussed the various contributing factors for arthritis, a burdened liver was one of the factors that hamper the immune system and create additional inflammatory responses. The reason why liver warnings are made on many drugs is that the liver must work harder to break down and process the various active and inactive chemicals contained within a drug. Because these chemicals are not nutritive in any way—in other words, the body has no current metabolic process for utilizing the chemicals; they are treated by the body as toxins. They can also form oxidative radicals and damage tissues. The clean up of these chemical metabolites can burden the liver's processes, dampening glutathione and enzymes that help break down and flush other toxins out of the body.

The various adverse effects from coxib use has been the subject of a number of lawsuits over the years, as people have died or suffered great difficulties following the use of these drugs. After 45,000 to 50,000 personal injury lawsuits had been filed against Merck by heart attack or stroke victims, a $4.85 billion dollar settlement was struck between Merck and the plantiffs (Associated Press, 2007). It is likely that for this reason, Pfizer—the manufacturer of Celebrex®—specifically states that celecoxib should be used at the lowest dose possible and for the shortest time needed.

Corticosteroids

The adrenal gland produces several types of corticosteroids. Corticosteroids are hormones naturally synthesized within the adrenal cortex. They play a wide range of important roles in metabolism and immunity throughout the body. The main corticosteroids are cortisol, aldosterone and corticosterone. These hormones are produced during times of stress in order to slow (and balance) the rate of inflammation and pain. But this is not their only purpose. They also enhance protein synthesis, insulin activity and glucose metabolism. For this later activity, corticosteroids are often also referred to as glucocorticoids.

It is their involvement in protein synthesis that motivates athletes to use steroids. The side effects of steroid use among athletes are well known, however: Rage, neanderthal appearance and over-built muscles are quite often seen among steroid-heads.

The side effects of pharmaceutical steroid use for reducing inflammation in arthritis are not limited to these types of effects, however. The long-term use of corticosteroid drugs also has many other side effects as listed below. These are in addition to the fact that with constant sreroid use, the adrenal gland begins to shut down and stop producing its own cortisol. Because natural cortisol is needed to slow inflammation, the body becomes unable to regulate inflammation without the steroids. After long-term use, if the body does not receive the drug, inflammation can spin out of control. This makes the transition out of long-term corticosteroid use a bit tricky.

Another problem with steroid drugs is that the body becomes deprived of the other adrenal functions. The result is a number of imbalances among the body's hormones, glucose utilization and other mechanisms. When the body's hormones are out of whack, an array of imbalances are created around the body. With continued dosing, the shutdown of the adrenal gland can create a domino effect of metabolic shortcomings. Steroid drugs might mimic cortisol's inflammation reduction mechanisms, but they do not replace the functions of the adrenal glands. And because the adrenal glands balance our body's stress response, we become more likely to over-react to psychological or physical stressors.

In addition, steroid injections made directly into sore joints can result in secondary injury. The pain-reduction from the injection allows the joint to be over-used, causing the possibility of additional damage to the joint.

In addition, clinicians have noted that the chronic use of steroids increases the risk of progression from rheumatoid arthritis to septic arthritis. The mechanism is not well known, but many believe that it is because corticosteroids lower the immune response, allowing opportunistic bacteria to grow unchecked.

Prednisone and methylprednisone (Deltasone®, Orasone®, Prednicen-M®, Liquid Pred®, Medrol®, Depo-Medrol®, prescription only): These drugs may be taken orally, injected directly into the site of inflammation or given intravenously. Prednisone and methylprednisone mimic the actions of cortisol produced by the adrenal gland with respect to its affect upon inflammation. Its main mechanism is to slow inflammation and suppress the immune system. It is used for a wide range of inflammatory conditions.

Adverse Side Effects: Because this steroid acts like a hormone, it significantly alters moods. This may begin with mild frustration or annoyance over trivial things. With consistent use, however, this can turn into rage, depression, mania, personality changes and psychotic behavior. Other side effects include weight gain, high blood pressure, sodium retention, headaches, ulcers, cataracts, irregular menstruation, elevated blood sugar, growth retardment, osteoporosis, wound healing impairment, moon face (puffiness of the face), glaucoma, bruising, buffalo hump (rounded upper back), and thinning of the skin.

Prednisolone (Pediapred®, Prednisolone®, Liquid Medrol®, prescription only): The effects of prednisolone are practically identical to prednisone, because prednisone is converted to prednisolone in the liver. This means that its actions are mechanically the same. Like prednisone, it is prescribed to reduce inflammation in a variety of conditions.

Adverse Side Effects: These are also similar to prednisone. Prednisolone also significantly alters moods. This may begin with mild frustration or annoyance over trivial things. With consistent use, this can also turn into rage, depression, mania, personality change and psychotic behavior. Other side effects also include weight gain, high blood pressure, sodium retention, headaches, ulcers, osteoporosis, elevated blood sugar, cataracts, irregular menstruation, growth retardment, wound healing impairment, moon face, glaucoma, bruising, buffalo hump, and again the thinning of the skin.

Dexamethasone (Decadron®, DexPak®, prescription only): Dexamethasone is another synthetic chemical prescribed to reduce inflammation. Its actions also imitate cortisol's ability to reduce inflammation. Like prednisone, it is used for a wide range of inflammatory conditions.

Adverse Side Effects: These are similar to prednisone and prednisolone. It also significantly alters moods. This may begin with mild frustration or annoyance over trivial things. Again, with consistent use, this can become rage, depression, mania, personality changes and psychotic behavior. Other side effects also include weight gain, high blood pressure, sodium retention, headaches, ulcers, cataracts, osteoporosis, elevated blood sugar, irregular menstruation, growth retardment, wound healing impairment, moon face, glaucoma, bruising, buffalo hump, and the thinning of the skin.

Immune System Modifying Drugs

Pharmaceutical companies are spending considerable resources, time and effort trying to shut off the pathways of the immune system in order to reduce the pain and inflammation associated with arthritis. This means shutting off immune triggers such as cytokines. Some of these strategies have become pretty successful in shutting down the process of inflammation, and to a degree, shutting down the swelling, pain and cartilage scarring. The problem of course, as we will see from their adverse effects, is that shunting these mechanisms also leaves the body vulnerable to other injury or infection—as critical features of the immune system are blocked.

Methotrexate: (Rheumatrex®, Trexall®, prescription only) Methotrexate has been prescribed to reduce the signs and symptoms of RA. It also seems to reduce joint damage caused from inflammation. It is also used for other forms of arthritis such as psoriatic arthritis and spondyloarthopathy. Methotrexate appears to interrupt adenosine and TNF pathways.

Adverse Side Effects: Methotrexate inhibits an enzyme that helps metabolize folic acid, so folic acid levels can become low. Other than this, liver injury, mouth ulcers, mild alopecia (balding), GI problems, reduced red blood cell count, and interstitial pneumonia have been seen in users of methotrexate.

Hydroxychloroquine: (Plaquenil®, prescription only) This is an anti-malarial drug also applied to the treatment of rheumatoid arthritis. No experience of reducing joint damage has been seen with either of these so far. The mechanism is somewhat mysterious.

Adverse Side Effects: Eye problems can result. Corneal deposits, extraocular weakness and light sensitivity have been reported. Retinopathy leading to irreversible loss of vision has also been seen, though rare.

Sulfasalazine (Azulfidine®, prescription only): This is often prescribed to reduce the symptoms of joint damage. It is often prescribed together with methotrexate and hydroxychloroquine in combination. Mechanism is unknown.

Adverse Side Effects: Folate depletion has been seen. Allergic reactions also have been seen, especially for those sensitive to sulfa drugs. Gastrointestinal discomfort, reduced red blood cell counts, and kidney damage have been observed. Sulfasalazine metabolizes into sulfapyridine—a withdrawn drug with a range of side effects including liver toxicity, immune cell reduction and male infertility.

Leflunomide (Arava®, prescription only): This is often prescribed to to slow joint damage in RA and psoriatic arthritis. It seems to work by inhibiting an enzyme called dihydroorotate dehydrogenase, and by modulating T-cells.

Adverse Side Effects: Liver enzymes have been seen to rise in laboratory examinations, so liver toxicity is suspected. Gastrointestinal upset, nausea, diarrhea, muscle cramping, lymph gland enlargement, hair thinning, back pain, headaches, mouth ulcers, numbness, dizziness and other side effects have also been seen.

Tumor necrosis factor (TNF) inhibitors

This is a subset of immune system modifying drugs. Tumor necrosis factor (TNF) is a cytokine produced by macrophages and lymphocytes. It stimulates inflammation and it initiates a cancerous cell death sequence—preventing tumors from forming.

Inflixmab: (prescription only) This drug sells under the brand name Remicade®. It is prescribed as a tumor necrosis factor-alpha (TNF-alpha) blocker. TNF-alpha is part of the inflammatory cascade that is stimulated when the body's immune system registers a possible tumor cell formation. Infliximab is prescribed with hopes of slowing the inflammation process and reducing the symptoms of RA. It is also used for inflammation response in Crohn's, psoriasis arthritis, ankylosing spondylitis and juvenile arthritis.

Infliximab is given intravenously in a doctor's office. After the initial dose, another will be given about two weeks later, followed by another six weeks later. Then maintenance doses every eight weeks are often given to continue its effects.

Adverse Side Effects: The drug comes with a number of side effects. The most common are related to infection. Because the TNF-alpha is critical to the processes of isolating and removing infections and infected cells throughout the body; infections of the lung and urinary tract, intestines and blood have been noted as the most common side effects. Thus, fevers, coughs, rashes, back pain, nausea, vomiting, abdominal pain and overall weakness are also listed as common side effects. Therefore, the manufacturer says that infliximab should not be used for anyone with serious infections, nor should it be continued if a serious infection occurs. Reactivation of tuberculosis has been seen among those with previous TB infections, for example.

Other side effects include low or high blood pressure, chest pain, breathing difficulties, chills, and itching shortly following the administration of the drug. Decreases in both white and red blood cell counts, and decreased platelet counts have also been reported from the research.

The manufacturer also states that patients with Crohn's or rheumatoid arthritis that take infliximab may be at a higher risk of contracting lymphoma.

Other cancers have been shown in open-label clinical studies. The rates of increase have been "several-fold." Because TNF-alpha is part of the body's anti-cancer process, blocking it naturally increases the risks of contracting cancer.

Etanercept: (Enbrel®, prescription only) is prescribed to reduce symptoms of RA and psoriatic arthritis, while slowing joint damage. Etanercept is a protein that binds to TNF inside joints to reduce its mechanism of action.

Adverse Side Effects: Etanercept comes with a risk of increased infections. This comes from inhibiting one of the body's most precious immune molecules. For this reason, lymphomas have been observed in patients. Patients with heart problems have been warned against use. White blood cell and other blood irregularities have also been seen.

Adalimumab: (Humira®, prescription only) This is another TNF antagonist. It is prescribed to reduce signs and symptoms of psoriatic arthritis, and ankylosing spondylitis. It is administered by injection weekly or every two weeks. It binds to TNF and blocks its interaction with cell surface receptors.

Adverse Side Effects: Infections are increased, as with other TNF antagonists. Respiratory tract infections such as bronchitis have been seen. Urinary tract infections have also been seen. Latent tuberculosis flair-ups have also been seen, and people with heart problems are discouraged from its use.

T-cell Co-stimulatory blockers

T-cells make up the most potent force in our immune system. T-cells have a variety of communications and signaling systems. These allow them to identify foreign pathogens or toxins, and then signal other T-cells to take immediate action. CD molecules are typically involved in the communication process—for this reason, they are also called co-stimulatory immune mechanisms.

Abatacept: (Orencia®, prescription only) This was the first of the T-cell co-stimulatory blockers. It is prescribed to block interactions between T lymphocytes and their antigens. This discourages the inflammatory cascade because the T-cell isn't activated. Abatacept binds a CD portion with an Fc portion of the T-cell. This stops the signalling process, ceasing T-cell stimulation.

Adverse Side Effects: Infections have been shown to increase, notably respiratory infections such as pneumonia—especially for patients with existing lung congestion.

B-Cell Depletors

B-cells are also extremely critical to the health of our bloodstream, intercellular region, and lymphatic system. B-cells cruise through these regions looking for invaders. The strategy of depleting the body's B-cells with pharmaceuticals is a new and controversial one, as it can open the body to a variety of infections.

Rituximab: (Rituxan®, prescription only) This is prescribed to deplete B-cells, slowing the inflammatory immune response. It modulates cytokine production and antibody-forming plasma cells. It is often prescribed to reduce symptoms of RA. It was originally developed to treat non-Hodgkin's lymphoma. Effects are not often seen for 90 days, but they have been shown to last from six months to two years after a single dose.

Adverse Side Effects: Infection increases have been seen. Reactivation of dormant viruses such as hepatitis has also been seen. Progressive multifocal leukoencephalopathy (PML)—a possibly lethal brain infection—has been seen. Immunizations may be interfered with, and the manufacturer advises they should be done before beginning therapy with rituximab. It is also contraindicated with live virus vaccinations. Decreased levels of important immunoglobulins IgG and IgM have been seen, and this is being studied for potential long-term harm. Some patients have experienced infusion reactions of itching, hives, swelling, fever, chills, difficulty breathing, and changes in blood pressure. These can be mild but also may be severe. Many of these are more commonly seen with the first injection.

Interleukin-1 (IL-1) Antagonists
IL-1 is a proinflammatory cytokine involved in wound healing— including RA inflammation. These antagonists block IL-1.

Anakinra: (Kineret™, prescription only) is a classic IL-1 receptor antagonist— blocking IL-1 activity by binding to the IL-1R.
Adverse Side Effects: Increased infections have been seen, especially if taken with TNF inhibitors (which it often is). Decreased neutrophil counts have been seen. About two-thirds of patients have injection site reactions such as itching and rash—which usually go away after a couple of months. However, more sensitive individuals may have more severe reactions.

Intramuscular Gold: (Myochrysine®, Solganal®, prescription only) This is prescribed to temporarily relieve RA pain when injected into the muscle. Intramuscular gold salts were used prior to the 1990's, but have now been largely replaced by other medications because of their slow and limited response.
Adverse Side Effects: Over a third of users discontinue the drug because of its side effects. Rash is common, and can lead to dermatitis. Ulcers in the mouth and throat have been seen. Up to 10% have mild proteinuria—excess protein in the urine—indicating the loss of protein. Anemia has also been seen. Lightheadedness, dizziness and fainting have been seen as well.

Other Immune Modulation Agents
New pharmaceutical strategies to alter the immune response have resulted in the development of other pharmaceuticals. Unfortunately, while they might block the immune system's joint activities, they also come with similar immunosuppressive side effects.

Azathioprine: (Imuran®, prescription only) This is prescribed to reduce inflammation and pain, but may take 8-12 weeks for any effect.

Adverse Side Effects: It reduces all blood cells (white, red, and platelets). This effect is increased with combined use of allopurinol or ACE inhibitors. Side effects also include nausea, immune suppression, and baldness.

Cyclosporine: (Sandimmune®, Neoral®, prescription only) This is prescribed for RA and psoriasis. It is an immunosuppressive agent that can also prevent kidney and liver transplant rejections. It blocks T-cell function through inhibition of IL-2 transcription.

Adverse Side Effects: Increased infections, kidney insufficiency, and increased blood pressure have been seen. It may also increase the risk of lymphoma and other malignancies.

Cyclophosphamide: (Cytoxan®, prescription only) This is another immunosuppressive for severe rheumatoid arthritis, lupus and vasculitis.

Adverse Side Effects: These include infection, bone marrow reduction, ovarian failure cystitis, premature ovarian failure, and increased bladder cancer risk.

d-Penicillamine: (Cuprimine®, Depen®, prescription only) This immunosuppressive has been prescribed for patients with persistent aggressive rheumatoid arthritis.

Adverse Side Effects: Severe rash and damage to kidney function. Lupus or other autoimmune diseases have also been seen.

Hyaluronic Acid or hylan: (Euflexxa®, Hyalgan®, Orthovisc®, Supartz®, Synvisc®, prescription only) This can be injected directly into the joint. Typical source of hylan is the comb (on the head) of roosters. Injecting this into the synovial fluid is thought that this will supplement the joint's own hyaluonan levels. Usually this is prescribed to a patient after other arthritis drugs have failed to offer pain relief. Meta data research (reviews of multiple studies) has shown that HA injection may provide some temporary pain relief, but these effects often do not last longer than six months (Medina, *et al.* 2006).

Adverse Side Effects: The injection of HA can cause pain and swelling. Allergic responses have also been seen.

Assessment of immunosuppressive effects among rheumatoid arthritis drug treatments found in the research.
(Adapted from Snowden 2007)

Drug	Immunosuppressive Effect
Cyclophosphamide and other cytotoxic drugs	"Severe" among T- and B-cells
Azathioprine	"Severe" primarily among T-cells
Ciclosporin, tacrolimus, sirolimus	"Severe" primarily among T-cells
Mycophenolate mofetil	"Severe" primarily among T-cells
Leflunomide	"Uncertain, probably severe" primarily among T-cells
Methotrexate	"Uncertain, probably moderate"
Anti-TNF drugs	"Highly selective: main risk is mycobacterial infection"
Rituximab	"Highly selective: likely to inhibit new antibody responses"
Corticosteroids	"Dose-dependent, but dose threshold for immunosuppression unclear"
Sulfasalazine, intramuscular gold	"No conventional immunosuppressive effect, but may cause impairment of antibody production in a small proportion of patients treated"

Gout Treatment: Hyperuricemia Drugs

Gout treatment currently aims to interfere with the conversion of uric acid that can crystallize and deposit in the joints. Note that this treatment does not halt the incoming purines that convert to uric acid, nor does it provide a permanent solution.

Allopurinol (Zyloprim®, Aloprim®): This drug is prescribed to temporarily block the enzyme that converts purine proteins into uric acid. This also serves to reduce the amount of trophi that is deposited in the joints, thereby temporarily relieving inflammation. However, once the drug is discontinued—if there is no change in the diet or alcohol consumption—the uric acid production will continue as before.

Adverse Side Effects: Most common adverse effects include diarrhea, skin rashes, fevers, nausea, itching, hepatitis, impaired kidney function, blood in the urine, toxic epidermal necrolysis (TENS), and eosinophilia (abnormally high red blood cell counts). Allopurinol can also cause gout flare-ups.

Surgical Treatments Used for Arthritis

Arthritis is an inflammatory process of the synovium. It can result in loss of joint function. Joint mobility is often the goal of surgery. Surgery on a joint is extremely complex, however. Total joint arthroplasty is prescribed most often for larger joints because of this complexity. Other surgical techniques include releasing nerve entrapments such as carpal tunnel syndrome, and the removal of a rheumatoid nodule. Synovectomy is sometimes done with osteoarthritis but typically not rheumatoid arthritis. Pain relief from surgery may also be temporary because the cause is not removed. Synovectomy for the wrist is sometimes done for intense synovitis.

Conclusion

Nearly every pharmaceutical drug listed in this chapter tries to *stop or alter the immune system* in one way or another. Some of these drugs are prescribed to interfere with the COX or LOX processes. They are given to block the production of prostaglandins. They are given to interfere with the activities of cytokines, TNF, T-cells or B-cells. While the work these scientists are doing is truly amazing and commendable, the blocking of the body's immune system can be inherently dangerous because these processes involve the body's repair mechanisms. By blocking these critical healing pathways, we interfere with the body's ability to correct other issues that may come up besides arthritis. Ironically, many of these pharmaceuticals also prevent the immune system from doing its job in repairing damaged joint tissues—the reason for the pain and inflammation in the first place!

Yes, we certainly commend the effort of these scientists and pharmaceutical companies. However, after this Herculean effort utilizing billions in investment dollars and the cost of many lives from side effects, we are left with only decades of failure in providing permanent solutions for arthritis.

Perhaps we need to investigate another strategy.

Chapter Five

The Botanical Solution

This discussion of herbs, spices and foods is for informational purposes only. Anyone suffering from arthritis or any other illness should consult their health professional before making changes to their diet, lifestyle, medications or botanicals. Furthermore, dosages are not given here, as each person may have unique requirements or sensitivities. Ones health professional should be consulted with to determine the appropriate dosages and combinations.

We know that arthritis—especially osteoarthritis—is not a new set of diseases. Remember the Iceman! While this may not have been the case for the Iceman (though they did find a small satchet containing herbs and foods), we know from traditional texts that arthritis has been treated with various degrees of success by a number of ancient cultures. Here we will examine these, and some of the recent science confirming medicinal effects of botanical agents.

Before we do this, let's compare the pharmaceutical drug statistics for death, disability and adverse side effects discussed in the previous chapter to the number of deaths, disability and adverse side effects of herbal medication usage—both prescribed and self-medicated. According to the FDA, a total of 184 deaths and 2,621 adverse reactions resulted from consumer use of herbal supplements *over a five-year period* from 1993 to 1998. Most of these deaths were associated with the incorrect use of ephedra weight-loss formulas. Still, this is an average of 37 annual herbal deaths, compared to the 106,000 annual deaths among pharmaceuticals. Also during this period, there was an average of 524 adverse side effects from medicinal herbs per year, compared to an estimated 36,000,000 adverse pharmaceutical reactions per year. For those who might think that these lopsided numbers reflect pharmaceutical use being much greater than herbal use, think again. Herbal supplementation use in the U.S. ranged from 27% to 36% of the population during that period. This nets out to about one-third of the population, which is actually higher than the range for prescription pharmaceutical use (Hirshon and Barrueto 2006).

For thousands of years, traditional healers, physicians and scientists carefully studied and documented particular botanicals associated with particular ailments. One of the earliest written records of herbal medicine is the *Pen Ts'ao*, written some 4500 years ago by a Chinese herbalist. The *Pen Ts'ao* recorded 366 different plants that had been used as medicines, along with their recommended uses. Ayurvedic texts have recorded the use of particular herbs for specific ailments beginning some 5,000 years ago. Sumerian Clay tablets over 4,000 years' old document using medicinal herbs. The Egyptian *Ebers Papyrus* of 2500-3000 B.C. also documented the use of botanicals as medicine. For some ancient cultures, the knowledge was passed down for centuries before being recorded. For others, the oral passing of the knowledge remained intact until modern herbalists learned it and subsequently recorded it. For some—especially applicable to South American and North American Indians—much of their knowledge of botanical medicine is lost forever. The short list of ancient cultures who had an advanced use of herbs included the Greeks, the Romans, the Polynesians, the New Zealand Maoris, the Aborigines, different North American Indian tribes, Indonesians, Mayans, Incas, Egyptians, North and South Afrikaans, Mesopotamians, early Arabs, various early Northern European cultures, and of course early Chinese, Tibetan and Indus Valley societies.

What all this means is that herbal medications are not only safe when compared to pharmaceutical use, but they have been used safely by billions of people over thousands of years.

A pharmaceutical drug might be approved based on a few studies of several hundred patients, managed by researchers paid by the pharmaceutical company. To this, we can compare the use of certain herbs for thousands of years by billions of people, and the knowledge of their use and possibly misuse being handed down through many generations. We must remember too, that there has been no financial conflict of interest in the study of traditional herbs—since they grow freely. In comparison, there is a giant conflict of interest in the study of pharmaceuticals—as pharmaceutical companies may spend billions of dollars on the development of a single drug. To abandon the drug is a proposal of mass proportions compared to not eating the leaves of a poisonous plant.

In addition, once a pharmaceutical company has designed a new drug, it can receive patent protection for that chemical combination, giving it up to twenty years of potential exclusivity for selling that drug—at least in the United States (patent laws are similar else-where). This means a guarantee of profits as long as doctors prescribe that drug. With a patent, there is protection from competition, guaranteeing salaries and profits for many years.

Without the doctor prescribing the medication, however, there is no continual use. Thus, control must include both the patent and the doctor. For this reason, pharmaceutical giants focus their attention on a combination of drug research, patent protection, regulation, and marketing to physicians.

In our modern medical institutions, pathology instruction relating to diagnosis also accompanies the use of specific pharmaceutical drugs. Western medical institutions synchronize with the pharmaceutical industry because of the financial relationships between pharmaceutical companies, medical schools, medical licensure and pathology documentation. Drug research by doctors—many of whom are also medical school professors—is often funded by the pharmaceutical manufacturers. There is thus a built-in incentive for a successful outcome. As the COX anti-inflammatory drug lawsuits and investigative reporting proved over the past few years, pharmaceutical manufacturers and medical researchers are often slow to disclose information damaging to a drug's income potential.

Even if a pharmaceutical results in an improved condition for a particular ailment, there are often dangerous side effects. Some of these can be worse than the original ailment. In addition, most medications stress the liver and kidneys in one respect or another—shortening the lifespan of these critical organs. Some medications, like aminoglycoside antibiotics streptomycin, kanamycin, garamicin and others have been shown to cause kidney damage in as many as 15 percent of patients. Others, such as acetaminophen, carbamazepine, atenolol, cimetidine, phenylbutazone, acebutolol, piroxicam, mianserin, naproxen, sulindac, ranitidine, enflurane, halothane, valproic acid, phenobarbital, isoniazid and ketoconazole can cause acute dose-dependent liver damage. This is because the liver and the kidneys work together to process most chemicals out of the body. Together these organs break down and excrete the chemical byproducts of medications, resulting in their hopeful extraction from the body. This chemical breakdown comes with a number of dangerous residual chemical derivatives as well.

The P450 liver enzyme process moves chemicals through the extraction pathway in many cases. This enzyme is effective in most healthy bodies for a few chemicals at a time. Yet multiple drugs can overwhelm and deplete this pathway. With the P450 pathway over-loaded by various chemicals, additional drugs can damage the body incrementally. For this reason, a higher number of liver enzymes in a blood analysis is seen by doctors as a dangerous sign.

This means that like most toxic chemicals, many pharmaceuticals put a burden on the liver. This is because the liver must work harder to filter and break down the chemicals—before sending them out through the kidneys, colon, lungs and/or sweat glands.

The central issue related to the burdening of liver is the fact that synthetic chemicals are foreign to the body. Most botanicals are quite the opposite. Botanicals are highly recognized by the body, simply because humans have been consuming these and similar botanicals for thousands of years. Thus, the body processes the constituents of a botanical with a very normal pathway.

In fact, many botanical herbs provide a broad spectrum of activity. They include antioxidant activity and immune stimulation. They may also be antiseptic and antibiotic as well. They might increase detoxification, stimulate the liver, increase kidney efficiency and stimulate the adrenal glands all at the same time.

While pharmaceuticals are isolated chemicals with often one central mechanism of action within the body, most botanicals have many—some even hundreds—of pharmacological constituents and complementary actions. For example, according to the research of James Duke, Ph.D. of the U.S. Department of Agriculture and Norman Farnsworth, Ph.D., a research professor at the University of Illinois, ginger contains at least 477 active constituents (Schulick 1996). While botanicals produce active biochemicals that act in a healing manner, they also produce active multiple constituents that buffer and balance each other.

Ginger is not alone. Research has confirmed that many other botanicals also have dozens if not hundreds of constituents.

Separately, one of ginger's active constituents might produce side effects along with its actions. The other constituents present a balance of mechanisms, however. Together these many constituents in ginger make it one of the most active and effective medicinal botanicals for many ailments. Many herbal medicine experts consider it one of the best anti-inflammatory botanicals. Like a number of other anti-inflammatory herbs, ginger has been shown to suppress the expression of both cyclooxygenase-1 and cyclooxygenase-2; yet without slowing down the immune system's healing mechanisms and GI mucosal lining secretions. Whole ginger also slows leukotriene production through the blocking of the 5-lipooxygenase enzyme (Grzanna *et al.* 2005) without adverse side effects.

Unlike the parade of adverse side effect-ridden COX inhibiting non-steroidal anti-inflammatory drugs introduced by the pharmaceutical industry over the past two decades, anti-inflammatory botanicals provide a level of safety and a myriad of nutritional benefits. We might add that these pharmaceuticals—some of which have been pulled from the market because they injured hundreds of thousands of people—have required billions of dollars of taxpayer investment in regulation and oversight. The complexity of these drugs is met with a double-complexity of regulation. If even a small amount of this wasted effort could be diverted to the growing and production of the anti-inflammatory botanicals discussed below, we could be saving billions of taxpayer dollars, not to speak of the damage to the environment from the dumping of toxic synthetics.

Further to this last point, on March 10, 2008, a water contamination report was released by the American Press National Investigation Team. This report confirms a 2002 report by the U.S. Geological Survey that pharmaceutical drugs are infecting many rivers and streams across the country. Together these reports confirmed that pharmaceutical drugs taken for pain, inflammation and other disorders have contaminated local water supplies in a number of cities and town across America. These pollutants now directly affect the drinking water supplies of over forty-one million Americans. Because most people flush their medications down the toilet (as advised by doctors and pharmaceutical manufacturers to prevent their getting into the wrong hands), these medications go right into the grey water of the community. They also arrive excreted through urine and stool. Unlike botanicals—which are easily broken down by the body and excreted as nutrients—most pharmaceuticals are foreign molecules not easily degraded. When and if they are degraded, many break down into toxic chemical byproducts.

Pharmaceutical drug residues slip through the filtration systems of municipalities, as these water treatment facilities were not designed for the treatment of pharmaceutical pollutants.

This disaster is compounded by the waste streams of pharmaceutical manufacturers. One report recently stated, for example, that a quite large and well-known pharmaceutical manufacturer generates some 2,400,000 pounds of hazardous waste every year, which escapes into the surrounding countryside and its waters. The report also stated this same manufacturing facility caused genetic mutation among a variety of crops near its manufacturing facility.

Up until 1996, the pharmaceutical industry had launched at least two hundred pharmaceuticals and spent over $70 billion aimed at reproducing the eicanosoidal-inhibitory effects that anti-inflammatory botanicals already produce. Today that number is much greater. Not only do botanicals act without side effects, but they also break down easily and even provide nutrition for the surrounding waters. How much better can nature get?

The issue modern medicine has with herbal medicine is the speed in which its therapeutic effects can be seen. This is also its benefit, however. While pharmaceuticals are fast acting, they also create imbalances within the body that require the body to work harder in other ways to detoxify the drug. Medicinal botanicals have no toxicity, but they work slower and more gradual. This forces the patient to be disciplined, and well, *patient*. It is because natural herbal medicines are complex and balanced that they tend to act more deeply. They also produce a result that is long-lasting, working with the body to strengthen its immunity and ability to resist the problem in the future.

Rather than causing negative side effects by blocking the immune system, anti-inflammatory botanicals produce *positive side effects*. While gradually reducing pain, fever and inflammation, they modulate eicanosoids and boost the immune system's activity. They also stimulate detoxification; increase healthy appetite; reduce nausea; protect against ulcers; increase liver vitality; stimulate circulation; calm nerves; balance endocrine function; encourage bone healing; improve lung and gum health; and neutralize oxidative (free) radicals. Many are also antiseptic, anesthetic, and antimetic— among so many other positive "side effects." Laboratory studies have also shown many of these to be protective against cancer as well (LaValle, 2001; Shukla and Singh 2007; Schulick 1996).

There are a number of other excellent botanical treatments for pain to consider before resorting to the array of increasingly toxic pharmaceutical analgesics. Botanicals such as *white willow tree bark* and *meadowsweet* are good examples. White willow tree bark and meadowsweet both contain a constituent called salicin. This of course is the natural version of the synthetic *acetyl-salicylic acid* we discussed in the last chapter, known by its expired patented trade-mark name of *aspirin*. As mentioned, acetyl-salicylic acid and its non-acetylated, isolated *salicylic acid* both come with a number of side effects, including internal bleeding and gastro-intestinal upset sometimes leading to ulceration and stomach bleeding.

Far from its natural origins, today's aspirin is usually manufac-tured from phenol, which can be derived from coal or isolated from other materials. The phenol is treated with sodium and then carbon dioxide under pressure, rendering salicylate. After acidification into salicylic acid, it is acetylated with acetic anhydride to yield the final product. The manufacturing facility hosting these reactions pro-duces pollutants to yield the synthetic result. Though it successfully relieves pain, aspirin also creates adverse side effects as we have discussed. We know that aspirin disrupts the cyclo-oxygenation (COX) process, which oxidizes arachidonic acid utilizing the en-zyme called cyclooxygenase. We have discussed this. By blocking COX, the production of prostaglandins and prostanoids such as thromboxane is interfered with. What we may not realize is that the original botanical sources of *salicylic acid*, white willow bark and meadowsweet flowers, also perform this same inhibition of COX. The difference, however, is that these botanicals also balance this inhibition by stimulating the immune system in other ways. This includes stimulating the detoxification process, which in turn speeds healing and removes the causative pathogens.

Aspirin's disruptive mechanisms are illustrated in its effective depletion of a number of nutrients from the body. These include iron, potassium, folic acid, and vitamin C. According to Kauffman (2000), death rates among populations of aspirin users are signifi-cantly higher than non-aspirin populations.

In contrast, the botanical versions contribute many of these nutrients. Botanicals not only relieve pain and boost the immune system. They also supply nutrients to balance the system.

In other words, white willow bark and meadowsweet—by nature's design—contain a biomolecular version of salicin, moderated by a variety of constituents to balance its effects. Subsequently, whole-plant salicin botanicals do not have a history of the negative side effects. Their molecular arrangements are synergistically oriented with a balance of constituents, which resonate with and stimulate our body's immune system while slowing the conversion of prostaglandins and leucotrienes to gradually ease inflammation. Unlike aspirin, willow and meadowsweet actually *promote* a healthy stomach lining, rather than cause gastrointestinal problems. In fact, traditional herbalists often recommend meadowsweet specifically for acid reflux, gastritis and ulcers.

While botanical pain relievers have the ability to gradually modulate the eicanosoid response in order to ease inflammation and pain, they also stimulate the body's own healing mechanisms to help solve the root problem.

In addition, pharmaceutical chemicals typically burden the liver and bloodstream with toxicity. Herbal medicines, on the other hand, stimulate detoxification and strengthen the liver. Nearly every medicinal botanical contains constituents that provide antioxidant and blood-purifying effects. They will thus neutralize toxic free radicals and stimulate glutathione scavenging. They will stimulate the immune system to respond more efficiently. In addition, many botanicals stimulate more efficient filtration and excretion among the kidneys, colon, liver, sweat glands and lungs to remove waste products from the blood and tissues. This means, frankly, that herbs are simply not comparable to pharmaceutical drugs. They are entirely different creatures. It would be like comparing a rocking chair to a helicopter.

Just as botanicals affect the body vastly different from pharmaceuticals, traditional health practitioners look at arthritis much differently than do medical doctors. Traditional health practitioners such as herbalists, naturopaths and acupuncturists are not focused upon naming the illness (diagnosis). They are focused upon the root cause of the imbalances that exist within the body, and thus seek to help rebalance the body's metabolism so that it will heal itself. They see joint inflammation and pain as a progression of internal toxicity and immune weakness that has just finally reached the joints. Whether the actual joint damage involves infection by microorganisms, acid-forming foods or chemical toxins, they seek to rebalance the system.

For example, herbalist Matthew Wood (1997) explains that the goldenrod herb illustrates a link between kidney health and the uric acid build up in gout. He explains that when the kidneys weaken, they can lose some of their sodium-pump ability—affecting their ability to pull uric acid from the bloodstream. As a result, uric acid builds up in the blood—acidifying the bloodstream and depositing crystals into the joints. One of goldenrod's effects is to help strengthen the glomular and sodium-pump capabilities of the kidneys, promoting increased uric acid excretion.

Medicinal qualities are not limited to the botanical herbs. Most botanical foods also have multifarious medicinal and disease-prevention capabilities. For example, as cancer researchers have spent billions upon billions of dollars on cancer research and probed for various anti-cancer strategies, the overwhelming evidence points to a conclusion that a number of botanical foods prevent cancer (or *chemo-protective*). In other words, the range of bio-chemicals contained within many botanical foods protect us against cancer before it forms. How do they do this? They are antioxidant. They prevent DNA mutation. They stimulate the immune system. They augment the process of detoxification.

The list of foods documented with anti-cancer properties is quite long. It includes apples, asparagus, barley, basil, beans, beets, various berries, broccoli, Brussels sprouts, buckwheat, bulgur wheat, cabbage, cantaloupe, carrots, cauliflower, celery, cherries, chili peppers, corn, fiber, flaxseed, garlic, grapefruit, grape juice, mangoes, milk, mushrooms, nuts, oats, olive oil, oranges, pears, peas, pectin, prunes, raisins, rhubarb, whole rice, soy, various spices, wheat, barley and many others (Yeager 1998).

Numerous constituents within these foods create their anti-cancer effects. The research is still unfolding. For example, new research indicates the intake of selenium—a mineral contained in nuts, grains and other foods—appears to protect the cell from the mutation of the p53 gene (Fischer *et al.* 2007). The p53 gene is now referred to as the *tumor suppressor gene.*

We are hard pressed to find edible botanicals that do not contribute to the immune system in one way or another. This lies in contrast to pharmaceuticals, where we are hard pressed to find medications without adverse side effects and liver toxicity.

Moreover, as researchers have investigated the causes of cancer, autoimmunity and other DNA-related disorders, overwhelmingly the biggest culprits appear to be synthetic chemical toxins and our generally pervasive chemical-laced environment. In addition to pharmaceuticals, we are exposed to air and water pollution, synthetic building materials, cleaning agents, chemical food additives, and many others. Many of these have been implicated as carcinogens and mutagens. Synthetic chemicals are often carcinogens and mutagens because their molecular structures become unstable within the body, and disrupt and damage cells. These include the vital cells within artery walls, the stomach, the intestines, the heart, and the brain—creating a basis for genetic mutation and the *switching off* of the protective p53 gene.

We must remember that plants are living organisms themselves. Therefore, they also have immune systems. They thus produce a number of biochemicals that protect them from invading bacteria, fungi, sun damage and injury. These same biochemicals become available to humans when we consume their leaves, bark and roots.

Because plants are stationary, they must protect themselves with their various biochemicals. This means the biochemicals they produce interact with environmental threats in the same way those biochemicals will interact with environmental threats within the human body.

One must wonder why there is not more information being made available about the many positive effects of botanical foods and medicines. There is one large glaring reason for the lack of rigorous clinical studies for many botanical products: Botanical medicine is simply not profitable enough for the financial appetites of many scientific institutions. Researchers have to be paid, and the pharmaceutical giants are very generous with their support of research, so long as that research illustrates the effectiveness of their drugs.

At least for now, natural botanical plants cannot be patented. (Genetically engineered plants can, however. So we need to keep an eye on this.) If we consider that hundreds of thousands of people die each year from medications, while very few if any die of herbal supplement use, the numbers do not imply any safety issue with botanicals. Yet every day research institutions are warning people about the dangers of using herbal medications. Ironically, much of these warnings are about problems caused by the *interactions* between herbs and pharmaceuticals.

Botanicals Used Traditionally for Rheumatism and Various Forms of Arthritis

Joint ailments and inflammation have been with humankind for thousands of years. However, it is apparent—from what we can tell from ancient texts and descriptions of life thousands of years ago—that the physically active lives of the ancients were far less encumbered by arthritis as we are today. We can see this among indigenous tribes living today: The elderly often stay quite active. They are not known for lying around with stiff, achy joints. Inflammation is quickly addressed with botanicals known to stimulate healing. Then they continue their activity—moderately but unrestrained—in contrast to the elderly in western society.

A number of botanicals have been used traditionally to treat different forms of arthritis. As we lay out the research, we should note that practically every study documents the safety of these botanicals. In those rare cases where there were a few adverse effects, the adverse effects were described as mild and not injurious. In fact, in many of those cases where (mild) adverse effects have been noted, the subject of the study was often a standardized or isolated extract of the botanical rather than a whole-herb extract or the more balanced whole herb itself.

Willow Bark *Salix alba, Salix spp.*

Some Active Constituents in Willow Bark

acetylated salicin
acetylsalicortin
catechin
catechin-3-O-ester
condensed procyanidins
dihydroxyflavone.
epicatechin
epicatechin-catechin
epicatechin-epicatechin-
  catechin
esters of salicylic acid
gallocatechin
gallotannins
helicon
isoquercitrin
isosalicin
isosalipurposide
isquercitrin
leonuriside A
luteolin
luteolin glucoside
matsudone A

methoxyflavone
naringenin
naringin
oligomeric procyanidins
picein
piceoside
populin
procyanidin B1 (dimeric)
procyanidin B3 (dimeric)
salicin
salicortin
salicoylsalicin
salicyl alcohol
salicylic acid
salidroside
saligenin
salinigrin
salipurposide
salireposide
sisymbrifolin
tremulacin
triandrin

(Li *et al.* 2008; Jürgenliemk *et al.* 2007; Kammerer *et al.* 2005; Wood 1997; Weiss 1988, Williard 1992; Schauenberg and Paris 1977; Potterton 1983; Hoffman 1990; Lininger *et al.* 1999; Ellingwood 1983; Mabey 1988; Foster and Hobbs 2002; Griffith 2000)

Traditional Uses and Characteristics of Willow Bark

The willow tree can grow to 75 feet tall, but many species are smaller trees and even shrubs. It has rough bark with narrow, glandular, pointed leaves and small yellow flowers. It grows along streams and fields—and often in neighborhood yards. There are some 450 species of the genus *Salix,* and most contain similar con-stituents. Willow species grow practically all over the world.

Willow bark has been used traditionally for over five thousand years for pain, rheumatism and inflammation. Sumerian Clay tablets some 4,000 years ago documented using willow leaves to treat fever and rheumatism. The 2500-3000 B.C. *Ebers-Edwin Smith Surgical Papyrus*—translated by James Breasted in the 1920s—documented the use of willow by the "Father of Medicine," Imhotep. He used willow for healing wounds and inflammation. The ancient Chinese also used willow to treat pain, wounds, goiter, hemorrhaging, and rheumatic fever. The ancient Greek physicians also used willow. Hippocrates, Celsius, Pliny the Elder, and Galen all recommended willow for pain and inflammation. Early western European physi-cian and herbalist Dioscoridies also documented its use for pain and inflammation.

Herbalists Steven Foster and Christopher Hobbs (2002) docu-mented that willow has "confirmed anti-inflammatory, pain-reducing, fever-lowering and antiseptic properties." The bark was often traditionally used, but famous herbalist Nicholas Culpeper suggested the sap from inside the bark—which also contains sali-cylic acid—can be used to "provoke the urine" or to "clear the face and skin from spots and discolourings." The leaves have also been defused (steeped into a tea) or even eaten raw to alleviate head-aches, arthritis, colds, flu and urinary tract infections. American Indians also chewed the bark to lower fevers, relieve sore throats and toothaches; and even to reduce tonsil inflammation.

Willow contains several salicin glycoside compounds. The salicin molecule will split off in the body, providing a good portion of willow's inflammation and pain reduction effects. Natural salicin from willow is slower acting than aspirin, but it does not come with aspirin's adverse gastrointestinal effects because of its constituent complex of buffers and digestive aid components. The bark is es-pecially high in certain tannins, which help reduce gastrointestinal discomfort.

Rafaele Piria, a university professor in Pisa and Turin, isolated salicin from willow bark in 1828. As we have discussed, this led to salicylic acid's isolation from meadowsweet and subsequent devel-opment of aspirin seventy years later.

Dr. Michael Tierra recommends willow bark for fever, headache, sciatic pain, arthritis, rheumatic conditions and neuralgic pain. Dr. Jethro Kloss advocated it for various types of fevers, chills, acute rheumatism, eczema, gangrene, nosebleeds, open wounds, and as a replacement to quinine. North American Indians also prepared poultices from willow for rashes, sores, itching, and cuts. Winter Griffith, M.D. notes that it may reduce symptoms of gout. Dr. Kloss and others describe it as tonic (immune system stimulant), antiperiodic (preventing relapses), astringent (contracts or constricts tissues and reduces bleeding), antiseptic, anodyne (soothing— relieves pain), diaphoretic (induces sweating), diuretic (increases urination), and antipyretic (reduces fever).

(Kammerer *et al.* 2005; Wood 1997; Weiss 1988, Williard 1992; Schauenberg and Paris 1977; Potterton 1983; Lininger *et al.* 1999; Ellingwood 1983; Mabey 1988; Foster and Hobbs 2002; Griffith 2000)

Some Research on Willow Bark

Probably the first clinical study on willow bark was performed by Reverend Edward Stone of Oxfordshire. In the 1760s, he gave 1 dram (1.8 gram) to 50 patients with rheumatic fever, and cured them all to one degree or another (Vane 2000).

While salicylic acid has been shown to inhibit both cyclooxygenase enzymes, other flavonoids in willow have also been shown to inhibit or moderate both cyclooxygenase enzymes COX-1 and COX-2 (Li *et al.* 2008). In one review of randomized human clinical studies on willow bark, three studies confirmed results with analgesic (pain-relieving) effects similar (and not inferior) to rofecoxib for backache; and one confirmed analgesic effects for osteoarthritis (Vlachojannis *et al.* 2009).

In another study of willow and its constituents (Khayyal *et al.* 2000) performed at the Cairo University, it was found that willow extract produces the same or greater ability to inhibit COX enzymes, reduce inflammatory cytokines, reduce leukocyte infiltration and suppress prostaglandins compared to aspirin and celecoxib. Willow extract also showed a greater ability to reduce malondialdehyde (a reactive species causing toxicity) levels, and significantly reduced oxidative free radical species compared to celecoxib. They found that several polyphenols in willow were responsible for this radical scavenging ability. This of course confirms the combined effects we've been discussing with respect to botanicals.

In a randomized, placebo-controlled double-blind clinical trial by researchers from the University of Sydney (Chrubasik et al. 2001), 228 outpatients with acute low-back pain took either willow bark extract or COX 2 inhibitor drug rofecoxib. After four weeks, 60% of the 114 patients that took a 240 mg extract from willow bark experienced more than a 30% improvement using the Total Pain Index, while 60% of the 114 patients that took rofecoxib (now withdrawn from the market) also responded "well." In other words, the two groups responded practically identically. The authors noted that the primary difference between the two treatments was the cost—the willow bark being cheaper.

In a study from researchers from the Eberhard Karls University in Germany (Taxis and Heide 2004), 127 outpatients with osteoarthritis and 26 patients with rheumatoid arthritis were tested in two trials of six weeks. Randomized patients took either 240 mg of salicin extracted from willow per day, diclofec or a placebo. In the OA trial, those taking the salicin extract averaged a 17% reduction in pain compared with 10% reduction in the placebo group. Among the RA patients, the mean pain reduction was 15% compared to 4% among the placebo group. It should be noted that this was a single extract of willow, salicin—less efficacious than the more active willow constituent, salicylic acid. In addition, a whole-herb extract containing the various other efficacious constituents would likely have fared better.

This was illustrated by a clinical trial from Germany's University of Tübingen (Schmid et al. 2001). Ten healthy volunteers took a whole willow bark extract with the equivalent of 240 mg of salicin in two doses three hours apart. Over the next 24 hours, the blood of the volunteers was tested for salicylates in the blood stream. Salicylic acid was 86% of the total salicylate content in the blood. Salicyuric acid was 10%. Gentisic acid was 4%. The amount of salicylic acid in the blood corresponded to 87 mg of synthetic acetylsalicylic acid. The researchers concluded that, "The formation of salicylic acid alone is therefore unlikely to explain analgesic or anti-rheumatic effects of willow bark."

Researchers from the University of Freiberg (Chrubasik *et al.* 2001), tested three groups of patients who used either 240 mg of willow extract supplemented with conventional pain drugs, 120 mg of willow bark supplemented with conventional pain drugs, or only conventional drugs. Only 18% of the 224 control patients who used only conventional drugs were pain-free after 18 months. On the other hand, 40% of the 115 patients who used 240 mg of willow extract plus conventional drugs were pain-free, and 19% of the 112 patients who used the 120 mg of willow extract were pain-free after 18 months.

In another randomized, double-blind study at the University of Tübingen (Schmid *et al.* 2001), 78 patients took either 240 mg of willow bark extract or placebo for two weeks. After the two week period, the average pain score (WOMAC standardized index) of the willow bark group was reduced by 14%, while the placebo group was reduced by 2%. The authors concluded that the study confirmed willow's analgesic effects.

Willow bark does cause a mild reduction in platelet aggregation like aspirin does, but nowhere near the sometimes-dangerous levels that aspirin produces. This is because willow bark contains a variety of other constituents that moderate these effects. In a study at the Rambam Medical Center in Israel (Krivoy *et al.* 2001), 51 patients were studied for platelet aggregating reduction—comparing willow bark extract with aspirin and a placebo. The mean platelet-aggregating factor from arachidonic acid was 78% (high baseline) in the placebo group. The aspirin group's platelet-aggregating factor was 13% in comparison. The platelet-aggregating factor was 61% for the willow bark extract group. This illustrated some blood thinning ability, but nowhere near the extreme reduction (that can cause internal bleeding) of aspirin.

In a randomized, double-blinded study from Israel's Rambam Medical Center (Crubasik *et al.* 2000) published in the *American Journal of Medicine*, 210 low-back pain patients were given willow bark in either 120 mg doses (67 patients) or 240 mg doses (65 patients), while 59 patients were given a placebo. After four weeks, 39% of the high dose (240 mg) willow treatment group was pain-free. Meanwhile, 21% of the 120 mg willow group was pain-free and 6% (four) of the placebo group was pain-free after the four weeks.

How does this compare with the pharmaceutical industry's COX-inhibitors for pain reduction? In another randomized, double-blinded low-back pain study by some of the same researchers (Chrubasik *et al.* 2002), 183 patients took either 240 mg willow bark extract or rofecoxib for four weeks. Both the willow extract group and the rofecoxib group had an identical 44% decrease in pain. This is a second clinical trial illustrating willow bark extract's nearly identical effect of COX-2 inhibitor rofecoxib.

As mentioned, botanical medicines have multiple *positive* side effects. Illustrating this was a study by researchers from the University Hospital in Zürich (Hostanska *et al.* 2007) that tested willow bark on the proliferation of colon cancer cells. It was found that the whole extract and many of willow's constituents inhibited the growth of cancerous cells.

Meadowsweet *Spiraea ulmaria, Filipendula ulmaria, Spiraea betulifolia, Filipendula glaberrima, Filipendula vulgaris*

Some Active Constituents in Meadowsweet

aglycon salicylaldehyde	opiraein
avicularin	other phenolic glycodides
coumarin	phenylcarboxylic acids
ellagitannins	pireine, methyl salicylate
ethereal oil	polysaccharides
ethylsalicylate	quercetin-4'-glucoside
eugenol	rugosin A
gallic acid	rugosin B
gaultherin	rugosin E
hydrolysable rugosin	rutin
hyperoside	salicin
isosalicin	salicylic aldehyde
meth-oxybenzaldehyde	spiraein
methylsalicylate	spiraeoside
monotropitin	tannic acid
mucilage	vitamin C

(Fecka 2009; Thieme 1996; Henih and Ladna 1980; Hoffman 1990; Lininger *et al.* 1999; Foster and Hobbs 2002; Griffith 2000; Hoffman 1990)

Traditional Uses and Characteristics of Meadowsweet

Also sometimes called *Queen of the Meadow*, this perennial bush grows throughout Europe and North America in damp grasslands and by streams in the forests. It has small, sweet-smelling white flowers that bloom in the summer. Its flowers, leaves and root extracts have been used to reduce fevers, aches, pains and inflammation for thousands of years. The Egyptians, Greeks, Romans and Northern Europeans were known to have utilized meadowsweet extracts for the treatment of rheumatism, infection of the urinary tract and abdominal discomfort. North American Indians used meadowsweet for bleeding, kidney issues, abdominal pain, colds and menstrual pain. Traditional herbalist Dr. Nicholas Culpeper wrote that meadowsweet "helps in the speedy recovery from cholic disorders and removes the instability and constant change in the stomach." [Cholic refers to increased bile acids.] According to herbalist Richard Mabey, the tannin and mucilage content in meadowsweet moderate the adverse gastrointestinal side effects of isolated salicylates. For this reason, it is often used for heartburn, hyperacidity, acid reflux, gastritis and ulcers. Meadowsweet has also been used to promote the excretion of uric acid. A purified version of salicin was isolated from meadowsweet in 1830 by Swiss Johann Pagenstecher. This led to the production of acetylsalicylic acid by the Bayer Company, now known by its common name of aspirin. The root of the word aspirin, "spirin" is derived from meadowsweet's genus name *Spiraea*.

The tannins within meadowsweet have been documented to have beneficial effects upon digestion as well. Thus, meadowsweet is often recommended for digestive disorders such as indigestion, diarrhea and colitis. Meadowsweet is also often recommended for the removal of excess uric acid because of its diuretic and detoxifying effects. It has thus been used for kidney stones. Herbalist David Hoffman documents its ability to reduce excess acidity in the stomach and ease nausea. Meadowsweet has been described as astringent, aromatic, antacidic, cholagogue (increasing bile flow), demulcent (soothing and providing mucilage), stomachic (tonic to

digestive tract), and analgesic. The German Commission E monograph suggests the flower and herb for pain relief.
(Gundermann and Müller 2007; Wood 1997; Weiss 1988, Miceli *et al.* 2009; Williard 1992; Schauenberg and Paris 1977; Potterton 1983; Ellingwood 1983; Mabey 1988; Lininger *et al.* 1999; Foster and Hobbs 2002; Griffith 2000; Hoffman 1990)

Some Research on Meadowsweet

Meadowsweet flower extracts exhibited liver-protective effects against toxic hepatitis. Meadowsweet was found to stimulate a normalization of liver enzymes, liver antioxidant effects. It also proved to normalize lipid peroxidation (cholesterol production) within the liver (Shilova *et al.* 2008).

Meadowsweet inhibited MMP-1 fibroblasT-cells, which promotes elastin production (Lee *et al.* 2007).

It has been shown to be antimicrobial (Radulović *et al.* 2007).

Meadowsweet extract was observed as hematoprotective (protects against liver damage) and exhibited significant antioxidant activity, with high levels of safety (Shilova 2006; Ryzhikov and Ryzhikova 2006).

It was observed being cytotoxic to cancer cells in research sponsored by the Russian Academy of Sciences (Spiridonov *et al.* 2005).

Meadowsweet's phenolic extracts were found to have significant antioxidant and free radical scavenging potential (Sroka *et al.* 2005; Calliste *et al.* 2001).

Meadowsweet extract decreased inflammation, which included suppressing proinflammatory cytokines, decreasing IL-2 synthesis, and eliminating hypersensitivity in mice (Churin *et al.* 2008).

Meadowsweet's antioxidant capacity was one of the highest levels in one test of 92 different phenolic plant extracts (Heinonen 1999).

Meadowsweet showed significant inhibition of several bacteria (Rauha *et al.* 2000).

Meadowsweet extract also exhibited the ability to reduce blood clotting. During *in vivo* and *in vitro* research, meadowsweet was determined to have anticoagulant (reducing clotting) and fibrinolytic (reducing the formation of fibrin, which can scar tissues) (Liapina and Koval'chuk 1993).

Meadowsweet's anticoagulant and fibrinolytic properties were considered similar to heparin in another study (Kudriasho *et al.* 1990).

Contrasting with NSAIDs, meadowsweet was also found to be curative and preventative for acetylsalicylic acid-induced ulcers in rats (Barnaulov and Denisenko 1980).

Furthermore, meadowsweet has been found to inhibit the growth of *H. pylori*—the microorganism thought to cause or contribute to the majority of ulcer disorders (Cwikla *et al.* 2009).

As far as side effects go, in a clinical study of 48 human patients with cervical dysplasia (small tumors) treated with a meadowsweet ointment, 67% (32 cases) had a reduction in the tumors and 52% (25 cases) had complete regression of the tumor. Ten patients were completely cured within a year (Peresun'ko *et al.* 1993).

Grapple Plant: *Harpagophytum procumbens, Harpagophytum spp.*

Some Active Constituents of Harpagophytum

acetylacteoside	galactopyranosylharpagoside
acteoside	harpagide
aucubinine B	harpagoside
beatrine A	harprocumbide A
beatrine B	harprocumbide B
beta-sitosterol	iridoid glycosides
caffeic acid	isoacteoside
cannamic acid	other phenolic glycosides
chlorogenic acid	pagoside
cinnamic acid	p-coumaroylharpagide
cinnamoylmyoporoside	procumbide
coumaroylharpagide	pyridine monoterpene
coumaroylharpagide	alkaloid (PMTA)
coumaroyl-procumbide	stigmasterol
diacetylacteoside	triterpenes
feruloylharpagide	verbascoside

(Abdelouahab and Heard 2008; Qi *et al.* 2006; Clarkson *et al.* 2006; Boje *et al.* 2003: Munkombwe 2003; Baghdikian *et al.* 1999; Weiss 1988; Mabey 1988; Lininger *et al.* 1999)

Traditional Uses and Characteristics of Harpagophytum

Harpagophytum is a creeper with long tuberous roots and large red flowers. The fruit is a large woody spectacle with branching fingers that end in barbs. The claw-like appearance of the fruit is why German herbalists gave harpagophytum the name *Teufelskralle*—translating directly to "devil's claw." The dreadful barbs have been known to trap and injure passing animals. The roots may grow up to several feet long. It is native to Africa, and is rare in any other part of the world. This often makes the herb rather expensive and not readily obtainable. Indigenous peoples of South Africa have used the dried roots of harpagophytum in decoctions for a variety of ailments, particularly rheumatic conditions and gastrointestinal problems. G. H. Mehnert, a German farmer in South Africa, noticed these qualities and introduced the herb into the medical institutions of Europe.

In the 1950's, harpagophytum underwent clinical study and application among herbalists, physicians and commercial pharmacists in Germany and France. Soon two popular extracts were being produced by European companies. It is considered a bitter—with a bitter value of about 6,000—matching that of gentian root. Over time, European herbalists came to use grapple for rheumatoid arthritis, osteoarthritis, backache, gallbladder disorders, diabetes, gastrointestinal upset, lumbago, headaches, backaches, gout and menstruation pain. Several herbalists have noted its ability to clear the bloodstream, and it has also been known to clear up skin ulcers with external use. Others have noted its ability to strengthen the liver and gall bladder. Dr. Rudoph Weiss notes that European physicians began injecting harpagophytum into sites around arthritic joints with good success. The effect has been compared to an injection with cortisone. Interestingly—and quite opposite to the effects of NSAIDs—harpagophytum also has been used in the treatment of ulcers, heartburn and gastritis.

(Wood 1997; Weiss 1988; Lininger *et al.* 1999; Ellingwood 1983; Mabey 1988; Balch and Balch 2000; Hoffman 1990)

Some Research on Harpagophytum

Harpagophytum (devil's claw) showed both analgesic and anti-inflammatory properties in a study done in Marseille France (Baghdikian *et al.* 1997).

In an 8-week, open study of 259 rheumatic patients by researchers from the Queen Margaret University in Edinburgh (Warnock *et al.* 2007), patents taking harpagophytum had a significant reduction in joint and limb pain. Quality of life measurements also significantly increased among the harpagophytum patients, and 60% either reduced or stopped other pain medications.

In another study out of Germany (Wegener and Lupke 2003), 50 mg of harpagophytum was given to 75 osteoarthritis patients. After twelve weeks, total pain improved 24.5%. Subscales included 23% improvement for stiffness, 45% improvement for pain upon palpation, 35% improvement in mobility, and 25% improvement in joint cracking (using the WOMAC pain scale).

In a double-blind, randomized placebo-controlled study also from Germany (Göbel *et al.* 2001), 31 patients with muscle pain were given 480 mg of harpagophytum twice daily while 32 patients received a placebo. After four weeks of treatment, the harpagophytum group experienced a significant improvement and lessening of pain.

In an open study from Germany (Laudahn and Walper 2001), 480 mg of harpagophytum extract was given to 130 patients twice a day. After eight weeks, the effectiveness of harpagophytum was tested using the Multidimensional Pain Scale and Arhus Back Pain Index. Using data from 117 of the harpagophytum treatment group, the researchers observed "a significant improvement of pain symptoms and mobility."

In vitro and *ex vivo* trials out of Germany (Loew *et al.* 2001) illustrated that harpagophytum extracts significantly inhibited levels of leukotriene and thromboxane.

In studies from researchers at the University of Metz in France (Lanhers *et al.* 1992), harpagophytum illustrated significant anti-inflammatory and analgesic properties *in vivo*.

A double-blind, randomized study by French researchers (Chantre *et al.* 2000) treated 122 osteoarthritis patients with either diacerhein (a European pharmaceutical arthritis drug) or 435 mg of harpagophytum powder. After four months, both groups were examined for pain and functional disability using the Lequesne Functional Index. Both groups experienced significant pain reduction. There was no difference in the treatment effectiveness between the two groups. Furthermore, patients tolerated harpagophytum better, and harpagophytum treatments produced far less side effects. The harpagophytum treatment was also favored by the patients.

In another randomized, double-blind placebo clinical study (Chrubasik et al. 1999), harpagophytum extract or placebo was given to 197 back pain patients. After four weeks, the 183 patients who completed the study were examined. The number of pain-free patients were double the number of placebo pain-free patients for the half-dose (50mg of harpagoside standardized harpagophytum), and there were 3.3 times the number of pain-free patients among the 100mg harpagoside-standardized harpagophytum treatment group.

In a review of studies from 1966 to 2003 done by the Faculty of Medicine at the University of Ontario (Gagnier et al. 2007), it was found that among the ten studies reviewed, harpagophytum illustrated the ability to significantly reduce pain and provide what the researchers described as "rescue medication."

In a study from France's Saint-Jacques Hospital (Moussard et al. 1992), harpagophytum was given to 25 healthy human volunteers for 21 days. Blood levels of PGE2, thromboxane, PGF-1 and leukotriene were tested before and after the dosage. None of the levels changed significantly, as other studies have indicated takes place among typical COX-inhibiting NSAIDs. Therefore, the researchers concluded that harpagophytum does not have the familiar mechanisms for reducing inflammation observed for other arthritic herbs and drugs. Given the reduction of inflammation, osteoarthritis pain, muscular pain and low-back pain as shown in the prior studies, another mechanism must be taking place.

Another study on the mechanisms for harpagophytum (Huang et al. 2006) illustrated that haragoside blocked the movement of NF-kappaB, which would inhibit the COX-2 enzyme with nicric oxide, "thereby inhibiting downstream inflammation and subsequent pain events," the researchers explained. In the situation where there is no critical process of pain occurring, blocking the cascade at the NF-kappaB point would likely not occur. This again indicates a different mechanism for harpagophytum outside of direct COX inhibition.

Herbalist Richard Mabey (1988) commented that while harpogoside and beta sitosterol are known to have anti-inflammatory properties, the actions of harpagophytum are best with the whole plant—as they are with most medicinal herbs.

Myrrh/Guggulu *Commiphora mukul, Balsamodendron myrrha*

cumic aldehyde	limonene
di-pentene	meta-cresol
eugenol	myrrhol
gugglesterones	pinene

(Nadkarni 1908; Mehra 1969; Chopra *et al.* 1956; Agarwal *et al.* 1999; Frawley and Lad 1988; Tonkal and Morsy 2008; Shishodia *et al.* 2008; Lininger *et al.* 1999)

Traditional Uses and Characteristics of Myrrh

Myrrh is from the gum oleoresin taken from the *Commiphora mukul* tree. This tree grows abundantly in India and Asia. In fact, many trees of the genus *Commiphora*—more than 200 species—have been called myrrh and used to treat pain, skin afflictions, inflammatory disorders, diarrhea, and periodontal diseases The frankincense and myrrh trade, along with gold and other spices, was an important commerce between the east, middle east and Africa thousands of years ago. Ayurvedic physicians consider it the most important medicinal resin used. "Guggul" is actually a general term meaning tree resins, but the widespread use of *Commiphora* has taken over the term. Myrrh has been widely used in India and the Middle East for thousands of years for a variety of ailments, including arthritis, rheumatism, gout, gastrointestinal problems, lumbago, nervousness, urinary tract issues, bronchitis, diabetes, asthma, obesity, phthisis, hemorrhoids, skin diseases, ulcers, infected gums, sore throat, intestinal worms, boils, liver disorders, vitiligo, edema, menstrual dysfunction, paralytic seizures and other ailments. It is applied both externally and taken internally. It is calming, considered an all-around tonic for the body, and slightly laxative. More recently, it has been recognized as significantly reducing serum triglycerides and cholesterol. It is considered stimulant, aromatic, expectorant, emmenagogue (stimulates menstruation flow), astringent (externally), antiseptic, antiparasitic, antineoplastic (preventing neoplasms), anesthetic (produces anesthesia), and anticarcinogenic.

(Nadkarni 1908; Mehra 1969; Chopra *et al.* 1956; Agarwal *et al.* 1999; Frawley and Lad 1988; Lininger *et al.* 1999; Tonkal and Morsy 2008; Shishodia *et al.* 2008; Hoffman 1990).

Some Research on Myrrh

A number of studies over the years have confirmed myrrh's immune-stimulating, antimicrobial and antitumor effects (Tonkal and Morsy 2008).

Research done by Banarus Hindu University researchers (Devaraj 1985) showed guggul resin had significant anti-inflammatory and anti-arthritic effects.

In 2008, laboratory testing (Raut *et al.* 2008) confirmed that myrrh oleoresin was effective at breaking down microcrystals that build up in the joints, kidneys and gallbladder.

In another study (Sumantran *et al.* 2007), myrrh proved effective in inhibiting hyaluronidase and collagenase. These are two enzymes that are involved in the breakdown of the cartilage around the bone. The researchers thus characterized myrrh as *chondroprotective*.

Researchers from the University of Kansas (Ding and Staudinger 2005), determined that the plant sterol pregnane X receptor inhibits the expression of the gene cytochrome Cyp2b10. Cyp2b10 apparently plays a role in liver metabolism. This illustrates not only one mechanism of myrrh in terms of its ability to protect the liver. It also shows the capability of botanicals to modulate human gene expression—for the better.

In an outcome study by researchers from the Southern California University of Health Sciences (Singh *et al.* 2003), 30 volunteers with osteoarthritis were given 500 mg of myrrh oleoresin extract for two months. After one month and two months of treatment, each participant was assessed for pain, mood and mobility, including a 6-minute walk test. At both one month and two months after treatment, significant improvement in mobility and secondary pain was achieved, with no side effects.

In an *in vivo* study from Glasgow's University of Strathclyde (Duwiejua *et al.* 1993), myrrh significantly reduced joint swelling. The researchers concluded myrrh was an anti-inflammatory agent.

An extract of myrrh, or pharmaceuticals phenylbutazone, ibuprofen were given to inflammatory arthritic rabbits daily. All three equally reduced the thickness of the joint swelling similarly among the rabbits. This indicated that myrrh extract had the same anti-inflammatory capacity as these two anti-inflammatory pharmaceuticals (Sharma and Sharma 1977).

Juniper *Juniperus communis, J. drupacea, J. communis var. saxatilis, J. oxycedrus subsp. oxycedrus, and J. oxycedrus subsp. macrocarpa*

Some Active Constituents in Juniper

abietane	isoscutellarein-hexosides
alpha-fellandren	izoquercitrin
alpha-pinen	junionone
alphapinene	juniper camphor
alpha-terpineol	kaempferol
amentoflavone	karotinoids
beta-pinen	labdane
bitter principal	limonene
cadinene	linol
calcium	linolen
camphene	magnesium
cupressoflavone	menthol
d-germacrene	methyl-biflavones
ferruginol	myrcene
flavonoids (16)	olein
gossypetin-hexoside	organic acids
gossypetin-hexoside-pentoside	palmithin
	pimarane
hydroxyluteolin	polyphenols (60)
hynokiflavone	polysaccharides
iron	potassium

quercetin-hexoside	terpineol
rutin	thymol methyl ether
sabinene	tocoferols
selenium	totarol
stearin	xlorofils

(El-Ghorab *et al.* 2008; Miceli *et al.* 2009; Samoylenko *et al.* 2009; Georgian Medical News 2009; Innocenti *et al.* 2007; Schepetkin *et al.* 2005; Angioni *et al.* 2003; Hoffman 1990; Lininger *et al.* 1999; Foster and Hobbs 2002).

Traditional Uses and Characteristics of Juniper

Juniper is a round evergreen bush that grows to about ten feet tall. It has short, pointed leaves, small yellow flowers, and produces small green or blue-black berries (actually small cones). Juniper grows throughout Europe, Asia, and the United States—among both plains and alpine regions. Traditional uses have included a variety of inflammatory diseases and infectious diseases including chronic and rheumatic arthritis, edema, gout, bronchitis, colds, fungal infections, hemorrhoids, wounds, gynecological diseases and general inflammation. It is known to purify and balance blood chemistry. It stimulates appetite and digestion. American Indians used juniper for tuberculosis, fevers, colds, coughs, sore throats, liver and kidney infections, and intestinal disorders. Tinctures from its berries and branches have been used for skin irritations and alopecia (baldness). It has also been used to combat urinary tract infections. In the Middle Ages, herbalists used juniper to prevent the contraction of various contagious diseases. When treating a person during the Black Death epidemic, many herbalists would keep a few juniper berries in the mouth to stave off infection—forming an antiseptic barrier of sorts. North American Indians used juniper berries as a liniment and an infusion for colds, sore throats and tuberculosis. Juniper is considered to be expectorant (detoxifying), analgesic, diuretic, stomach tonic, carminative, rubefacient (irritant when rubbed on), and disinfectant (antimicrobial). Rudolf Weiss, M.D. pointed out that along with chronic arthritis and gout; juniper is indicated for "the large group of neuralgic-muscular rheumatic diseases, including tendopathies [tendon problems] and myogeloses [muscle disorders]." Michael Tierra, N.D. documents juniper's traditional uses for gout, rheumatism, arthritis and urinary infections. Culpeper wrote, "They [the berries] strengthen the brain, fortify the sight by strengthening the nerves, are good for agues, gout and sciatica, and strengthen the limbs." He also said that juniper was good for coughs, shortness of breath, consumption, pains in the belly, rupture, cramps, convulsions, hemorrhoids, worms, palsies and to increase appetite. The *American Materia Medica and Pharmacognosy* says that in addition to its renal and nephritic uses, juniper is a gastric stimulant and catarrhal detoxifier. Juniper is also part of the Ayurvedic *Indian Materia Medica*, as it is quite commonly found in the Himalayan mountains and valleys of India. In Ayurveda, juniper is suggested for urinary issues, digestive ailments, rheumatism, and as an antiseptic. Today herbalists frequently use juniper for cystitis, gout, and rheumatic joints. The German Commission E monograph recommends the dried fruit on a daily basis for rheumatic disorders.

(Weiss 1988, Miceli *et al.* 2009; Tierra 1980; Williard 1992; Schauenberg and Paris 1977; Potterton 1983; Ellingwood 1983; Mabey 1988; Foster and Hobbs 2002; Griffith 2000; Hobbs 1998; Nadkarni 1908; Lininger *et al.* 1999; Hoffman 1990)

Some Research on Juniper

In a study from the Karl-Franzens-University's School of Pharmacognosy, juniper extract inhibited LOX activity—the enzyme conversion process involved in the production of pro-inflammatory leucotrienes (Schneider *et al.* 2004).

Researchers from the University of Zagreb tested juniper essential oil against sixteen different bacterial species, seven different yeast-like fungi, three different yeast species, and four dermatophytes. Juniper illustrated antibacterial properties against both gram-positive and gram-negative bacteria; showed fungicidal activity; and significantly inhibited dermatophytes (Petlevski *et al.* 2008).

The berry extract showed significant antimicrobial ability against gram-positive bacteria. Studies show significant prostaglandin-2 inhibition, producing an anti-inflammatory effect and the blocking of pain (Akkol *et al.* 2009).

Juniper berries also stimulate hydrochloric acid production in the stomach (Williard 1992).

A study from Italy's University of Cagliari (Angioni *et al.* 2003) determined that juniper inhibited *Staphylococcus aureus*.

Tests have shown juniper's essential oils produce a number of different antifungal effects (Pepeljnjak *et al.* 2005).

Juniper's insecticidal properties have shown to be more productive than malathion in agricultural studies (Wedge *et al.* 2009).

Bioassay fraction tests illustrated that juniper berries have showed antiparasitic qualities, nematicidal properties, antibacterial and antifungal properties in a number of other studies (Samoylenko *et al.* 2009; Cavaleiro *et al.* 2006; Filipowicz *et al.* 2003).

Juniper extract exhibited significant antimicrobial effects upon *Candida albicans, Aspergillus niger,* and others (El-Ghorab *et al.* 2008).

In a study from Turkey's Gebze Institute of Technology (Karaman *et al.* 2003), juniper inhibited 57 different strains of bacteria, including those of *Xanthomonas, Staphylococcus, Enterobacter, Cinetobacter, Bacillus, Brevundimonas, Brucella, Escherichia, Micrococcus* and *Pseudomonas.* Eleven *Candida albicans* species were also shown to be inhibited by juniper.

Juniper was shown effective against tumor cells (Moujir *et al.* 2008). This chemoprotective quality seems to relate to the lignans.

In tests against a variety of viruses, juniper essential oils were found to inhibit replication of the SARS-CoV and HSV-1 (herpes simplex) viruses (Loizzo *et al.* 2008; Sassi *et al.* 2008).

Juniper leaves and berries also contain a significant amount of antioxidant potency and free radical scavenging abilities. (Al-Mustafa 2008; Lim *et al.* 2002).

Juniper's safety has been established in a number of reports (Petlevski *et al.* 2008; Wang *et al.* 2002; Schilcher and Leuschner 1997).

Juniper extract also appears to increase the level of phosphorylation in adipose tissue with increased AMP-activated protein kinase—in mice studies this reduced obesity and increased the efficiency of insulin and leptin (Kim *et al.* 2008).

The polysaccharides in juniper stimulated macrophage and mononuclear phagocyte activity in a study by researchers from the Montana State University (Schepetkin *et al.* 2005).

Some of the terpenoids in juniper displayed anti-malarial effects (Okasaka *et al.* 2006).

Researchers from the University of California's Department of Pediatric Nephrology in Davis (Butani *et al.* 2003) found that juniper oil given to rats increased prostaglandin F excretion, associated with lowering inflammation and speeding up insulin clearance. Both are associated with lower inflammation and increased immune system efficiency.

Juniper's essential oils were found to inhibit bone resorption—the primary mechanism in osteoporosis (Mühlbauer *et al.* 2003).

Juniper proved to be toxic to cells infected with HIV-1 and HIV-3 at 50% concentration (Salido *et al.* 2002).

Juniper also showed antimicrobial activity against *Fusobacterium necrophorum*, *Clostridium perfringens*, *Actinomyces bovis* and *Candida albicans* in research performed at Oregon State University (Johnston *et al.* 2001).

Juniper's diterpenes and sesquiterpene showed activity against *Mycobacterium tuberculosis* (Topcu *et al.* 1999).

In an *in vivo* study, juniper oil resulted in higher levels of TNF (stimulated immune system) and lower levels of PGE2 and cytokines IL-6 and IL-10 (reduced inflammation) compared to controls (Chavali *et al.* 1998).

In another study, juniper oil reduced liver damage and increased liver microcirculation and bile flow, illustrating that juniper was liver-protective (Jones *et al.* 1998).

Goldenrod: *Solidago virgaurea, Solidago altissima, Solidago canadensis*

Some Constituents in Goldenrod

alpha-tocopherol-quinone
beta-amyrin acetate
beta-dictyopterol
cadinene
caffeic acid
caffeoylquinic acids
ent-germacra
erythrodiol-3-acetate

glucopyranosyl-
   butyrrophenone
kaempferol
kaempferol-3-O-
   rutinoside
limonene
methyl caffeoyl

neochlorogenic acid
oleanolic acid
pumiloxide
quercetin
quercetrin
quinate
rutin
saponins

sesquiterpenes
solicanolide
tannins
trans-phytol
trans-phytol labdane
trien-1alpha-ol
trien-1beta-ol

(Bradette-Hébert *et al.* 2008; Choi 2004; Vila *et al.* 2002; Sung *et al.* 1999; Bader *et al.* 1996; Bongartz and Hesse 1995; Hoffman 1990)

Traditional Uses and Characteristics of Goldenrod

Belonging to the daisy family, goldenrod is a perennial bushy plant indigenous to North America and many other places in the world. It has beautiful summer yellow panicle-oriented flowers that grow at the tops of stiff stems that stand upright. It grows in meadows, woods and moorlands. Its Latin name is derived from "solido" which means to make whole or strengthen. The leaves and flowers have been used for medicinal purposes. Goldenrod has been used for many centuries in the treatment of the kidneys; for inflammation; and for urinary tract infections. It was used by early Americans and North American Indians for rheumatism, colds, headaches, sore throats, and neuralgia (pain). American Indians also used a mouthwash of goldenrod for toothaches. The flowers were chewed for sore throats. Herbalist David Hoffman documented goldenrod's anti-inflammatory effects and wound-healing abilities. It has also been used traditionally for arthritis, gout, prostatitis, rheumatism, flatulence and eczema. Goldenrod has been observed increasing glomerular filtration and decreasing albumin levels. It has been used for issues of nephritis, unuria and oliguria. Goldenrod's medicinal properties are considered anti-inflammatory, antimicrobial, diaphoretic, antidiarrhoeic, carminative, stimulant, diuretic (increases urine output), analgesic, antiseptic, antispasmodic (reduces spasms), antioxidant, antifungal and antiedematous (reduces swelling). The flowers are typically used for medicinal purposes.

(Melzig 2004; Gundermann and Müller 2007; Wood 1997; Weiss 1988, Miceli *et al.* 2009; Tierra 1980; Williard 1992; Schauenberg and

Paris 1977; Potterton 1983; Ellingwood 1983; Mabey 1988; Foster and Hobbs 2002; Griffith 2000; Hoffman 1990).

Some Research on Goldenrod

A German review of multiple clinical studies indicated that significant anti-inflammatory and pain-relieving effects were accomplished when dosages of goldenrod were comparable to NSAID use—with a fraction of the adverse effects of NSAIDs (Klein-Galczinsky 1999).

Goldenrod illustrated significant anti-inflammatory activity, reducing swelling and pain among rats with various degrees of rheumatoid arthritis (el-Ghazaly *et al.* 1992).

Goldenrod proved to have significant antifungal properties when tested against twenty-three different yeast species. (Webster *et al.* 2007).

Goldenrod was also found to boost immune response and promote cytotoxicity to tumor cells (Wu *et al.* 2008, Plohmann *et al.* 1997).

In several open, randomized, placebo-controlled and double-blind clinical studies, goldenrod significantly reduced pain and inflammation in rheumatic diseases (Gundermann and Müller 2007).

Goldenrod proved spasmolytic (reduced spasms), antihypertensive and diuretic in other investigations (von Kruedener *et al.* 1995).

Goldenrod showed antifungal properties against five different strains of fungi (Vila *et al.* 2002).

Goldenrod proved to be a potent free radical scavenger in a study from Canada's McGill University (McCune and Johns, 2002).

A 60% ethanol extract of goldenrod showed anti-inflammatory activity similar to diclofenac (a well-known NSAID also marketed as Voltaren®).

Goldenrod extracts have been used with clinical success in urinary infections and stones, but use is contraindicated for persons with renal failure (Yarnell 2002).

Goldenrod stimulated glutathione activity in rats (Apáti *et al.* 2006).

The essential oil from goldenrod produced antimicrobial activity against a number of bacteria and yeasts (Morel *et al.* 2006).

Dandelion *Taraxum officinale, Taraxum mongolicum, Taraxum spp.*

Some Constituents in Dandelion

aesculetin
aesculin
arabinopyranosides
arnidiol
artemetin
B vitamins
benzyl glucoside
beta amyrin
beta-carboline
  alkaloids
beta-sitosterol
bitter principle
boron
caffeic acid
caffeic acid ethyl
  esters
calcium
chicoric acid
chlorogenic acid
chlorophylls
choline
cichoriin
coumaric acid
coumarin
deacetylmatricarin
diglucopyranoside
dihydroconiferin
dihydrosyringin
dihydroxylbenzoic
  acid
esculetin
eudesmanolides
faradiol
four steroids

furulic acid
gallic acid
gallicin
genkwanin-lutinoside
germacranolide acids
glucopyranosides
glucopyranosyl-
arabinopyranoside
glucopyranosyl-
glucopyranoside
glucopyranosyl-
xyloypyranoside
guaianolide
hesperetin
hesperidin
indole alkaloids
inulin
ionone
iron
isodonsesquitin A
isoetin
isoetin-glucopyranosyl
lactupicrine
lupenol acetate
lutein
luteolin
luteolin-7-O-
  gluccoside
magnesium
mannans
mongolicumin A
mongolicumin B
monocaffeyltartaric
  acid

monoterpenoid
myristic acid
pyridine derivative
palmitic acid
pectin
phi-taraxasteryl acetate
phosphorus
p-hydroxybenzoic acid
p-hydroxyphenylacetic
    acid
polyphenoloxidase
polysaccharides
potassium
quercetins
rufescidride
scopoletin
sesquiterpene
sesquiterpene ketolac-
    tone
sesquiterpene lactones
seventeen antioxidants
several caffeoylquinic
    acids
several luteolins
silicon
sodium
sonchuside A

steroid complexes
stigmasterol
syringic acid
syringin
tannins
taraxacin
taraxacoside
taraxafolide
taraxafolin-B
taraxasterol
taraxasteryl acetate
taraxerol
taraxinic acid beta-
    glucopyranosyl
taraxinic acid
    derivatives
taraxol
thirteen benzenoids
trime-thyl ether
triterpenoids
violaxanthin
vit. A (7000 IU/oz)
vitamin C
vitamin D
vitamin K
xyloypyranosides
zinc

(Williams *et al.* 1996; Hu and Kitts 2003; Hu and Kitts 2004; Seo *et al.* 2005; Trojanova *et al.* 2004; Leu *et al.* 2005; Kisiel and Michalska 2005; Leu *et al.* 2003; Michalska and Kisiel 2003; Kisiel and Barszcz 2000; Hoffman 1990; Lininger *et al.* 1999)

Traditional Uses and Characteristics of Dandelion

Taraxum is derived from the Greek words "taraxos" for "disorder" and "akos" meaning remedy. Dandelion is a common weed with a characteristic beautiful yellow flower that assumes a globe of seeds to spread its humble yet incredible medicinal virtues. Its hollowed stem is full of milky juice, with a long, hardy root and leaves that taste good in a spring salad. Dandelion is one of the most well known traditional herbs for all sorts of ailments that involve toxicity within the blood, liver, kidneys, lymphatic system and urinary tract. Dandelion has been listed in a variety of formularies and codeces around the world since the tenth century. Its use was expounded by many cultures from the Greeks to the Northern American Indians, who used it for stomach ailments and infection. It is also used for the treatment of viral and bacterial infections as well as cancer. The latex or milky sap that comes from the stem has a mixture of polysaccharides, proteins, lipids, rubber and metabolites such as polyphenoloxidase. The latex has been used to heal skin wounds and protect wounds from infection—also its function when the plant is injured.

Dandelion is known to protect and help rebuild the liver. Culpeper documented that it "has an opening and cleansing quality and, therefore, very effectual for removing obstructions of the liver, gall bladder and spleen and diseases arising from them, such as jaundice." It is known to stimulate the elimination of toxins and clear obstructions from the blood and liver. This is thought to be the reason why dandelion helps clear stones and gravel from kidneys, gallbladder and bladder. It has also been used to treat stomach problems, and is thought to reduce blood pressure. In ancient Chinese medicine, it has been recommended for issues related to "liver attacking spleen-pancreas"—describing the imbalance between liver enzymes and pancreatic enzymes. It has been used in traditional treatments for hypoglycemia, hypertension, urinary tract infection, skin eruptions and breast cancer. It has also been used traditionally for appetite loss, flatulence, dyspepsia, constipation, gallstones, circulation problems, skin issues, spleen and liver complaints, hepatitis and anorexia.

Dr. Michael Tierra notes that, "even the most serious cases of hepatitis have rapidly been cured, sometimes within a week with dandelion root tea taken in cupful doses four to six times daily..." In Chinese medicine, dandelion is known to clear heat, more specifically in the liver, kidney and skin. These effects are consistent with dandelion's traditional uses for rheumatism, gout, eczema, cardiac edema, dropsy and hypertension. Dandelion is also said to increase the flow of bile. Dandelion root has also been used to heal bone infections. Dandelion has been used to increase urine excretion, and reduce pain and inflammation. Yet it also contains an abundance of potassium—which balances its diuretic effect (as potassium is lost during heavy urination). It has been documented as a blood and digestive tonic, laxative, stomachic, alterative, cholagogue, diuretic, choleretic, anti-inflammatory, antioxidant, anti-carcinogenic, analgesic, anti-hyperglycemic, anti-coagulatory and prebiotic.

(Shi *et al.* 2008; Schutz *et al.* 2006; Melzig 2004; Gundermann and Müller 2007; Wood 1997; Weiss 1988, Miceli *et al.* 2009; Tierra 1980; Williard 1992; Schauenberg and Paris 1977; Potterton 1983; Ellingwood 1983; Rodriguez-Fragoso *et al.* 2008; Mabey 1988; Foster and Hobbs 2002; Griffith 2000).

Some Research on Dandelion

Among 222 different medicinal extracts, dandelion was one of ten that regulated and inhibited the differentiation of osteocytes to osteoclasts—associated with the resorption process that results in bone loss and bone remodeling (bone spurs and growths) (Youn *et al.* 2008).

A study by researchers at the University of British Columbia in Canada (Hu and Kitts 2004) found that dandelion extract suppressed prostaglandin E2 (PGE2) without causing cell death. Further tests indicated that COX-2 was inhibited by the luteolin and luteolin-glucosides in dandelion.

In another study from Canada (Hu and Kitts 2005), nitric oxide was inhibited. Reactive oxygen species—free radicals—were also significantly inhibited by dandelion—attributed to the plant's phenolic acid content. This in turn prevented lipid oxidation—one of the mechanisms in heightened LDL (bad cholesterol) levels and artery inflammation.

Tests against several types of tumor cell lines resulted in inhibition of cancer cells (Sigstedt 2008).

In a 2007 study from researchers at the College of Pharmacy at the Sookmyung Women's University in Korea (Jeon *et al.* 2008), dandelion was found to reduce inflammation, leukocytes, vascular permeability, abdominal cramping, pain and COX levels among exudates and *in vivo*.

Dandelion was found to stimulate fourteen different strains of bifidobacteria—important components of the immune system that inhibit pathogenic bacteria (Trojanova *et al.* 2004).

Another study found that dandelion extract significantly prevented cell death in Hep G2 (liver) cells, while stimulating TNF and IL-1 levels—illustrating its ability to arrest or slow liver disease and stimulate healing (Koo *et al.* 2004).

Other studies have illustrated that dandelion inhibits both interleukin IL-6 and TNF-alpha—both inflammatory cytokines (Seo *et al.* 2005).

Dandelion was shown to stimulate the liver's production of glutathione (GST)—an important antioxidant (Petlevski *et al.* 2003).

Another study by University of British Columbia researchers showed that dandelion extract was capable of reducing copper radicals—showing its ability to reduce heavy metals in the body (Hu and Kitts 2003).

Dandelion increased the liver's production of superoxide dismutase and catalase, increasing the liver's ability to purify the blood of toxins (Cho *et al.* 2001).

UDP-glucuronosyl transferase, another important detoxifying liver enzyme, was increased 244% from controls *in vivo* by dandelion extract (Maliakal and Wanwimolruk 2001).

Leukotriene production was decreased with an extract of dandelion (Kashiwada *et al.* 2001).

The lupeol trierpenes in dandelion illustrated antitumor effects in mice (Hata *et al.* 2000).

Dandelion illustrated the ability to inhibit IL-1 and inflammation in Kim *et al.* (2000) and Takasaki *et al.* (1999).

In a study of 96 chronic hepatitis B cases at the Beijing TCM Hospital (Chen 1990), 46 controls were compared to 51 patients given a mix of herbs that included a dandelion species. After five months of use, the medicinal herb group had a total effective rate of 74.5% compared to 24.4% in the control group.

In another study at the Jiangxi Medical College (Zheng 1990), 472 traditional medicinal herbs were screened against the type 1 herpes simplex virus. After repeated screens, ten "highly effective herbs" included dandelion.

In a study of 24 patients with chronic colitis, pains in the large intestine vanished in 96% of the patients by the 15th day after being given a blend of herbs including dandelion (Chakŭrski *et al.* 1981).

Nettle *Uritca urens*

Some Active Constituents in Nettle:

beta-sitosterol	kaempferol
carotene	polysaccharides
formic acid	quercetin
glucoquinine,	rutin
histamine	vitamin C
iron	

(Newall *et al.* 1996; Schottner *et al.* 1997; Konrad *et al.* 2000; Hoffman 1990; Lininger *et al.* 1999)

Characteristics and Traditional Uses for Nettle

Nettle is a low creeper found among open fields and disturbed ground. Its leaves have tiny hairs that produce an acid, which can 'sting' the skin on contact. Only the fresh plant will sting, however. This acid breaks down when cooked, so the plant may be eaten steamed or boiled. The taste is not unlike steamed or boiled spinach greens. The famous herbalist Dioscorides discussed using nettle for pneumonia, pleurisy and a number of other disorders. Nettle's use for cleansing the blood, kidneys and the urinary tract is famous. The famed nineteenth century English herbalist and physician James Compton Burnett recorded that nettles removed gouty deposits and uric acid wastes from the body. The fresh juice of nettles or a tincture was often used. He wrote in *Gout and Its Cure* (1895): "[when] under the influence of Urtica urens [they] passed grit and gravel pretty freely for the first time in their lives, I came to the conclusion that Urtica possesses the power to remove urates..." He also wrote later, "I then proceeded to employ Urtica urens in the classic attacks of genuine gout, and that [met] with very great satisfaction indeed.

Within a few hours after beginning its use the urine becomes fairly free, of a high colour, and the bottom of the vessel is often found more or less covered with urates in the form of grit and gravel, and simultaneously herewith the gouty attack begins to subside."

Applying fresh stinging nettles to the skin above arthritic pain has been anecdotal for centuries. In 1994, C.F. Randall, M.D., a physician from Cornwall, England, reported in the prestigious *British Journal of General Practice* of an 81 year old male patient whose x-rays showed osteoarthritis of the hip. His prognosis was not good, and it prevented him from riding his bike or walking up hills. Dr. Randall prescribed ibuprofen. Two months later the patient returned to inform Dr. Randall that the ibuprofen had not helped, but for several weeks, the man had been applying stinging nettle leaves onto the skin above his left hip. The man said that after a few weeks, the pain had gone away and he only had to apply the leaves to the skin every few days. The patient reported that he was walking just fine, and riding his bike 10 miles every day without pain. Dr. Randall visited with an elderly woman sometime after, and the woman told of her swollen, red and inflamed finger joints being relieved by the application of fresh nettles as well. This jounal report was followed up by Dr. Adrian White, Chairman of the Centre for Complementary Health Studies/Postgraduate Medical School from the University of Exeter. Dr. White documented research and clinical experience with the treatment of osteoarthritis with botanical liniments and rubefacient ointments that redden and irritate the skin.

Dr. White explained that the active ingredient causing this irritation—formic acid—has stimulated pain relief for arthritis and other inflammatory conditions for centuries when the fresh leaves were applied externally. He described how Galen and Hippocrates applied counter-irritation techniques with topical applications of nettle. Dr. White also explained and provided references for the efficacy of the ancient Chinese treatment of moxibustion—the burning of a botanical herb next to the skin to produce irritation and erythema (pinkness in the skin)

(Hoffman 1990; Lininger *et al.* 1999; Fisher and Hobbs 2002; White 1995; Wood 1997; Randall 1994).

Boswellia/Frankincense: *Boswellia serratta, Boswellia thurifera, Boswellia spp.*

Some Constituents in Boswellia:

boswellic acids
keto-beta-boswellic acid
acetyl-keto-beta-boswellic
  acid
acteyl-beta-boswellic acid
acetyl-11-keto-beta-
  boswellic acid

alpha-boswellic acids
cembrane-type diterpenes
e-beta-ocimene
e-caryophyllene
incensole acetate
limonene
lupeolic acids

(Banno *et al.* 2006; Takada *et al.* 2006; Krüger *et al.* 2009; Al-Harrasi and Al-Saidi *et al.* 2008; Moussaieff *et al.* 2008; Lininger *et al.* 1999)

Traditional Uses and Characteristics of Boswellia

The genus of *Boswellia* makes up a group of trees that grow in Africa and Asia, known for their fragrant sap resin. Frankincense was used in ancient Egypt, India, Arabia and Mesopotamia thousands of years ago as an elixir that relaxed and healed the body's aches and pains. The gum from the resin was applied as an ointment for rheumatic and nervous ailments, urinary tract disorders, to help grow hair, and on the chest for bronchitis and general breathing problems. It is considered in Ayurveda to be bitter, astringent, and pungent. Orally, boswellia has been used for a wide variety of ailments, including bronchitis, asthma, arthritis, rheumatism, anemia, liver sluggishness and a variety of infections. Its properties include being a stimulant, diaphoretic, anti-rheumatic, tonic, analgesic, antiseptic, diuretic, demulcent, astringent, expectorant, and antispasmodic.
(Nadkarni 1908; Mehra 1969; Chopra *et al.* 1956; Agarwal *et al.* 1999; Frawley and Lad 1988; Newmark and Schulick 2000)

Some Research on Boswellia

Boswellia has undergone extensive study over the past few decades. Most of these studies have focused upon boswellia's ability to reduce inflammation and pain. A meta-study from the UK's Peninsula Medical School and the Universities of Exeter and Plymouth published in the *British Medical Journal* (Ernst 2008) reviewed 47 clinical studies on boswellia. Seven met their control criteria, including rheumatoid arthritis research. The researchers concluded that, "B. serrata extracts were clinically effective."

In one double-blind, randomized and placebo-controlled study (Sengupta *et al.* 2008), 75 osteoarthritis patients were given either 100 mg of boswellia extract, 250 mg of boswellia extract, or a placebo for 90 days. Of the 70 patients that completed the study, patients who took either dose of boswellia had significantly lower pain scores and mobility throughout the trial. Furthermore, levels of metalloproteinase-3—the enzyme matrix thought to be present during the cartilage breakdown process—were significantly lower in the boswellia treatment group.

In two other studies, boswellic acids extracted from boswellia were found to have significant anti-inflammatory action. The trials revealed that boswellia inhibited the LOX enzyme (5-lipoxygenase) and thus reduced leukotriene production (Singh *et al.* 2008; Ammon 2006).

Another study (Takada *et al.* 2006) showed that boswellic acids inhibited cytokines and suppressed cell invasion through NF-kappaB inhibition. This enhances the immune system's ability to stop cell mutation and suppress osteoclast (deranged bone cells) production.

In an *in vivo* study by researchers from the University of Maryland's School of Medicine (Fan *et al.* 2005), boswellia extract illustrated "significant anti-arthritic and anti-inflammation effects." The report also concluded that, "these effects may be mediated via the suppression of pro-inflammatory cytokines."

In an *in vitro* study also from the University of Maryland's School of Medicine (Chevrier *et al.* 2005), boswellia extract proved to inhibit Th1 cytokines while potentiating Th2 cytokines. This illustrated boswellia's ability to modulate the immune system in the face of inflammation.

In a study of 29 dogs with degenerative osteoarthritis, boswellia extract significantly reduced osteoarthritis severity and significantly increased mobility in 71% of the 24 dogs that completed the study (Reichling *et al.* 2004).

In a randomized, placebo-controlled, double-blind study from India's Indira Medical College (Kimmatkar *et al.* 2004), 30 patients with osteoarthritis of the knee were given either boswellia extract or a placebo. The boswellia-treated patients had significantly less swelling of the knee, decreased knee pain, increased knee flexion and increased walking distance at the end of the study.

Boswellia extracts also illustrate significant inhibition against microorganisms. In one study (Schillaci *et al.* 2008), *Staphylococcus epidermidis, Staphylococcus aureus,* and *Candida albicans* were effectively inhibited by boswellia extracts.

A Few Honorable Mentions

There are other botanical herbs that have been shown in research to have anti-inflammatory effects. These also have multiple actions, including the modulation of COX and/or LOX enzymes through various means and immune system stimulation.

Lei Gong Teng (*Tripterygium wilfordii Hook F* (or TwHF): This is a Chinese herb that has been used traditionally to treat inflammatory conditions, including rheumatoid arthritis. A recent multicenter study (Goldbach-Mansky *et al.* 2009) of 121 rheumatoid arthritis patients illustrated that this herb reduced swelling and inflammation significantly greater than sulfasalazine. However, this study had some limitations, requiring further confirmation.

Feverfew (*Tanacetum parthenium*): Research from Louisiana State University and the UK's University of Reading has confirmed COX-2 inhibition through constituents parthenolide and melatonin.

Bakial Scullcap (*Scutellaria baicalensis*): Research from Barcelona University confirmed COX-2 inhibition.

Hops (*Humulus lupulus*): The University of Tokushima's School of Medicine has confirmed that the constituent humulone significantly inhibits the COX-2 enzyme.

Selected Herbal Formulations

Most herbalists combine botanicals into a formulation to take advantage of their multiple and synergistic effects. Because there are so many botanicals that have properties of purifying the blood and detoxifying the liver, kidneys and urinary tract, there are also a number of different traditional herbal formulations for arthritis that have been met with success. For many traditional herbalists, their formulations were dependent upon the types of plants that grew around them at the time. Today, of course, we can ship in seeds and herbs grown from around the world—allowing herbalists to formulate based upon the research. Illustrating this, here is a quick survey of a few botanical combinations recommended by traditional herbalists of yesterday and today.

Traditional Joint Remedy
By Jethro Kloss:
Infusion of whole herbs (tea):
Black cohosh (*Cimicifuga racemosa*)
Gentian root (*Gentianaceae spp.*)
Angelica (*Apiaceae spp.*)
Columbo (*Frasera caroliniensis*)
Skullcap (*Scutellaria lateriflora*)
Valerian (*Valeriana officinalis*)
Rue (*Ruta angustfolia*)
Buckthorn bark (*Rhamnus spp.*)

Comment

This formula used local herbs from the wilderness around Dr. Kloss' family farm in Minnesota during the early-mid 1900s. Herb selection was likely developed using information passed down from fellow herbalists, combined with clinical success at Dr. Kloss' famous treatment center.

Arthritis Remedy
By Michael Tierra:
<u>Infusion of whole herbs:</u>
Oregon grape root (*Mahonia aquifolium/M. repens*) (6 parts)
Parsley root (*Petroselinum sativum*) (6 parts)
Sassafras (*Sassafras offinale*) (3 parts)
Prickly ash bark (*Zanthoxylum americanum*) (3 parts)
Black cohosh (*Cimicifuga racemosa*) (3 parts)
Guaiacum (*Guiacum officinale*) (3 parts)
Ginger root (*Zingiber officinale*) (2 parts)

Comment
This formula was chosen among herbs prevalent or available in the western United States three decades ago. Dr. Tierra is an herbalist with naturopathic and acupuncturist training who also mentored under native American healers.

Classic Ayurveda Anti-Inflammatory Formula
<u>Whole herb extracts (capsules):</u>
Ashwaghanda (*Withania somnifera*)
Boswellia (*Boswellia serrata*)
Ginger (*Zingiber officinale*)
Turmeric (*Curcuma longa*)

Clinical Study
In a 32-week randomized, double-blind and placebo-controlled study from the Center for Rheumatic Diseases at the Bharati Hospital Medical College (Chopra *et al.* 2004), a placebo or a formula consisting of ashwaghanda, boswellia, ginger and turmeric was given to 358 patients with osteoarthritis of the knees. After 16 and 32 weeks, the patients were examined, and at both points the botanical-formula group demonstrated significant pain reduction and clinical improvement over the placebo.

In a randomized, double-blind, placebo-controlled study (Kalkarni *et al.* 1991) of 42 osteoarthritis sufferers, patients took either a placebo or a formula containing ashwaghanda, boswellia, turmeric and zinc. After a one-month washout period and a three-month trial period, patients who took the botanical formula had a significant reduction in pain and stiffness compared to the placebo group. Joint mobility, grip strength and disability index levels were significantly higher in the botanical group as well.

Modern Botanical Arthritis Formula
By Mark Lubin
Whole herb extracts (capsules):
Juniper (*Juniperus communis*)
Goldenrod (*Solidago virgaurea*)
Dandelion (*Taraxum officinale*)
Meadowsweet (*Filipendula ulmaria*)
Willow Bark (*Salix alba*)
Whole Grape (*Vitis vinifera*)

Clinical Study:
In a randomized, double-blind and placebo-controlled study (Mongomery and Duncan, 2006), 75 arthritis patients were given either placebo or this formulation of juniper, goldenrod, dandelion, meadowsweet, willow and whole grape extract for 30 days. No rescue medications (other pain medications) were taken during the study. Patients were interviewed at the start and end of the treatment with regular monitoring in between. Both groups began with extreme pain—rated at levels 9 to 10 using the Comparative Pain Scale (10 is "unbearable"). The placebo group experienced no change in pain during the treatment period. In the botanical treatment group, by the fourth day only 53% had pain in the 9-10 range. On the seventh day of treatment, only 6% still had pain in the 9-10 range, and 10% were reporting no pain at all. During the second week, no patients reported pain in the 9-10 range among the botanical formula treatment group. By the tenth day of treatment, 86% of the patients were reporting no pain at all. After day 14, an astounding 100% of the botanical treatment group was reporting *no pain at all.*

Foods and Spices for Arthritis

There are a number of foods and spices that research has shown will reduce inflammation and pain symptomized by arthritis, and possibly even turn around the cartilage and synovial membrane damage associated with arthritis. Like the botanical herbs, these foods have a multitude of constituents that all play a role in curbing pain and inflammation. In fact, the line between some foods and herbs can become quite blurry. In order to have a complete balance of constituents, it is recommended that botanicals in general be consumed in their whole form, with a minimum of heating. For some herbs, this is neither possible nor palatable. For those botanicals that can be eaten or used as spices, it is therefore recommended to consume them in whole form.

Ginger (*Zingiber officinalis*)

Ginger is one of the most versatile food/spice/herb known to humanity. In Ayurveda—the oldest medicine still in use—ginger is the most recommended medicine among any other. As such, ginger has been referred to as *vishwabhesaj*—meaning "universal medicine" by Ayurvedic physicians. As mentioned earlier, an accumulation of studies and chemical analyses in 2000 determined that ginger has at least 477 active constituents. As in all botanicals, each constituent will stimulate a slightly different mechanism—often moderating the mechanisms of other constituents. This tremendous number—477 active constituents—illustrates the beauty of botanical medicine. Furthermore, a number of these constituents—and perhaps a combination of them—cause an inhibition of the COX and LOX enzymes, reducing inflammation and pain. Ginger also stimulates circulation, inhibits various infections, and strengthens the liver.

Traditionally, Ginger has been considered as a treatment for rheumatoid arthritis, respiratory ailments, fevers, nausea, colds, flu, hepatitis, liver disease, headaches and all sorts of gastrointestinal and digestive ailments to name a few. Herbalists classify ginger as analgesic, tonic, expectorant, carminative, antiemetic, stimulant, anti-inflammatory, and antimicrobial.

(Frawley and Lad 1986; Hobbs 1988; Newmark and Schulick 2000; Lininger *et al.* 1999; Hoffman 1990).

A Few of the Thousands of Studies on Ginger

In a six-week randomized, double-blind and placebo-controlled study by researchers from the Miami Veterans Affairs Medical Center and the University of Miami (Altman and Marcussen 2001), 261 osteoarthritis patients were either given ginger extract or a placebo for six weeks. After the study, 63% of the ginger group experienced a reduction in knee pain. The patients were also examined for standing knee pain and pain after walking. In the ginger group, pain after walking improved 173% more than the control group. The ginger group had significantly more reduced pain in each parameter, including the Western Ontario and McMaster Universities Arthritis Composite Pain Index. It should be noted also that 59 patients of the ginger group and 21 patients of the control group experienced mild gastrointestinal upset.

As for this mild stomach upset (not ulcers or bleeding), the logical rationale for this is the use of the ginger extract rather than fresh ginger. In fact, ginger is actually clinically proven as a treatment for nausea, stomachache, ulcers and many other gastrointestinal problems. With at least 477 constituents, whole ginger has the ability to provide these effects along with the inflammation-reduction effects. Through extraction, many constituents are often lost. Some are sensitive to heat and light. Others are sensitive to ethanol or methanol extraction methods. Therefore, during the pulverization, dehydration and extraction process to make ginger extract, there is a great likelihood that some balancing constituents will not remain in the extract. This is the major reason we put ginger into our food category rather than the herb category.

In other words, it is suggested that ginger be consumed only in its raw form. Fresh ginger root can be purchased at practically any grocery or health food store. It then can be washed like any other fresh food, and then grated onto a salad or other dish. If it is put onto a cooked dish, it is recommended that it be put in after the cooking. Just grate onto the food just before serving. Ginger root can also be bitten into and chewed raw, and it can also make a nice tea—not steeped too long of course. It would seem this inexpensive food-medicine would be a *must* addition to meals for any chronic arthritis sufferer.

A randomized, double-blind and placebo-controlled study by researchers from the Tel Aviv University and Medical Center (Wigler *et al.* 2003) gave 29 arthritis patients ginger extract or a placebo. After six months of treatment, the ginger group "showed a significant superiority over the placebo group."

Cayenne *Capiscium frutescens* or *Capiscium annum*

This red pepper contains the alkaloid capsacin—known to reduce the amount of substance P in nerves, thereby reducing pain transmission. Cayenne also has other healing effects, which help to mitigate arthritis symptoms as well. Capiscium contains capsaicinoids; various carotenoids such as zeaxanthin, beta-cryptoxanthin, and beta-carotene; steroid glycosides, vitamins A & C and volatile oils; and at least twenty-three flavonoids including quercetin, luteolin and chysoeriol. These constituents work together to provide a number of joint benefits. Cayenne is known to increase circulation; increase detoxification; stimulate appetite; increase liver and heart function; stimulate the immune system and increase metabolic function. It is also a recognized antibacterial and antiviral agent. Some consider cayenne's antiseptic abilities at the level of an antibiotic. Its actions have been described as carminative, alterative, hemostatic, anthelmintic, stimulant, expectorant, antiseptic and diaphoric.

Cayenne is also useful as a topical cream. In a review by the Faculty of Medicine at the University of Ontario (Gagnier *et al.* 2007) of studies from 1966 to 2003, it was concluded that when applied as a topical treatment, cayenne consistently reduced low-back pain more than placebo. For this reason, capiscium is now an active ingredient in a number of over the counter topical creams for arthritis and other aches.

Turmeric *Curcuma longa*

Turmeric can also either be considered a medicinal herb or a food-spice. It is a root (or rhizome) and a relative of ginger in the *Zingiberaceae* family. Just as we might expect from a botanical, turmeric has a large number of active constituents. The most well known of those are the curcuminoids, which include curcumin (diferuloylmethane), demethoxycurcumin, and bisdemethoxycurcumin). Others include volatile oils such as tumerone, atlantone, and zingiberone, polysaccharides, proteins, and a number of resins. We describe turmeric as a food because it is often recommended by Ayurvedic physicians and naturopaths to be included into the daily diet as a food rather than an herb. For this reason, Indian curried dishes are eaten nearly daily by indigenous Indians. Indeed, the whole herb or encapsulated turmeric powder is preferred over curcumin extracts.

As stated in a recent review from the Cytokine Research Laboratory at the University of Texas (Anand 2008), studies have linked turmeric with "suppression of inflammation; angiogenesis; tumor genesis; diabetes; diseases of the cardiovascular, pulmonary, and neurological systems, of skin, and of liver; loss of bone and muscle; depression; chronic fatigue; and neuropathic pain."

Indeed, turmeric has been used for centuries for arthritis, inflammation, gallbladder problems, diabetes, wound-healing, liver issues, hepatitis, menstrual pain, anemia, and gout. It is considered alterative, antibacterial, carminative and stimulant. It also is known for its wound-healing, blood-purifying and circulatory powers, and has the ability to, as Dr. Tierra puts it, "relieve pains in the limbs." Indeed, studies have illustrated that curcumin has about 50% of the effectiveness of cortisone, without its damaging side effects.

(Jurenda 2009; Frawley and Lad 1986; Newmark and Shulick 2000; Tierra 1990; Hobbs 1998; LaValle 2001)

A Sampling of Turmeric Research

A number of studies have proved over the past decade that turmeric or its constituents halt or inhibit both COX enzymes and LOX enzymes (Aggarwal and Sung 2009; Thampithak et al. 2009; Sompamit et al. 2009).

In a randomized, double-blind clinical study from the Medical College at India's University of Poona (Kulkarni et al. 1991), 42 osteoarthritis patients were given either a placebo or a combination of boswellia and turmeric. During and after three months of treatment, the boswellia and turmeric group experienced a significant drop in pain severity and disability score compared to the placebo group.

In a blinded, randomized study done at the UK's University of Reading (Bundy 2004), 500 human volunteers with irritable bowel syndrome took either one or two tablets of a standardized turmeric extract for 8 weeks. After the 8-week period, the prevalence of IBS dropped by 53% for the one-tablet group and 60% for the two-tablet group. Pain severity scores also dropped significantly. Because both arthritis and IBS are considered autoimmune inflammatory diseases, the relevancy seems appropriate.

In another study on 45 patients with peptic ulcers (Prucksunand 2001), ulcers were completely resolved and absent in 76% of the group taking turmeric powder in capsules.

Other studies have also shown similar positive gastrointestinal effects of turmeric. We can conclude that not only is turmeric a known anti-inflammatory, but it has *positive* gastrointestinal side effects.

Turmeric can certainly be taken in a capsule as the above studies mention. However, because turmeric is readily available as a delicious spice, there is every reason to conclude that adding it (along with ginger) to our daily meal-plans is appropriate for arthritis sufferers. This said, some herbalists, such as James LaValle, R.Ph, N.M.D., suggest that for best results turmeric should also be taken as a supplement.

Other Significant Anti-inflammatory Foods & Spices

Basil (*Osimum basilicum*) contains ursolic acid and oleanolic acid, both shown in laboratory studies to inhibit COX-2 enzymes and inflammation in general.

Rosemary (*Rosmarinus officinalis*) contains ursolic acid, oleanolic acid and apigenin—a few of the many constituents in this important botanical—have been shown to inhibit COX-2 enzymes in laboratory studies.

Oregano (*Origanum vulgare*) contains at least thirty-one anti-inflammatory constituents, twenty-eight antioxidants, and four significant COX-2 inhibitors (apigenin, kaempherol, ursolic acid and oleanolic acid).

Reishi mushroom (*Ganoderma spp.*) has illustrated a number of anti-inflammatory effects. Studies have shown its ability to modulate cytokine production, specifically among rheumatoid synovial fibroblasts (Ho *et al.* 2007).

Garlic (*Allium sativum*) probably deserves a more expansive section, but that section would likely encompass a book in itself. Garlic is an ancient medicinal plant with a wealth of characteristics and constituents that stimulate the immune system, protect the liver, purify the bloodstream, reduce oxidative species, reduce LDL, reduce inflammation, and stimulate detoxification systems throughout the body. This is supported by a substantial amount of rigorous scientific research. Garlic is also one of the most powerful antibiotic-antimicrobial plants known. A fresh garlic bulb has at least five different constituents known to inhibit bacteria, fungi and viruses. This antibiotic capability, however, is destroyed by heat and oxygen. Therefore, eating freshly peeled bulbs are the most assured way to retain these antibiotic potencies. Cooked, aged or dehydrated garlic powder also has a variety of powerful antioxidants, but little of its antibiotic abilities. Garlic is also a tremendous sulfur donor, as we'll discuss in the next chapter. The combination of garlic's antibiotic, antioxidant, anti-inflammatory and sulfur donor characteristics make it a *must* daily food for any inflammatory condition.

Antioxidants

Colorful Fruits

Over the past few years, research has discovered that red, purple and blue fruits have tremendous antioxidant, protective and anti-aging benefits. Continued studies have concluded that oxidative species—free radicals—are at the root of much of the damage caused to the cartilage and synovial membranes around joints. Oxidative species come from poor diets and chemical toxins—exacerbated by stress. The greatest and most efficient ability to neutralize these oxidative radicals comes from fresh botanical foods. The method scientists and food technologists have come to measure the ability a particular food has to neutralize free radicals is the "Oxygen Radical Absorbance Capacity" test (or ORAC). These technical laboratory studies are performed by a number of scientific bodies, including the USDA and specialized labs such as the Brunswick Laboratories in Massachusetts.

Research from the USDA's Jean Mayer Human Nutrition Research Center on Aging at Tufts University has suggested that a diet high in ORAC value may slow aging, may prevent memory loss, may increase mental response time, may protect blood vessels from damage and may slow damage to many other functioning tissues in the body (Sofic *et al.* 2001; Cao *et al.* 1998). This is relevant to arthritis because it is widely considered that cartilage damage and a weakened or deranged immune system is directly related to higher levers of circulating oxidative species or free radicals.

This research and others have implicated that damage from free radicals also contributes to cardiovascular disease, cancer, liver disease, kidney problems, gastrointestinal issues, Alzheimer's and many other ailments. Although antioxidants cannot be considered treatments for any disease, many studies have suggested that increased antioxidant intake decreases our risk of contracting both infectious and degenerative disease by supporting immune function and detoxification. Many researchers have agreed that consuming 3,000 to 5,000 ORAC units per day can have protective benefits. We would add that reducing free radical content also allows the immune system to operate more effectively, helping to prevent arthritis.

ORAC Values of Selected (Raw) Fruits (USDA, 2007-2008)

Cranberry	9,382		Pomegranate	2,860
Plum	7,581		Orange	1,819
Blueberry	6,552		Tangerine	1,620
Blackberry	5,347		Grape (red)	1,260
Raspberry	4,882		Mango	1,002
Apple (Granny)	3,898		Kiwi	882
Strawberry	3,577		Banana	879
Cherry (sweet)	3,365		Tomato (plum)	389
Gooseberry	3,277		Pineapple	385
Pear	2,941		Watermelon	142

There is tremendous attention these days on two unique fruits from the Amazon rain forest and China called *acai* and *goji berry* (or wolfberry) respectively. A recent ORAC test documented by

Schauss *et al.* (2006) gives acai a score of 102,700 and a test documented by Gross *et al.* (2006) gives goji berries a total ORAC of 30,300. However, subsequent tests done by Brunswick Laboratories, Inc. gives these two berries 53,600 (acai) and 22,000 (gogi) total-ORAC values. In addition, we must remember that these are the dried berries being tested in the later case, and a concentrate of acai being tested in the former case. The numbers in the chart above are for fresh fruits. Dried fruits will naturally have higher ORAC values, because the water is evaporated—giving more density and more absorbance per 100 grams. For example, on the USDA database, dried apples have a 6,681 total-ORAC value, while fresh apples range from 2,210 to 3,898 in total-ORAC value. This equates to a two-to-three times increase from fresh to dried. In another example, fresh red grapes have a 1,260 total-ORAC value, while raisins have a 3,037 total-ORAC value. This comes close to an increase of three times the ORAC value following dehydration.

One of the newest additions to the new high-ORAC superfruits is the *maqui superberry*. This is small purplish fruit grown in Chile. It is about the size of an elderberry (another good antioxidant fruit).

Part of the equation, naturally, is cost. Dried fruit and concentrates are often more expensive than fresh fruit. High-ORAC dried fruits or concentrates from acai and/or gogi will also be substantially more expensive than fruits grown domestically (for Americans that is). Our conclusion is for the best value and greater fiber content, consider local or in-country grown fruits with high total-ORAC values to obtain the best value for free radical scavenging ability (and support for your local farmers).

By comparison, spinach—an incredibly wholesome vegetable with a tremendous amount of nutrition—only has a fraction of the ORAC content of some of these fruits, at 1,515 total-ORAC. It should be noted, however, that some (dehydrated) spices have incredibly high ORAC values. For example, USDA's database lists ground turmeric's total-ORAC value at 159,277 and oregano's at 200,129. However, while we might only consume a few hundred milligrams of a spice per day, we can eat many grams—if not pounds—of fruit per day.

Red Tart Cherries

One of the more effective fruits for arthritis sufferers—especially for gout—is red tart cherries. Sour cherries have some special attributes that apparently clear out uric acid crystals from the joints, and speed up the process of clearing them from the urinary tract. Like cranberries, cherries have a pH that gives them antiseptic effects in the urinary tract to reduce microbial growth. They also have unique constituents that help purify the bloodstream and joints. The ORAC value of red tart cherries are in the range of sweet cherries, but now many manufacturers are selling the juice in a concentrate form—giving it a higher ORAC value and greater uric acid clearing potential.

Montmorency (red tart) cherries also have a number of powerful phytonutrients, including melatonin, anthocyanins 1, 2 and 3, perillyl alcohol, quercetin, SOD (super oxide dismutase) and many others. Melatonin has been connected to relaxation, sleep and healthy circadian rhythms. Anthocyanins have been linked to helping protect arteries from plaque build-up and other tissues from oxidative damage. Perillyl alcohol and ellagic acid have been studied for their cancer-protective qualities, while quercetin and SOD have been shown to support detoxification and healthy immune function.

In the 1950's, Texan Ledwig Blau, Ph.D. decided to try eating cherries as part of a diet intended to heal his crippling gout. He subsequently reported in a medical journal that six cherries per day turned things around for him, and soon he was up walking. A survey by *Prevention Magazine* polled 700 respondents who took cherries for their gout. 67% said the cherry protocol helped them. Steve Schumacher, M.D. from Kentucky has confirmed this protocol for his gouty patients. Robert Giller, M.D. wrote that cherries (along with other dark red and blue berries) contain compounds that help prevent collagen destruction—rendering more collagen available for cartilage repair (Yaeger 1998).

Botanical Anti-inflammatory Nutrition

Any discussion of preventing excess oxidative radicals cannot be complete without a review of antioxidant phytonutrients. Antioxidants are extremely important in arthritis because antioxidants protect against DNA damage caused by oxidation from free radicals. There are a number of different foods that contain varying degrees of antioxidant potential. The common denominator is that they are whole, raw or minimally processed plant foods.

Botanical constituents known to be significant antioxidants and blood-purifying elements include *lecithin* and *octacosanol* from whole grains; *polyphenols* and *sterols* from vegetables; *lycopene* and other phytochemicals from tomatoes; *quercetin* and *sulfur/allicin* from garlic, onions and peppers; *pectin, rutin* and quercetin from apples; *phytocyanidins* and antioxidant *flavonoids* such as *apigenin* and *luteolin* from various greenfoods; and *anthocyanins* from various fruits and even oats.

Some sea-based botanicals like kelp also contain antioxidants as well. Consider a special polysaccharide compound from kelp called *fucoidan.* Fucoidan has been shown in animal studies to significantly reduce inflammation (Cardoso *et al.* 2009; Kuznetsova *et al.* 2004).

Nearly every botanical has some measure of these botanical constituents. The goal is to alkalize the blood and increase the detoxification capabilities of the liver, and help clear the blood of toxins. Foods that are particularly detoxifying and immune-strengthening include fresh pineapples, beets, cucumbers, apricots, apples, almonds, artichokes, avocado, banana, lima beans, greens, berries, casaba, celery, coconuts, corn, cranberries, dandelion greens, grapes, raw honey, kale, citrus fruits, lettuce, mango, mushrooms, oats, okra, onions, papaya, parsley, peas, radishes, raisins, spinach, chard, tomatoes, walnuts, watermelon, watercress, zucchini and many more.

Diets with significant fiber levels also help clear the blood and tissues of toxins to support the immune system. Fiber in the diet should range from about 35 to 45 grams per day. Six to ten servings of raw fruits and vegetables per day should accomplish this. This means raw foods can be at every meal. Good fibrous protein sources and sources of healthy lignans and phytoestrogens (that help balance hormone levels) include peas, garbanzo beans, soybeans, kidney beans and lentils. Garlic, cayenne and onions can be added to cooked dishes too. These contain inflammatory-inhibiting quercetin and other antioxidant constituents. Cooked beans or grains can be spiced with turmeric, ginger, basil, rosemary and other anti-inflammatory spices such as cayenne.

The extract of *vitis vinifera* seed (grapeseed) is one of the highest sources of bound antioxidant proanthrocyanidins and leucocyanidines called *procyanidolic oligomers*, or "PCOs." Research has demonstrated that PCOs from grapeseed extract have a protective and strengthening effect on tissues by increasing enzyme conjugation (Seo *et al.* 2001). They also encourage greater collagen fiber crosslinking and prevent proteolytic damage (Robert *et al.* 2002). PCOs also increase glycoprotein and sulphated glycosaminoglycan synthesis (Drubaix *et al.* 1997), which is necessary to replace cartilage. PCOs also inhibit hyaluronan-varicosis (Cahn and Borzeix 1983) and increase vascular wall strength (Robert *et al.* 2000). PCOs also reinforce vascular connective tissue (Corbe *et al.* 1988). PCOs also were shown to decrease proteinuria—making them especially good for gouty conditions (Melcion *et al.* 1982).

Over the past few years an increasing amount of evidence is pointing to the conclusion that foods with *reservatrol* and *quercetin* help protect the body not only against free radical damage, but also inhibit inflammation and prevent inflammatory and autoimmune derangement. In a new study out of Italy's Catholic University, researchers (Crescente *et al.* 2009) found that both reservatrol and quercetin inhibited arachidonic acid-induced platelet aggregation. This means that these botanical polyphenols naturally slow down the process of inflammation. Foods high in reservatrol include purple grape juice, blueberries, cranberries and peanuts. The Japanese knotweed plant (*Polygonum cuspidatum*) is particularly high in reservatrol. Whole red grapes are particularly high in reservatrol.

Foods rich in quercetin include onions, garlic, apples, capers, grapes, leafy greens, tomato and broccoli. In a study from the University of California-Davis' Department of Food Science and Technology (Mitchell *et al.* 2007) documented flavonoid levels between organic and conventional tomatoes over a ten-year period. Their research concluded that quercetin levels were 79% higher for tomatoes grown organically under the same conditions.

Oxygenated carotenoids such as lutein and astaxanthin also have been shown to exhibit strong antioxidant activity. Astaxanthin is derived from microalga *Haematococcus pluvialis,* and lutein is available from a number of foods, including spirulina.

Arthritis Therapy Diet

Paavo Airola, N.D., Ph.D., documented his decades of clinically successful natural treatments in 1974. For any type of arthritis, Dr. Airola recommended a therapy diet complete with a detoxification program. The therapy diet included avoiding meat, fowl, milk, cheese, bread, salt and sugar. Here is a summary of his anti-arthritis diet:

Paavo Airola's Arthritis Therapy Diet

Juice Fast	First 4-6 weeks, with vegetable juices and broths
Vegetable Juices	carrot, celery, red beet juice, raw potato
Fruit Juices	bananas, sour cherries, pineapples, tart apples
Vegetable broth	potatoes, carrots, celery, beet tops, turnip tops, parsley, garlic, onions, herb spices to taste
Vegetables	wheat grass, watercress, potatoes, yams, celery, parsley, garlic, comfrey and endive
Alfalfa	dehydrated tablets and raw if possible
Raw Potato Therapy	Peel and slice one raw potato; put in glass of water overnight. Drink water on empty stomach in the morning.

Dr. Bernard Jensen was also a big proponent of the potato-vegetable broth prescribed by Dr. Airola. Here is Dr. Jensen's recipe (2001):

"**Potato Peeling Broth....** for extreme rheumatism and arthritic problems, excess catarrh in the body, and neutralizing the body's acids is potato peeling broth. This is a high potassium broth. Use two good-sized potatoes and one and a half pints of water. Simmer for fifteen minutes, strain, and drink just the broth. Take one or two cups a day over a period of a month. I have seen many rheumatic pains leave with this."

Essential Fatty Acids

The types of fats we eat relates to arthritis primarily because arachidonic acid fats are pro-inflammatory and others are anti-inflammatory. The fat content of our diet is also important because our cell membranes are made of lipids and lipid-derivatives like phospholipids. An imbalanced fat diet therefore can lead to weak cell membranes, which leads to cells that are less protected and more prone to damage by oxidative radicals.

Arachadonic acids in moderation are important fatty acids, and we all need them. They are important factors in the inflammatory process—in the right quantity of course. For this reason, our bodies convert linoleic acid to arachadonic as needed. However, we can also obtain arachidonic acid directly from meat and fish. Unfortunately, a heavy meat and fish diet can cause an overload of arachidonic acid. Because arachidonic acid stimulates the production of pro-inflammatory prostaglandins and leucotrienes in the COX and LOX enzyme conversion process, too much of it leads to a tendency for our bodies to over-respond during an inflammatory event. Worse, a system overloaded with arachidonic acid makes halting the inflammatory process more difficult.

Interestingly, carnivorous animals cannot or do not readily convert linoleic acid (found in many common plants) to arachidonic acid, but herbivore animals do convert linoleic acid to arachidonic acid. Humans convert linoleic acid to arachidonic acid.

Here is a quick review of the major fatty acids and the foods they come from:

Major Omega-3 Fatty Acids (EFAs)

Acronym	Fatty Acid Name	Major Dietary Sources
ALA	alpha-linolenic acid	walnuts, soybeans, flax, canola, pumpkin seeds, chia seeds
SDA	stearidonic acid	hemp, spirulina, blackcurrant
DHA	docosahexaenoic acid	Body converts from ALA; also obtained from certain algae, krill and fish oils
EPA	eicosapentaenoic acid	converts in the body from DHA
GLA	gamma-linolenic acid	borage, primrose oil, spirulina

Major Omega-6 Fatty Acids (EFAs)

Acronym	Fatty Acid Name	Major Dietary Sources
GLA	gamma-linolenic acid	borage, primrose oil, spirulina
LA	linoleic acid	many plants, safflower, sunflower, sesame, soy, almond especially
AA	arachidonic acid	meats, salmon
PA	palmitoleic acid	macadamia, palm kernel, coconut

Major Omega-9 Fatty Acids

Acronym	Fatty Acid Name	Major Dietary Sources
EA	eucic acid	canola, mustard seed, wallflower
OA	oleic acid	sunflower, olive, safflower
PA	palmitoleic acid	macadamia, palm kernel, coconut

Major Saturated Fatty Acids

Acronym	Fatty Acid Name	Major Dietary Sources
Lauric	lauric acid	coconut, dairy, nuts
Myristic	myristic	coconut, butter
Palmitic	palmitic acid	macadamia, palm kernel, coconut, butter, beef, eggs
Stearic	stearic acid	macadamia, palm kernel, coconut, eggs

Essential fatty acids—or EFA's—are fats necessary for adequate health. Eaten in the right proportion, they can also lower inflammation and speed healing. EFA's are long-chain polyunsaturated fatty acids—longer than the linolenic, linoleic and oleic acids. The major EFAs are omega-3s—primarily *alpha linolenic acid* (ALA), *docosahexanoic acid* (DHA) and *eicohexanoic acid* (EPA); and omega-6s—primarily *linoleic acid,* (LA), gamma-linoleic acid (GLA), palmitoleic acid (PA) and arachidonic acid (AA). The term *essential* was originally given with the assumption that these types of fats could not be assembled or produced by the body—they had to be taken directly from our food supply.

This assumption, however, is not fully correct. While it is true that we need *some* of these from our diet, our bodies readily convert linoleic acid to arachidonic acid, and ALA to DHA and EPA. Therefore, these fats can be considered essential in some sense, but we do not necessarily have to consume each one of them.

Monounsaturated oils are high in omega 9 fatty acids like oleic acid. A monounsaturated fatty acid has one double carbon-hydrogen bonding chain. Oils from seeds, nuts and other plant-based sources have the largest quantities of monounsaturates. Oils that have large proportions of monounsaturates such as olive oil are known to lower heart disease when replacing high saturated fat in diets. Monounsaturates also aid in skin cell maintenance; improve glycemic tolerance by increasing the glucagon-like peptide GLP-1; and moderate insulin levels as needed.

Polyunsaturated fats have at least two double carbon-hydrogen bonds. They come from a variety of plant and marine sources. DHA and EPA simply have longer chains with more double carbon-hydrogen bonds. ALA, DHA and EPA are known to lower heart disease and increase artery-wall health. The omega-6 polyunsaturates are also considered healthy for the heart and arteries, assuming they are not converted to trans-fats.

Saturated fats, or fats with high levels of fatty acids without double bonds (the hydrogens "saturate" the carbons), are found among animal fats and tropical oils such as coconut and palm. Milk products such as butter and whole milk contain saturated fats, along with a special type of healthy linoleic fatty acid called CLA or *conjugated linoleic acid.*

The saturated fats from coconuts and palm differ from animal saturates in that they have shorter chains. This actually gives them—unlike animal saturates—an antimicrobial quality.

Trans-fats are oils that either have been overheated or have undergone hydrogenation. Hydrogenation is produced by heating while bubbling hydrogen ions through the oil. This adds hydrogen and repositions some of the bonds. The "trans" refers to the positioning of part of the molecule on the other side—as opposed to "cis" positioning. The cis positioning is the bonding orientation the body's cell membranes work best with. Trans-fats have been known to be a cause for increased radical species in the system; damaging artery walls; contributing to heart disease, high LDL levels, liver damage, diabetes; and other metabolic dysfunction (Mozaffarian *et al.* 2009). It should be noted that CLA is also a trans-fat, but this is a trans-fat the body works well with—it is considered a healthy fat.

Omega-6 fatty acids are the most available form of fat in the plant kingdom. Linoleic acid is the primary omega-6 fatty acid and it is found in most grains and seeds. A healthy body will convert linoleic acid into GLA readily, utilizing the same delta-6 desaturase enzyme used for ALA to DHA conversion. From GLA, the body produces *dihomo-gamma linoleic acid,* which cycles through the body as an eicosinoid. GLA aids in skin health, assists in joint movement and healthy synovial fluid, and is critically important to nerve conduction. Limited conversion of both LA to GLA and ALA to DHA is thought to be caused by trans-fat consumption, smoking, pollution, stress, infections, and various chemicals that affect the liver. For those who may not convert easily, GLA can be also obtained from the oils of borage seeds, evening primrose seed, hemp seed, and from spirulina. Excellent food sources of LA include chia seeds, seed, hempseed, grapeseed, pumpkin seeds, sunflower seeds, safflower seeds, soybeans, olives, pine nuts, pistachio nuts, peanuts, almonds, cashews, chestnuts, and their respective oils.

Research has supported the observation that increased GLA oil consumption can reduce inflammation in arthritis. In a double-blind, randomized and placebo-controlled study of 37 patients with rheumatoid arthritis from the University of Pennsylvania (Leventhal *et al.* 1993), supplementation with 1.4 grams per day of GLA reduced the tender joint score by 45% and the swollen joint score by 41%. The placebo group showed no improvement. Other studies have shown similar results (Brzeski *et al.* 1991; Horrobin 1989).

Omega-9 fatty acids are technically not "essential," as the body manufactures a limited amount. However, monounsaturated fatty acids like oleic acid have been shown in studies to lower heart attack risk, aid blood vessel health, and offer anti-carcinogenic potential. The best sources of omega-9s are olives, sesame seeds, avocados, almonds, peanuts, pecans, pistachio nuts, cashews, hazelnuts, macadamia nuts, several other nuts and their respective oils.

In a meta-study by researchers from the University of Crete's School of Medicine (Margioris 2009), multiple studies showed that omega-3s tend to be anti-inflammatory while omega-6s tend to be pro-inflammatory.

Because much of the early research on the link between fatty acids and inflammatory disease was performed using fish oil, it was assumed that both EPA and DHA fatty acids reduced inflammation. Recent research from the University of Texas' Department of Medicine/Division of Clinical Immunology and Rheumatology

(Rahman *et al.* 2008) has clarified it is DHA that is primarily impli-cated in reducing inflammation. DHA inhibited osteoclast differentiation (thought to be one of the first steps leading to carti-lage damage) by expressing certain genes. DHA also inhibited RANKL-induced proinflammatory cytokines, and a number of inflammation steps.

Alpha linolenic acid (ALA) is the primary omega-3 fatty acid the body can most easily assimilate. Once assimilated, the healthy body will convert ALA to eicosapentaenoic acid (EPA) and docosahex-aenoic acid (DHA) at a rate of about 7-15%, depending upon the health of the liver. One study of six women performed at England's University of Southampton (Burdge *et al.* 2002) published in 2002 in the *British Journal of Nutrition* showed a conversion rate of 36% from ALA to omega-3 fatty acids (EPA, DHA and other omega-3). A follow-up study of men at Southhampton showed ALA conver-sion to EPA and other n-3 fatty acids occurred at levels of 16%.

The process of converting ALA to DHA and EPA requires an enzyme produced in the liver called *delta-6 desaturase*. Some people—especially those who have a poor diet, are immune-suppressed, or burdened with toxicity such as cigarette smoke—may not produce this enzyme very well. As a result, they may not convert as much ALA to DHA and EPA. For those with low levels of DHA—or for those with problems converting ALA and DHA—DHA microalgae can be supplemented. These algae produce significant amounts of DHA. They are the foundation for the DHA molecule all the way up the food chain, including fish. This is how fish come to have DHA. Three algae species—*Crypthecodinium cohnii, Nitzschia laevis* and *Schizochytrium spp.* —are now in commercial production and available in oil and capsule form. Microalgae-derived DHA is pref-erable to fish or fish oils. Fish and fish oils typically contain saturated fats and may also—depending upon their origin—contain toxins such as mercury and PCBs. We should note that salmon con-tain a considerable amount of arachidonic acid as well (Chilton 2002).

Research has illustrated that like fish oils, DHA algal oils have il-lustrated significant therapeutic and anti-inflammatory effects. One study (Aterburn *et al.* 2007) measured pro-inflammatory arachidonic acid levels after a dosage of algal DHA. It was found that arachidonic acid levels decreased by 20% following a dose of 100 milligrams. In a randomized open-label study (Aterburn *et al.* 2007), researchers gave 32 healthy men and women either algal DHA oil or cooked salmon for two weeks. After the two weeks, plasma levels of circulating DHA were bioequivalent. In a study by researchers from The Netherlands' Wageningen University Toxicology Research Center (van Beelan *et al.* 2007), all three species of commercially produced algal oil showed equivalency with fish oil in their inhibition of cancer cell growth. Another study (Lloyd-Still *et al.* 2007) of twenty cystic fibrosis patients concluded that 50 milligrams of algal DHA was readily absorbed, maintained DHA bioavailability immediately, and increased circulating DHA levels by four to five times.

DHA readily converts to EPA by the body, or is produced directly from ALA. Although fish contain both EPA and DHA, EPA degrades quickly if unused in the body anyway. It is easily converted from DHA as needed. Our bodies store DHA and not EPA.

We emphasize omega-3 here instead of DHA/EPA, because ALA also produces anti-inflammatory activity. In studies at Wake Forest University (Chilton *et al.* 2008), for example, flaxseed oil also produced anti-inflammatory effects, along with borage oil and echium oil (both also containing GLA).

This, however, probably simplifies the equation too much. Most of the research on fats has shown that omega-6s are healthy oils. Perhaps there is another factor. Let's dig a little deeper:

In a study by researchers from the University of Guelph in Ontario (Tulk and Robinson 2009), eight middle-aged men with metabolic disorder were tested for the inflammatory effects resulting from changing their fat content proportion between omega-3 and omega-6. The men were divided into two groups, one eating a high saturated fat diet with a proportion of 20:1 between omega-6 and omega-3, and the other eating a diet of 2:1 (high omega-3 diet). Both groups were tested before and after the diet change. Testing after the diet change showed that the high omega-3 diet did not change the inflammatory marker tests.

The proportion between omega-6s and omega-3s is thus recommended to be about one or two to one (1-2:1). The current western American diet has been estimated to be about twenty to thirty to one (20-30:1) for the proportion between omega-6 and omega-3. This imbalance (of too much omega-6 and too little omega-3) has been associated with a number of inflammatory diseases, including arthritis, heart disease, ulcerative colitis, Crohn's disease, and others. When fat consumption is out of balance, the body's metabolism will trend towards inflammation. This is because omega-6 oils convert more easily to arachidonic acid than do omega-3s. AA seems to push the body toward the processes of inflammation (Simopoulos 1999).

It appears that the anti-inflammatory effects of DHA in particular relates to a modulation of a gene factor called NF-kappaB. The NF-kappaB is involved in signaling among cytokine receptors. With more DHA consumption, the transcription of the NF-kappaB gene sequence is reduced. This seems to reduce inflammatory signaling (Singer *et al.* 2008).

The drivers for both of these effects involve the liver. The stearoyl-coenzyme A desaturase 1 (inhibits inflammation) is produced by a healthy liver; and NF-kappaB activity is stimulated in the presence of a weak liver. We also know that saturated fatty acids burden the liver, as they elevate LDL cholesterol and total cholesterol, and increase the incidence of diabetes, artery inflammation, and high blood pressure. We also know that reducing dietary saturated fats and increasing omega-6 polyunsaturated fats reduces inflammation, cardiovascular disease, high cholesterol and diabetes (Ros and Mataix 2008). This relationship appears to lie not in the inflammatory cascade, but the ability of the liver to properly modulate lipid content and enzyme content. Increased LDL cholesterol, of course, is associated with an increase in free radical species that damage arteries, cartilage and many other tissue systems.

This relationship was cleared up in a study performed at Sydney's Heart Research Institute (Nicholls *et al.* 2008). Here fourteen adults consumed meals either rich in saturated fats or omega-6 polyunsaturated fats. They were tested following each meal for various inflammation and cholesterol markers. The results showed that the high saturated fat meal blocked the anti-inflammatory capacity of the liver's production of HDL cholesterol, whereas HDL's anti-inflammatory capacity was increased after the omega-6 meals.

What this tells us is that the omega-3/omega-6 story is complicated by the saturated fat content of the diet and subsequent liver function. High saturated fat diets increase (bad) LDL content and reduce the anti-inflammatory and antioxidant capacities of the liver. Diets lower in saturated fat and higher in omega-6 and omega-3 fats encourage antioxidant and anti-inflammatory activity.

We also know that diets high in monounsaturated fats—such as the famous Mediterranean Diet—are also associated with significant anti-inflammatory effects. Mediterranean diets contain higher levels of monounsaturated fats like oleic acids (omega-9) as well as higher proportions of fruits and vegetables, and lower proportions of saturated fats (Basu *et al.* 2006).

High saturated fat diets are also associated with increased obesity, and a number of studies have shown that obesity is directly related to inflammatory diseases—including arthritis. High saturated fat diets and diets high in trans fatty acids have also been clearly shown to accompany higher levels of inflammation and inflammatory factors such as IL-6 and CRP (Basu *et al.* 2006).

Noting the research showing the relationships between the different fatty acids and inflammation, and the condition of the liver (which can be burdened by too much saturated fat), we can logically arrive at a model for dietary fat consumption for a person who is either dealing with or wants to prevent inflammation-oriented diseases such as arthritis:

Omega-3	25%-30% of dietary fats
Omega-6+Omega 9	40%-50% of dietary fats
Saturated	5%-10% of dietary fats
GLA	10%-20% of dietary fats
Trans-Fats	0% of dietary fats

Fibrinolytic Enzymes

When cartilage is damaged by oxidative LDL, toxins or other radical species leading to arthritis, the immune system responds by activating thrombin and fibrinogen along with inflammation and pain. Thrombin and fibrinogen stimulate the production of fibrin to scab the wound and promote the healing process. As this healing cascade matures, the body activates plasminogen, which produces the plasmin enzyme. Plasmin is called a fibrinolytic enzyme because it breaks down the fibrin after it is no longer needed. Inhibited plasmin genesis can result in excess fibrin and thrombin, which results in the build-up of scar tissue within the cartilage region.

Several botanical-derived enzymes are available to assist the fibrinolytic process. The *nattokinase* enzyme, produced by the bacterium *Bacillus natto,* has been lauded for its fibrinolytic effects. Natto is a preparation of soybeans, a traditional food in Japan. The resulting enzyme has fibrinolytic and proteolytic properties, delaying clotting, thrombosis and platelet aggregation (Suzuki *et al.* 2003). In a randomized, placebo-controlled study of 92 high-risk deep vein thrombosis patients traveling by airplane—when acute deep vein thrombosis is more likely—the nattokinase group experienced 60% less thrombosis than the control group (Cesarone *et al.* 2003).

Bromelain is another botanical enzyme with fibrinolytic, proteolytic and anti-inflammatory properties. Naturally derived from pineapple, *in vivo* and *in vitro* studies have shown bromelain's effectiveness in inhibiting thrombosis and platelet-aggregation by modulating plasmin-activator (Maurer 2001; Taussig and Batkin 1988; Felton 1980). *Papain,* the enzyme contained in papaya, is also considered to have similar fibrinolytic properties.

These fibrinolytic plant enzymes have also had some respectable clinical success for arthritis. One study on bromelain resulted in improved joint mobility and decreased swelling, while another allowed rheumatoid arthritis patients to decrease their anti-inflammatory medications (Stengler 2008).

Conclusion

Nature's botanicals are quite complex. They contain hundreds of different compounds that provide a balance of benefits to prevent and help relieve arthritis. All this research on natural botanicals underscores the ability of botanicals to not only control and moderate the process of inflammation—as pharmaceutical drugs do—but can accomplish a turnaround of the mechanisms at the root of arthritis.

Here is a summary of the benefits of the botanicals we have discussed in this chapter:

❖ They protect joint tissues and cartilage from damage due to oxidative species

❖ They help neutralize toxins before they damage cells

❖ They stimulate and strengthen the liver and help protect the liver from toxicity damage

❖ They create a more alkaline blood and urine pH—discouraging the entry and growth of microorganisms

❖ They protect cells from mutation

❖ They speed up the process of healing by stimulating the immune system

❖ They modulate the inflammatory process to balance injury repair with inflammation shut-down

❖ They speed up the process of clearing scarring with fibrinolytic and plasminogen shunting

❖ They balance the tumor necrosis factor (TNF) so it is active against tumor cells, yet not overactive against healthy cells

❖ They modulate cytokines — stimulating them against invaders yet reducing their behavior against healthy cells

❖ They stimulate the rebuilding of healthy cartilage and synovial membrane tissues

❖ They stimulate and invigorate the thymus gland

❖ They strengthen the adrenal glands, and modulate their production of corticosteroids

❖ They moderate the endocrine system to balance the various hormones and their receptors

❖ They invigorate the heart and heart muscles

❖ They help strengthen arteries and veins

❖ They help balance cholesterol and bile

❖ They stimulate and purify the urinary tract

❖ They modulate nerve cells, to relax and tune them by balancing neurotransmitter fluid content

❖ They stimulate restful sleep

❖ They strengthen the immune system (listed again for emphasis)

❖ They provide nutrients—minerals, vitamins, proteins and numerous phytonutrients needed to rebuild synovial membranes and cartilage

Chapter Six

Fallacies of Glucosamine and Chondroitin

Glucosamine and chondroitin have both received considerable attention from consumers and researchers over the past few years.

Sales of both products—alone, together, or within other formulations—have skyrocketed over the past decade.

Yet there is still a growing epidemic of arthritis. Some claim they help, and some say they are a waste of money. Do they work or not?

Contradictions in Research

Many studies have been done on both chondroitin and glucosamine. Some have resulted in some decrease in pain among patients. But some have shown no difference whatsoever between treatment groups and placebo groups. Many researchers have pointed out that many of the studies showing improvement were not placebo-controlled or properly randomized.

To clear the air, physicians and researchers at Switzerland's University of Berne (Reichenbach *et al.* 2007) reviewed twenty clinical trials on glucosamine and chondroitin. After screening for protocols, methods and study criteria, the researchers concluded that chondroitin and glucosamine were no better than placebo. Some of the studies indicating positive results had inherent problems with protocols. Other positive results, the researchers determined, could have just as well been the result of chance.

These researchers also concluded that, "Large-scale, methodologically sound trials indicate that the symptomatic benefit of chondroitin is minimal or nonexistent. Use of chondroitin in routine clinical practice should therefore be discouraged."

In another review from the University of Kentucky's College of Pharmacy (Morris and Smith 2009), the researchers concluded that, "Despite the news of aid from chondroitin sulfate, recent research has questioned its efficacy in treating osteoarthritis."

Even the results from large-scale trials on chondroitin-glucosamine have been dubious. For example, in a placebo-controlled clinical trial (the Glucosamine/chondroitin Arthritis Intervention Trial or GAIT—Clegg *et al.* 2006) from the University of

Utah's School of Medicine, 1583 patients were assessed with osteoarthritis of the knee. There were five treatment groups: one group took glucosamine alone (1500 mg), one group took chondroitin alone (1200 mg); another group took both chondroitin and glucosamine (1500+1200 mg); one group took celecoxib (Celebrex®); and the last group took a placebo. After 24 weeks, the celecoxib group experienced 70% pain relief while the placebo group experienced 60% pain relief. Overall, all the other groups—the chondroitin and glucosamine and combined groups—experienced no greater pain relief than the placebo.

However, in one smaller subgroup of patients—those with moderate-to-severe osteoarthritis pain, the combined therapy produced moderately higher levels of pain relief than the placebo group. The combination glucosamine-chondroitin group experienced 79% pain relief while the placebo group experienced 54% pain relief.

This result appears to be the hat rack that glucosamine-chondroitin promoters are currently hanging on, noting the reviews of the previous studies. The reviewers and others had recommended a large-scale study like this to settle the debate.

Did this study really settle the debate? Again, when we look at the study group as a whole, neither glucosamine, chondroitin nor the combination of the two was any better than placebo. Only when the subgroup of the severe pain sufferers was extracted could we see that the combined therapy had any benefit? What does this mean? It must mean, statistically, that the placebo group had *better* pain relief than the glucosamine-chondroitin group in the mild-to-moderate pain cases. This simply does not make sense. Why would the severe group have an effect while the mild-to-moderate group would not? Furthermore, why would the mild-to-moderate group have a worse effect than the placebo group? This would also mean that the placebo group in the severe cases had far less pain reduction than the placebo group in the moderate-to-severe cases.

This puzzle may partly be explained by the fact that the entire study allowed patients to take what is called *rescue analgesia*—in other words, patients were able to take up to 4000 mg of acetaminophen daily in addition to the test product, which was being tested for pain relief! This is why the placebo group's pain relief was so high (50-

60%) in general. So let's consider this ramification for a moment. The severe pain group could take both 4000 mg of acetaminophen as well as the placebo or glucosamine-chondroitin combination. Why did the placebo part of this group have less pain relief than the placebo group overall? Could it have something to do with the subjects' ability to take up to 4000 mg of acetaminophen? Is it not more likely that the severe group took the 4000 mg maximum? In other words, there was a higher chance of interaction between the acetaminophen and the glucosamine and chondroitin, because the severe group most likely took more acetaminophen than the mild-to-moderate group.

Another possibility is that more pain relief could have been accomplished with the maximum dose of acetaminophen in the mild-to-moderate group. In other words, the mild-to-moderate group could have had more relief from the 4000 mg of acetaminophen than the severe group could have had.

These are of course puzzles in the study that are currently unanswered. Even the study authors—twenty-five of them—concluded that: "Glucosamine and chondroitin sulfate alone or in combination did not reduce pain effectively in the overall group of patients with osteoarthritis of the knee. *Exploratory analyses* suggest that the combination of glucosamine and chondroitin sulfate may be effective in the subgroup of patients with moderate-to-severe knee pain." [Italics added] Note the difference between the major conclusion of the study, and the idea of an "exploratory analysis." The controls of a study are typically designed to test a particular hypothesis. An exploratory analysis is a proportional recalculation of a study's results that occurred outside of the design of the study. It was an exploration: A "what if" scenario.

The fact is—just as the research history has been on these two supplements—the results of this study are unconvincing. The overall conclusion (that they do not provide any pain relief) of the study's main result appears solid. Aren't we reaching a bit when we have to deny the study's overall results? The "exploratory analysis" of a group subsection could have been caused by other factors. There are a number of statistical possibilities, including the possibility raised that glucosamine and chondroitin may be interacting somehow with the "rescue" acetaminophen dose.

We do know there is an interaction between glucosamine-chondroitin supplementation and warfarin (Scott 2004). Warfarin is an anticoagulant agent—known for thinning the blood and preventing clotting. Aspirin is also an anticoagulation agent, and so is acetaminophen to a lesser degree. A subtle interaction—perhaps one that could be problematic in larger doses—is possible.

In early 2008, Drs. Knudsen and Sokol reported in *Pharmacotherapy* magazine of a 71-year-old man who was taking warfarin and glucosamine-chondroitin supplements. He was prescribed the warfarin for arterial fibrillation. A test called the *international normalized ratio* (or INR) was given periodically to make sure the patient stayed within a certain clotting risk range. He had been taking small dosage glucosamine-chondroitin supplements (500/400 mg) for five years with the warfarin. His INR averaged 2.3. He then increased his glucosamine-chondroitin dosage to 1500/1200mg (the level of the GAIT study above). After three weeks, his INR increased to 3.9. This alarmed his physician and he asked that the man reduce his glucosamine-chondroitin dosage. After the man cut his glucosamine-chondroitin dose to 750/600 mg, the INR kept going up. After two more weeks, his INR was 4.7. The doctor advised his patient to completely curtail his glucosamine-chondroitin supplementation. After 16 days off the glucosamine-chondroitin supplements, the man's INR returned to 2.6.

This experience underscores the possibility that glucosamine-chondroitin can interact with anticoagulant and/or analgesic drugs. Could this interaction be the reason for the slight reduction in pain among the severe group in the GAIT study?

The results of this study indeed are also contradicted by a later larger-scale study at the University of Utah—by some of the same researchers (Sawitzke *et al.* 2008) who had conducted the GAIT trial two years earlier. This double-blind, placebo-controlled study enrolled 572 osteoarthritis patients who took either glucosamine-chondroitin supplements separate or combined, celecoxib or placebo for 24 months. The trial was intended to show whether there was a difference in the progressive joint space loss between the different groups. In other words, this study would show whether glucosamine-chondroitin supplements actually improved joint and cartilage conditions (which has been the hypothesis of the glucosamine-chondroitin proponents). After the two years, there was no difference in the joint space loss between the glucosamine-chondroitin supplement groups, the celecoxib group and the placebo group. In other words, after two years of glucosamine-chondroitin supplementation, either alone or combined, there was no discernable improvement in the joints. The glucosamine-chondroitin does not help rebuild cartilage or other joint membranes as theorized by their proponents.

Furthermore, if these supplements truly work, why do they not work alone? Almost all of the research to date—including the above one—has concluded that taken alone, these supplements have no effect. But for some mysterious reason, when taken together they suddenly work?

It would be one thing if there were any understanding about the mechanism of such a benefit. Researchers have come to understand the mechanism for nearly every medicine and even most herbal medicines and nutrients. Today's researchers understand inflammatory and pain mechanisms quite well. In the case of glucosamine-chondroitin, they draw a blank.

To illustrate this lack of mechanism, Dr. Robert Lauder from Lancaster University's School of Health and Medicine notes that the chondroitin molecule is an extremely complex molecule that varies dramatically, depending upon its source. He points out medical science's inability to understand the mechanism involved in the product. He stated, "…it is clear that significant challenges remain in the identification of composition, sequence and size impacts on function, understanding how the consumed material is altered during uptake and travels to a site of action and how it exerts an influence on biological processes." (Lauder 2009)

We should note as well that chondroitin/glucosamine supplementation has not been proven effective for rheumatoid arthritis, and it is for this reason they are primarily studied on persons with osteoarthritis.

Finally, we should also add that glucosamine does not come without adverse side effects. In a review (Barclay *et al.* 1998) of studies on glucosamine between 1965 and 1997 (which concluded mostly flaws in study design), the researchers noted that the side effects most often reported included "mild gastrointestinal problems, drowsiness, skin reactions, and headache."

Nutrient Absorption and Utilization

Absorption and utilization is a central problem with chondroitin and glucosamine. Our bodies manufacture these molecules from raw nutrients. The chondrocytes pull together the raw molecules and build the cartilage structure.

We might compare these supplements to getting a piece of animal skin, and slapping it onto the skin and assume our skin will absorb the animal skin. The body just does not work this way. Our cells assemble their own proteins and build most tissue systems using basic nutrients like minerals and amino acids.

Anything we orally ingest must be absorbed through the intestinal tract first. In order for a molecule to be absorbed into the bloodstream, it must clear the oral cavity and empty into the stomach somewhat biochemically intact. It must endure amylase enzymes, probiotic bacteria and immunoglobulins lining the mucosal membranes. These are intended break down recognized toxins. Amylase and other salivary acids are intended to break down starches (polysaccharides), for example. This means that many polysaccharides (glucosamine is part polysaccharide and part amino acid) will break down even before reaching the stomach.

Once the substance empties into the stomach, it must endure gastrin, peptic acids and various enzymes intended to break down proteins and starches in the stomach. The resulting slurry of amino acids, polypeptides, fats, vitamins and minerals are dumped into the duodenum and jejunum of the upper intestines. Here they are further broken down by bile, enzymes and probiotics, in preparation for their journey across the mucosal brush membrane of the intestinal walls.

Assuming they have been sufficiently broken down, oriented molecularly and cleared immunologically for absorption, the resulting nutrient components cross the intestinal brush barrier into the blood stream. By this time, their molecular structures will be simplified. The nutrients will exist in the form of amino acids or small polypeptide sequences, simple sugars, mineral ions, vitamin substrates and fatty acid chains.

Once in the blood stream these nutrients will counter the processes of the liver to further break them down into the raw elements needed by cells. In addition, various lymphocytes, immunoglobulins and antioxidants will latch on to and clear out any foreigners that made it through. Here the pressure of being identified correctly by the body's immune system is even greater.

Once through this myriad of screens, nutrients needed by chondrocytes are fed from the canaliculi between the osteocytes through bone marrow capillaries. Here the nutrients are further screened for size and usefulness. At the chondrocyte level, only the most elemental nutrients are utilized to produce the unique polysaccharide-protein matrix—unique to each of us, like a fingerprint—that makes up our cartilage.

Botanical-based nutrients are readily recognized and broken down by the intestinal tract. Plants yield basic minerals, amino acids and phytonutrients including sulfurated molecules for use by the tiny cells of the body. A plant nutrient contains genetic markers and biomolecular structures that the body recognizes. Plant-based foods and herbs have been consumed for hundreds of thousands of years by humankind and related species. Our immune systems and enzymatic processes are thus geared to ingest and assimilate herbal constituents with a minimum of reactivity or rejection. Botanical-based nutrients are more likely to pass all the barriers and immune system screens and be broken down into the molecules that support metabolic processes. They are less likely to produce an immune response that stimulates the inflammatory process.

Protein is a good example. Our bodies are made of many complex proteins some with hundreds of amino acids. Nearly all the proteins we eat are broken down into their elemental amino acids or small combinations of polypeptides. These make the building blocks for the RNA inside the cells to build their own specialized protein molecules.

The body also builds most of its other tissue structures the same way. All of the components of tissue are built through a process dictated by the DNA and executed by protein-constructing RNA molecules. These molecules, together with special enzymes and the raw materials, assemble the building blocks from basic nutrients.

There are different types of cells in the body, and each type produces and forms unique tissue structures. For example, muscle fiber cells assemble special protein filaments called myosin. Myosin is bound to another protein called nebulin, and these molecules together create elasticity and contractibility in the muscle.

Bone material is produced by osteoblasts. These specialized cells assemble bone tissue utilizing boron, vitamin D, calcium and several other basic nutrients. They produce a special protein called *osteoid*. Osteoids are mineralized through an enzyme (alkaline phosphatase—also produced by the osteoblasts) process. Osteoblasts work conjunctively with osteocytes and osteoclasts to cycle in and out the raw materials needed to shape and model the bones.

Cartilage is the same way. Cartilage is made up of special cells called chondrocytes. Chondrocytes produce *chondrin*. Cartilage is a network of fibers of collagen woven together with chondrin. Chondrin is a guey substance made up of about 80% polysaccharides and 20% protein. These proteins are made of unique amino acids, and their structure is unique. The ending combination has often been referred to as a *mucopolysaccharide*.

The chondrocytes utilize various raw molecules to assemble cartilage. They utilize glucose, amino acids, vitamin C, zinc, magnesium and copper, as well as others to build the matrix. These are all readily available in a botanical diet. Using these raw elements, the chondrocytes repair and replace damaged cartilage. *Without these basic nutrients being available from the diet, the chondrocytes will not have the raw materials to manufacture effective cartilage.*

When cartilage is boiled, *condrigen* is separated. This can be further broken down to gelatin and chondrotin ions. Chondroitin is often found bound or can be synthetically bound to sulfate ions to form chondroitin sulfate. The quality of the chondroitin ions and those that properly bond to sulfate can range from manufacturer to manufacturer, and from source to source. Chondroitin is derived from a variety of sources, including shark cartilage and cow cartilage.

Furthermore, many commercial sources of glucosamine-chondroitin are considered unassimilable. In a laboratory study (Barnhill 2006) of various glucosamine-chondroitin supplements, it was determined that, "No commercially available chondroitin product was deemed appropriate." (The lab was investigating sources for product to be used in the GAIT study). They also identified, among the commercial products, "the consistent appearance of an unidentifiable contaminant..."

The Sulfur Connection

It would be irresponsible for us to completely ignore some of the studies that have shown some benefit from glucosamine and/or chondroitin. There could be, however, another explanation for the few inconsistently positive study results. There is a strong likelihood that there could be effects from sulfur ions separated from glucosamine and chondroitin supplements during digestion and absorption. It is rather curious that the sulfate versions (glucosamine-sulfate and chondroitin-sulfate) seem to have the positive results among those studies.

Furthermore, MSM (methylsulfonylmethane) has also been demonstrated to relieve joint inflammation and pain. In one randomized, double-blind and placebo-controlled study (Kim et al. 2006), 50 patients with knee osteoarthritis were given either 6 grams per day of MSM) or a placebo for 12 weeks. The Western Ontario and McMaster University Osteoarthritis Index was used to gauge pain and mobility. After the 12 weeks, the MSM group had significantly less pain and significantly more mobility than the placebo group.

Other studies (and reviews) have confirmed that MSM reduces inflammatory symptoms for arthritis and other ailments, including allergic rhinitis.

Where does MSM come from? Most organisms—especially plants and animals—produce and circulate MSM. Commercial MSM supplements, however, are synthetically produced, using a variety of substrates. The sulfur in MSM is readily absorbed by the intestines, and this sulfur is readily used by many of the body's cells to assemble various tissues and molecules.

DMSO, or dimethyl sulfoxide, is another supplement with readily available sulfur. DMSO is a byproduct of the wood pulp industry. Its use dates back to 1953, when it was used as a solvent. In 1961, Stanley Jacob, M.D. noticed that DMSO readily penetrated the skin and seemed to relieve pain. Since then, thousands of medical papers and even some clinical studies and veterinary use have confirmed DMSO's ability to reduce pain and inflammation.

Reports have confirmed that DMSO blocks nerve transmission (Evans *et al.* 1993), relieves pain and inflammation in chronic musculoskeletal injuries such as rotator cuff tendonitis and tennis elbow injury (Lockie and Norcross 1967; Percy and Carson 1981), urinary tract inflammation (Shirley *et al.* 1978), and even rheumatoid arthritis (Matsumoto 1967).

In one double-blind, placebo-controlled study (Kneer *et al.* 1994) of 157 patients with arthritic musculoskeletal issues (periarthropathia humeroscapularis or lateral epicondylitis); DMSO topical gel was applied three times a day. At three days, pain relief was noticeable in some of the patients. After 14 days on DMSO, 44% of the DMSO-treatment group was pain free, while 9% of the placebo-group reported being pain-free.

Why is this important? Sulfur is the third most prevalent mineral in the body by weight (Parcell 2002). It is utilized as a component in many enzymes, and is a central component of many cellular structures, including those of the skin, bones and cartilage. Sulfur is also utilized in an enzyme used by chondrocytes to produce cartilage. Without adequate dietary sulfur intake (as we discussed in our botanical chapter), the content and quality of our cartilage can erode, as the body works to balance critical extracellular sulfur content.

However, because sulfur is heat-sensitive, and degrades rather quickly in challenging environments, many sources of sulfur are compromised before we have the chance to eat them. Amino acids methionine, cysteine, cystine, homocysteine, homocystine, and taurine also contain sulfur. These are critical amino acids as the research has shown. Glutathione, one of the central antioxidant elements produced by the liver, is made primarily of cysteine and glutamate. Other important sulfur compounds are S-adenosylmethionine (SAMe), taurine, homocysteine, alpha-lipoic acid, coenzyme A, biotin, heparin and N-acetylcysteine (NAC). These are all involved in important metabolic processes, including modulating inflammation. However, free sulfur is another matter. While we can likely draw free sulfur from these amino acids as they combine or break apart, we readily obtain free sulfur from various plants—which also utilize sulfur for building tissues.

While sulfur amino acids are critical to many body processes, free sulfur is also critical for the health of our tissues. Sulfur is typically consumed bound within a complex molecule. Once within the body it can be freed as sulfonate, sulfide or sulfate. The bottom line, as explained by Dr. David Baker (2005), is that our understanding of sulfur and sulfur amino acid nutrition is still in its infancy.

Let's not forget that cartilage contains sulfate woven in with collagen, elastin, chondroitin and proteoglycan. Sulfur is thus an important raw material used by chondrocytes to build cartilage.

Because sulfur's existence is so ubiquitous within the body, there are few obvious signs of sulfur deficiency. That is, unless you want to include most degenerative diseases. Certainly, the fact that sulfur is so needed by the body, yet its availability in foods is quite small in processed diets because of sulfur's heat-sensitivity—would equate to the logic that many of us are sulfur-deficient. This would especially be the case for those on heavy western diets. Perhaps this is the reason the studies have illustrated that diets with more fruits and vegetables lowers joint inflammation and pain. In other words, the less fresh fruits and vegetables we eat, the less sulfur we are getting in our diet. This lower sulfur dietary consumption also corresponds to the lower sulfur content in cartilage found among many elderly persons.

There is decent evidence that sulfur levels in many adults—especially as they age—are low, and this has been confirmed by testing sulfur amino acid levels. For example, the RDAs for sulfur amino acids for adults are lower than that for pigs, primarily because of oxidation testing methods (Parcel 2002; Baker 2005).

The subject of sulfur mineral deficiency usually gets lost within the discussion of sulfur amino acids. As Dr. Parcel noted in his 2002 paper: "Most nutrition textbooks ignore the contribution free sulfate and sulfate bound to parent molecules as sulfoesters make to total available sulfur, because their contribution to total sulfur intake is considered negligible by comparison." This, statement, however, is based upon tests that show that "free" inorganic sulfate and sulfoester fractions contribute less than 5% of *breast milk* (McNally *et al.* 1991). We would contend firstly that 5% of breast milk is a rather significant percentage, noting how important breast milk is to the health of a newborn. We should note that once breast milk feeding is over, it is time for us to begin getting our sulfur from food sources. Five percent of breast milk and the third most prevalent mineral in the body: These are not proportions to scoff at.

Foods high in sulfur are called *thiols*. Some, like cruciferous vegetables, contain sulforaphanes, and others, like garlic, contain diallyl sulfide and many other free sulfur donors. Garlic, for example, contains at least 18 different sulfur compounds (Bergner 1996).

Researchers from the Keimyung University's School of Medicine (Woo and Kwon 2007) found that sulforaphanes from cruciferous vegetables such as broccoli and cabbage specifically suppressed COX-2 enzyme conversion activity. NF-kappaB and other cytokine signaling mechanisms were involved in the "down-regulation" of COX-2 related inflammation. So we find that sulfur has yet another benefit for arthritis sufferers.

Here is a listing of some known sulfur-containing botanicals:

avocado	leeks
asparagus	lentils
barley	mustard
beans and bean sprouts	nuts
blueberries	oats
broccoli	onions
cabbage	parsley
carob	peas
carrots	radishes
Brussels sprouts	red peppers
cherries	rutabaga
chives	soybeans (tofu, soymilk)
coconuts	seeds
corn	shallots
garlic	Swiss chard
grapes	tomatoes
horseradish	watercress
leafy green vegetables	wheat

Sulfur's involvement in the structure of cartilage utilizes a special enzyme and carrier molecule—both produced by the body. 3'-

phosphoadenosine 5'-phosphosulfate (PAPS) fuels sulfotransferase reactions, using PAPS-synthase (or PAPSS). There are two forms of PAPSS in humans: PAPSS1 and PAPSS2. PAPSS1 enzymes are present in skin and the brain. PAPSS2 is utilized in the liver, cartilage and adrenal glands. Perhaps this illustrates how the body must uniquely assemble its own cartilage.

Conclusion

There is little consistent research evidence that glucosamine and chondroitin reduce inflammation and pain in arthritis. Many of these studies have either been invalidated with protocol reviews or invalidated by other, even larger and more controlled studies. This indicates at the very least, a possible interactive or indirect benefit from the sulfur in chondtroitin-sulfate and glucosamine-sulfate. Furthermore, there is little evidence, nor a verifiable mechanism that chondroitin or glucosamine molecules are useful in themselves in the building of healthy cartilage.

At the same time, there is a rather solid base of evidence supporting the those kinds of results—pain and inflammation reduction—among other sulfur donor molecules like MSM and DMSO, as well as evidence that sulfur foods specifically reduce inflammation.

It appears likely that any positive results derived from glucosamine and chondroitin are created by the donation of free sulfur.

More importantly, the sulphur within botanicals is readily absorbable and assimilable. Because the body readily recognizes botanical forms of sulfur, dosage is no problem, and just about the only side effects to most of these foods would be getting full eating them. Still, it is advisable to consult a health professional trained in natural foods and medicinal botanicals before embarking on a change in diet or one that utilizes any specific botanical to any extreme.

Illustrating the body's ability to readily absorb sulfur does not end at the studies on the topical application of DMSO discussed earlier. Illustrating this further is the traditional application of *balneotherapy,* an ancient practice that utilizes sulfur-rich baths (such as from the Dead Sea) for joint therapy.

Recently, researchers from the Faculty of Health Sciences of Israel's Ben-Gurion University and Soroka University Medical Center conducted a randomized, controlled and single-blinded study to test whether sulfur baths offered any real benefit to osteoarthritis patients. Forty-four osteoarthritis of the knee patients were divided into two groups. The first took two baths per week for six weeks in a sulfur-treated pool heated to 35-36 degrees Celsius (about 96-97 degrees Fahrenheit). The other group took two baths per week for six weeks in a pool at the same temperature but filled with tap water. The group treated with sulfur baths had significantly less pain that lasted six months following the treatment period.

Assuming a diet rich in fresh sulfur foods and essential sulfur-containing amino acids (and sulfur baths if we are fortunate), we will have the ingredients—together with the right combination of botanical herbs and foods—to be able to moderate inflammation and give our cartilage and joint tissues the ability to heal, begin to rebuild, and remain healthy.

Chapter Seven
Other Arthritis Considerations

There are a number of ways we can encourage our bodies to heal faster and reduce inflammation and pain when it comes to joint pain and arthritis. Here are a few ways:

(Like any information offered in this book, a medical professional should be consulted prior to any radical lifestyle changes.)

Sunshine

Sunshine is necessary for supporting joint health.

The Australian National University has found a strong relationship between various autoimmune diseases and ultraviolet radiation exposure. One of the most prominent results of the study was evident among those with multiple sclerosis, rheumatoid arthritis and insulin-dependent diabetes mellitus. The research also analyzed photo-immunology trials that showed that UV-B radiation seems to reduce the Th-1 cell-mediation process, which stimulates inflammatory responses. This new perspective was considered a factor incremental to the metabolic effects of vitamin D production (from sunshine) in the body (Ponsonby *et al.* 2002).

Other researchers have confirmed the relationship between vitamin D and various arthritic conditions (Holick 2008).

In a study performed at the Rheumatology Unit of Internal Medicine at the University of Pisa (Di Munno *et al.* 2004), systemic lupus erythematosus (SLE) was associated with *"sunshine avoidance with consequent vitamin D deficiency."*

Most arthritis sufferers experience ups and downs with pain related to the weather. Some debate these relationships. To settle this, researchers have investigated the associations between arthritic pain and weather conditions.

Researchers from Argentina (Strusberg *et al.* 2002) studied 151 outpatients with arthritis for one year. Fifty-two patients had osteoarthritis, while 82 had rheumatoid arthritis and 17 had fibromyalgia. Thirty-two healthy subjects were used as a control group. Low temperatures with high atmospheric pressure and high humidity were associated with more pain in rheumatoid arthritis. Low temperatures and high humidity was associated with pain in osteoarthritis. Low temperatures and high atmospheric pressure was associated with greater pain in fibromyalgia. The control group had no associations. Let's see how this maps out on a chart:

Condition	Low temps	High pressure	High humidity
Osteoarthritis	Greater Pain		Greater Pain
Rheum Arth	Greater Pain	Greater Pain	Greater Pain
Fibromyalgia	Greater Pain	Greater Pain	

The common denominator appears to be colder temperatures in all three conditions. High pressure and humidity increased pain among the rheumatoid arthritis patients; but higher atmospheric pressure was not associated with greater pain among the osteoarthritis patients (indeed many complain that low pressure increases osteoarthritis pain).

Other studies have found the common denominator to be humidity—ameliorated by local conditions. In 2004, researchers from the University of Groningen in The Netherlands (Patberg and Rasker 2004) reviewed arthritis research from 1985 to 2003 for correlations between weather conditions and arthritis. They found amongst the research that rheumatoid arthritis pain increased with greater humidity. While some localities experienced higher humidity during hot weather, others experienced higher humidity (rain for example) during lower temperatures. In those regions where lower temperatures were associated with higher humidity, RA pain was worse during lower temperatures. For areas where humidity was associated with hotter weather, RA pain worsened during higher temperatures.

For this reason, many arthritis sufferers—osteoarthritic, rheumatoid and others—have found their inflammation, pain and progression of arthritis eases when they live in warmer, drier and sunnier locations.

We should note (as the researchers have) that excess humidity (and mold) can exist within indoor environments as well. In other words, humidity can come from within the home—due to humidifiers, wet air conditioners or wet basements.

The bottom line is that sunshine stimulates the immune system and reduces inflammation. More research on this topic can be found in the author's book, *Healthy Sun* (2009).

Motion and Exercise

Exercise is necessary for a number of reasons.

The first is circulation. Exercise increases the rate of circulation amongst all tissues. This brings nutrients to regions of the body that are not always well served when we sit or sleep. When we exercise, the arteries expand and nutrient molecules can squeeze through the tiny capillaries that serve some of our body parts—including fingers, toes, bones, and indirectly, joints.

Exercise increases detoxification processes. The expansion of arteries, the increase in oxygen-CO2 exchange, sweating, and energy production all drive toxic molecules out of cells and tissues. Exercise increases the body's main excretion pathways—lungs, skin, kidneys, colon and mucus.

Most of us know the heart pumps blood throughout the arteries. But did we know that tiny venous pumps are strategically placed up and down the venous system, which practically vacuum blood back to the heart? These venous pumps are also stimulated and kept healthy by muscle contraction—exercise.

Do we know what pumps lymphatic fluid around the body? The lymphatic fluid carries immune cells around the body, and carries out the various toxins and broken down pathogens. And it is the flow of lymph that will accelerate our body's (and joints) healing mechanisms. The lymph vessels are also driven by muscle contraction. In other words, we "pump" our lymphatic system when we move around and exercise.

Exercise also increases joint mobility. It pushes the joints to commit to a larger range of motion. This larger range of motion in turn helps stimulate internal circulatory mechanisms and stimulates the flow of fluids and nutrients into the cartilage and synovial fluid.

There are three essential elements in exercise to consider for arthritis sufferers: Diversification, mobility, strenuousness and weight bearing.

Diversification means that we are not simply doing one single exercise over and over, such as riding a bike or swimming. Rather, we are doing a variety of exercises that work opposing muscles. A repetitive motion exercise can in fact lead to more complications for arthritis sufferers.

Mobility means *range of motion.* This is not limited to exercise. Throughout the day, we should be moving our fingers, wrists, shoulders, ankles, hips, knees and feet in a variety of ways. This means we keep the joints active. Gardening and other household chores are excellent for this. There are also a lot of activities that we can choose to do in our everyday tasking—such as sweeping rather than vacuuming, taking the stairs instead of the elevator, and cleaning up around the house instead of waiting for others to clean up after us.

Periodic strenuousness is important because this temporarily stresses and raises the heart and breathing rates—increasing circulation and oxygen content; contracting muscles rigorously (pumping the lymphatic system); and pushing the body to be more adaptive and resilient.

Weight-bearing exercises are critical to mild arthritis cases because these put a little stress on the joints, stimulating a response with increased tensility and capacity over time. This stimulates the growth of new bone and new cartilage. Weight-bearing exercises include walking, running, weight lifting, tennis, squash, racquetball, basketball, soccer, baseball and so on. Biking is partially weight bearing. Swimming is non-weight bearing. One can moderate the exercise by doing different exercises on different days, while maintaining a minimal joint pain threshold.

Of course, arthritis sufferers can also take advantage of non-weight bearing exercises like swimming. Non-weight-bearing exercises can increase mobility and diversification while allowing the healing process to continue.

Hydration

Without an ample supply of water, the joints and the spinal discs are among the first regions of the body to be deprived of fluid resources. This is because these anatomical regions do not have direct vascular circulation. Joints do not draw fluids and nutrients directly from arteries like many tissues do. Chondrocytes and cartilage receive their fluid and nutrients from *lacunae*—tiny spaces between osteocytes. Tiny bone space canals called canaliculi feed this network, and draw from larger delivery canals called Haversian canals.

Fluids from arteries are prioritized towards the production of red blood cells in the bone marrow. Should there be sufficient hydration in the diet, there will be enough water left over to supply the cartilage. A lack of hydration will deprive the cartilage and discs first—to reserve water for marrow red blood cell manufacturing.

When the cartilage is deprived of water, chondrocytes cannot build healthy cartilage because water is a critical component of the matrix. What cartilage matrix does get produced may also be deficient in fluidity. In this condition, as the joint moves, the increased friction can cause the cartilage to further break down (Batmanghelidj 1991).

The question is how much water is necessary? Most health professionals suggest optimal water volume around six to eight 8-oz glasses per day. In 2004, the National Academy of Sciences released a study indicating that the average woman requires approximately 91 ounces of water per day, while men meet their needs with about 125 ounces per day. This study also indicated that approximately 80% of water intake comes from water and beverages and 20% comes from food. Therefore, we can assume a minimum of 73 ounces of fresh water for the average adult woman and 100 ounces of fresh water for the average adult man should cover our minimum needs. That is significantly more water than the standard eight glasses per day (64 ounces)—especially for men. It is not surprising that some health professionals suggest that 50-75% of Americans have chronic dehydration. Dr. Batmanghelidj, one of the world's most respected researchers on human hydration, suggests 1/2 ounce of water per pound of body weight. Anna Maria Sapugay, M.D. (2007) recommends up to an additional 32 ounces (after 64 ounces) for each forty-five minutes to an hour of strenuous activity. She suggests consuming 16 ounces of water before and 16 ounces after exercising, in addition to taking a few sips during exercise. Extremes in temperature and elevation increase our water requirements. Additional water is also required in the case of fever or increased sweating.

Most experts agree that as soon as we feel thirsty, our bodies are already experiencing dehydration. Becoming consciously thirsty is the point where tissue and cell damage is occurring. Our thirst sensation decreases as we age, so it is much easier to become dehydrated in our later years. Water is critical for the smooth running of all of our cells. Areas likely to suffer first during dehydration include our digestive tract, joints, eyes and liver. Some health experts have estimated as little as a 5% loss of body water will decrease physical performance by up to 30%. Dr. Sapugay suggests watching our urine to make sure we are getting enough water. Our urine color should range from light yellow to clear. Darker urine indicates dehydration.

The best water, as several World Health Organization studies have determined over the past decade, is natural spring or well water. These contain important minerals needed for building healthy cartilage.

Massage and Aromatherapy

Massage and aromatherapy are two proven methods to reduce stress and tension and increase the body's healing response. Massage is yet another way to increase circulation to deliver nutrients to the joints.

There are other benefits. The touch of a caring living being upon another radiates a number of subtle energies. The first of these is infrared. Each of us radiates unique infrared waves through our skin. This is why we can heat up a small bottle of liquid by just wrapping our hands around it. In the same way, by massaging, the masseuse radiates infrared waves deep into the dermal layers of their subject. Deep into the epidermal tissue, infrared radiation opens up small capillaries to increase blood flow, and relaxes nerve fibers. Increasing blood flow can increase nutrient delivery to the joints. Relaxing muscles also eases the tension on the joint, giving the tendons that attach to it better balance and support.

Massage also produces more subtle effects. Inflammation is associated with the body's production of stress hormones like cortisol. When anxiety is lessened, tension decreases. Decreased tension is often accompanied by an increase in the neurotransmitter gamma-aminobutyric acid (or GABA), which decreases pain sensation and strengthens the immune system (Abdou *et al.* 2006).

In one study (Field *et al.* 1997), children with juvenile rheumatoid arthritis were massaged by their parents for 15 minutes per day for 30 days with a control group receiving relaxation therapy. After the 30 days, the massaged children had lower levels of arthritic pain (incidence and severity), along with reduced anxiety levels.

Rubbing the joints in a circular fashion can increase circulation. A certified massage therapist is a good place to start. A good therapist can also show us some techniques to continue at home.

Accupuncture is also a good therapy for arthritis.

One type of massage therapy easily done at home is *skin brushing*. A soft, natural-fiber brush is recommended. Strokes can be circular around the joints, in the direction of the back flow of lymph (in towards the thymus or other larger glands). Again, a knowledgeable massage therapist or naturopath can illustrate the technique.

In addition to these general effects of massage, we can consider a number of botanical *essential oils* that have been used traditionally to reduce pain and encourage mobility for arthritis sufferers.

This has been supported by research. In one double-blind, placebo-controlled study (Yip and Tam 2008), 59 elderly persons with moderate-to-severe knee pain received the same massage, with olive oil only, ginger/orange essential oil, or no massage at all. One week after six massage sessions over a three week period, those patients receiving the essential oil combination massage had significantly less knee pain intensity, less stiffness, and enhanced mobility.

In another study (Atsumi, *et al.* 2007), smelling lavender and rosemary increased the body's free radical scavenging capacity and increased cortisol levels (which reduces inflammation).

Other aromatherapy essential oils used traditionally for arthritis and joint pain include:

Chamomile oil	Myrrh oil
Cypress oil	Pimento oil
Eucalyptus oil	Orange oil
Fennel oil	Pine oil
Frankincense oil	Rose oil
Ginger oil	Rosemary oil
Juniper oil	Tea tree oil
Lavender oil	Wintergreen oil
Lemon grass oil	Yarrow oil

(Tisserand 1979; Keville and Green 1995; Selby and Albright 1996; Ryman 1991, Worwood 1991)

It is probably best to choose three of these that attract us upon smelling. A maximum of three essential oils is advised. Two drops of each can be put into a hot bath. Two or three drops of each can also be put into two tablespoons of carrier oil such as olive oil or walnut oil and massaged onto the skin. Alternatively, a couple of drops of each may be put into the palm and rubbed into the skin. This latter method should be done with caution, however, because certain essentials may irritate the skin, especially for sensitive skin types. The carrier oil is good for this purpose. Even so, it is possible we might be sensitive to a particular botanical oil. Testing with one small drop first would be advisable.

Probiotics

We have discussed a number of scenarios relating to the infection of joints by invasive and pathogenic bacteria, fungi and viruses. While a strong immune system will defend against these, healthy probiotic colonies can help attack and crowd out pathogenic bacteria before they can advance through the body. This has been confirmed in numerous studies (see the author's book and published articles on probiotics for more specifics). In addition, research (such as Baharav *et al.* 2004) has illustrated that probiotic supplementation can reduce inflammation associated with arthritis.

Stress and Sleep

What would stress and sleep have to do with arthritis? Arthritis often occurs in those who are immunosuppressed. As we have discussed, immunosuppressed means that our immune system has become overloaded or depleted. Depletion of the immune system is directly associated with stress and sleep. A strong immune system depends upon rested and active adrenal glands, thymus gland, liver, kidneys and many other functional organs. Stress depletes adrenal response because it accelerates the adrenaline and cortisol cycles. Stress reduces thymus activity. Lack of sleep depletes circulating melatonin levels. Melatonin is an important component for the immune system, endocrine system and liver.

As we have discussed at length, arthritis is a symptom of a dysfunctional and overburdened immune system. Adequate sleep and reduced stress levels are important components to immune health.

Conclusion

The Bottom Line

The literature provides a substantial amount of data about arthritis. As we review the data logically, we come to different conclusions about arthritis than assumed by conventional medicine.

Determining the causes of a disease is not the same as determining the mechanisms of its symptoms. Modern medical research has advanced significantly in determining the mechanisms of inflammation and pain. These, however, are the *symptoms* of arthritis. Thus, the mechanisms of inflammation might be part of the causes for arthritis symptoms, but they are not the root causes of arthritis.

For this reason, much of the medical research has taken us off the track of discovery. It has focused us upon how to stop the symptoms. In most cases, this means somehow blocking the immune system. The problem with this strategy is that once the immune system is blocked, the body is left open to a variety of other opportunistic infections and injuries. Stopping the immune system also does not allow the body to complete the job of healing the damage or infection at the root of the problem.

This is not to say that pharmaceuticals are not effective at their intended purpose—to stop the symptoms.

However, the pharmaceutical solution also comes with a price. There are many adverse side effects that have been demonstrated in pharmaceutical research and from drug use in general. Because most pharmaceuticals have been ingeniously developed with one or two active constituents, they often imbalance the body's metabolic functions. Their chemical compositions are also often treated as toxins by the body, which further burdens the immune system.

In comparison, botanical medicines come with a very long history of successful use for ailments such as arthritis and inflammation. Most have a long history of safety among billions of people over thousands of years. This history can be added to a record of safety and clinical success in recent years, using modern research protocols.

Despite a lack of financial motive (as botanicals cannot be patented), botanical medicines are increasingly being studied side by side with pharmaceuticals, using the same methodology and protocols that pharmaceuticals have been studied with. We certainly commend and appreciate this research, but we also question the narrow bandwidth within which these studies are conducted. Botanicals deserve a much wider research perspective because they produce a wide spectrum of whole-body benefits. They stimulate various metabolic functions in different parts of the body, and strengthen different organs.

Yes, this research has proven that botanical medicines and foods can decrease pain and inflammation comparable to the effects of some of the most successful anti-inflammatory and pain-relieving pharmaceuticals. So we know that there is a botanical solution to the symptoms of arthritis—pain and inflammation.

However, the remaining question is whether a botanical diet combined with botanical medicines will do more than simply reduce pain and inflammation. Can botanicals cure arthritis?

The thesis presented here proposes the answer is *no*. The correct botanical herbs together with the appropriate mix of botanical foods, supported by a healthy combination of hydration, sunshine, exercise and sleep may not in themselves cure arthritis.

However, we propose that the right mix of botanical herbs and foods can stimulate the body *to repair itself*.

In other words, botanical medicines and foods, water, sunshine and exercise can stimulate and support the immune system's ability to repair the body. People do recover from disease, so we know the immune system has this ability. The right mix of botanicals will stimulate the immune system's ridding joint tissues of toxins and pathogens. Botanicals will stimulate the clean up of scarred and damaged cartilage. They will nourish chondrocytes, strengthen the liver, neutralize oxidative radicals, and quite possibly stimulate a regeneration of healthy cartilage and synovial tissues.

Botanical or herbal *medicine* is actually somewhat of a misnomer. Herbs and other botanicals do not cure disease in themselves. They stimulate the body's own healing abilities. The cells of the body are dying and being replaced constantly. This miracle we call the human body is designed to regenerate under certain environmental conditions and with certain inputs: *Natural conditions and botanical inputs.*

Our intention is to synchronize with that beautiful design.

References and Bibliography

Abdelouahab N, Heard C. Effect of the major glycosides of Harpagophytum procumbens (Devil's Claw) on epidermal cyclooxygenase-2 (COX-2) in vitro. *J Nat Prod.* 2008 May;71(5):746-9.

Abdelouahab N, Heard CM. Dermal and transcutaneous delivery of the major glycoside constituents of Harpagophytum procumbens (Devil's Claw) in vitro. *Planta Med.* 2008 Apr;74(5):527-31.

Abdou AM, Higashiguchi S, Horie K, Kim M, Hatta H, Yokogoshi H. Relaxation and immunity enhancement effects of gamma-aminobutyric acid GABA. *Biofactors.* 2006;26(3):201-8.

Abebe W. Herbal medication: potential for adverse interactions with analgesic drugs. *J Clin Pharm Ther.* 2002 Dec;27(6):391-401.

Abou-Seif MA. Blood antioxidant status and urine sulfate and thiocyanate levels in smokers. *J Biochem Toxicol.* 1996;11(3):133-138.

Adam O, Beringer C, Kless T, Lemmen C, Adam A, Wiseman M, Adam P, Klimmek R, Forth W. Anti-inflammatory effects of a low arachidonic acid diet and fish oil in patients with rheumatoid arthritis. *Rheumatol Int.* 2003 Jan;23(1):27-36.

Adam O. Nutrition as adjuvant therapy in chronic polyarthritis. *Z Rheumatol.* 1993 Sep-Oct;52(5):275-80.

ADAPT Research Group. Cardiovascular and cerebrovascular events in the randomized, controlled Alzheimer's Disease Anti-Inflammatory Prevention Trial (ADAPT). *PLoS Clin Trials.* 2006 Nov 17;1(7):e33.

Aderinto J, Knight D, Keating JF. Early syphilis: a cause of mono-arthritis of the knee. *Ann R Coll Surg Engl.* 2008 Jul;90(5):W1-3.

Agarwal SK, Singh SS, Verma S. Antifungal principle of sesquiterpene lactones from Anamirta cocculus. *Indian Drugs.* 1999;36:754-5.

Aggarwal BB, Harikumar KB. Potential therapeutic effects of curcumin, the anti-inflammatory agent, against neurodegenerative, cardiovascular, pulmonary, metabolic, autoimmune and neoplastic diseases. *Int J Biochem Cell Biol.* 2009 Jan;41(1):40-59.

Aggarwal BB, Sung B. Pharmacological basis for the role of curcumin in chronic diseases: an age-old spice with modern targets. *Trends Pharmacol Sci.* 2009 Feb;30(2):85-94.

Aho K, Koskenvuo M, Tuominen J, *et al.* Occurrence of rheumatoid arthritis in a nationwide series of twins. *J Rheumatol.* 1986;13(5): 899-902.

Airola P. *How to Get Well.* Phoenix, AZ: Health Plus, 1974.

Akkol EK, Güvenç A, Yesilada E. A comparative study on the antinociceptive and anti-inflammatory activities of five Juniperus taxa. *J Ethnopharmacol.* 2009 Jun 6.

Al-Ahaideb A. Septic arthritis in patients with rheumatoid arthritis. *J Orthop Surg Res.* 2008 Jul 29;3:33.

Albert LJ, Inman RD. Molecular mimicry and autoimmunity. *N Engl J Med.* 1999;341:2068-2074.

Alexandre P, Darmanyan D, Yushen G, Jenks W, Burel L, Eloy D, Jardon P. Quenching of Singlet Oxygen by Oxygen- and Sulfur-Centered Radicals: Evidence for Energy Transfer to Peroxyl Radicals in Solution. *J. Am. Chem. Soc.,* 120 (2), 396 -403, 1998.

Al-Harrasi A, Al-Saidi S. Phytochemical analysis of the essential oil from botanically certified oleogum resin of Boswellia sacra (Omani Luban). *Molecules.* 2008 Sep 16;13(9):2181-9.

Al-Mustafa AH, Al-Thunibat OY. Antioxidant activity of some Jordanian medicinal plants used traditionally for treatment of diabetes. *Pak J Biol Sci.* 2008 Feb 1;11(3):351-8.

Al-Tawfiq JA. Bacteroides fragilis bacteremia associated with vertebral osteomyelitis in a sickle cell patient. *Intern Med.* 2008;47(24):2183-5.

Altman RD, Marcussen KC. Effects of a ginger extract on knee pain in patients with osteoarthritis. *Arthritis Rheum.* 2001 Nov;44(11):2531-8.

American Conference of Governmental Industrial Hygienists. *Threshold limit values for chemical substances and physical agents in the work environment.* Cincinnati, OH: ACGIH, 1986.

American Dietetic Association; Dietitians of Canada. Position of the American Dietetic Association and Dietitians of Canada: vegetarian diets. *Can J Diet Pract Res.* 2003 Summer;64(2):62-81.

Ammon HP. Boswellic acids in chronic inflammatory diseases. *Planta Med.* 2006 Oct;72(12):1100-16.

Anand P, Thomas SG, Kunnumakkara AB, Sundaram C, Harikumar KB, Sung B, Tharakan ST, Misra K, Priyadarsini IK, Rajasekharan KN, Aggarwal BB. Biological activities of curcumin and its analogues (Congeners) made by man and Mother Nature. *Biochem Pharmacol.* 2008 Dec 1;76(11):1590-611.

Andermann A. Physicians, Fads, and Pharmaceuticals: A History of Aspirin. *McGill J Med.* 1996:2(2).

Anderson RC, Anderson JH. Acute toxic effects of fragrance products. *Arch Environ Health.* 1998 Mar-Apr;53(2):138-46.

Angioni A, Barra A, Russo MT, Coroneo V, Dessi S, Cabras P. Chemical composition of the essential oils of Juniperus from ripe and unripe berries and leaves and their antimicrobial activity. *J Agric Food Chem.* 2003 May 7;51(10):3073-8.

Anim-Nyame N, Sooranna SR, Johnson MR, Gamble J, Steer PJ. Garlic supplementation increases peripheral blood flow: a role for interleukin-6? *J Nutr Biochem.* 2004 Jan;15(1):30-6.

Anonymous. Cimetidine inhibits the hepatic hydroxylation of vitamin D. *Nutr Rev.* 1985;43:184-5.

Aoki, T. *et al.* Low natural killer syndrome: Clinical and immunologic features. *Natural Immunity.* 1987;6: 116-128.

Apáti P, Houghton PJ, Kite G, Steventon GB, Kéry A. In-vitro effect of flavonoids from Solidago canadensis extract on glutathione S-transferase. *J Pharm Pharmacol.* 2006 Feb;58(2):251-6.

Argento A, Tiraferri E, Marzaloni M. Oral anticoagulants and medicinal plants. An emerging interaction. Ann Ital Med Int. 2000 Apr-Jun;15(2):139-43.

Armstrong D. How the New England Journal Missed Warning Signs on Vioxx. *Wall Street J.* 2006 May 15, A1. http://online.wsj.com/article/SB114765430315252591.html.

Arterburn LM, Oken HA, Hoffman JP, Bailey-Hall E, Chung G, Rom D, Hamersley J, McCarthy D. Bioequivalence of Docosahexaenoic acid from different algal oils in capsules and in a DHA-fortified food. *Lipids.* 2007 Nov;42(11):1011-24.

Arterburn LM, Oken HA, Bailey Hall E, Hamersley J, Kuratko CN, Hoffman JP. Algal-oil capsules and cooked salmon: nutritionally equivalent sources of docosahexaenoic acid. *J Am Diet Assoc.* 2008 Jul;108(7):1204-9.

Arthanari S, Yusuf S, Nisar M. Tuberculosis of the knee complicating seronegative arthritis. *J Rheumatol.* 2008 Jun;35(6):1227-8.

Associated Press. Merck to Pay $4.85B Vioxx Settlement. *Newsvine.com.* 2007 Nov 9. 6:57 AM EST. http://www.newsvine.com/ _news/2007/11/09/1084627-merck-to-pay-485b-vioxx-settlement. Accessed August 19, 2009.

Atcheson SG, Ward JR. Acute hematogenous osteomyelitis progressing to septic synovitis and eventual pyarthrosis: the vascular pathway. *Arthritis Rheum.* 1978;21:968–971.

Atsumi T, Tonosaki K. Smelling lavender and rosemary increases free radical scavenging activity and decreases cortisol level in saliva. *Psychiatry Res.* 2007 Feb 28;150(1):89-96.

Avery RK. Vaccination of the immunosuppressed adult patient with rheumatologic disease. *Rheum Dis Clin.* 1999 Aug;25(3):567-84, viii.

Azumagawa K, Kambara Y, Murata T, Tamai H. Four cases of arthritis associated with Mycoplasma pneumoniae infection. *Pediatr Int.* 2008 Aug;50(4):511-3.

Bachmann KA, Sullivan TJ, Jauregui L, *et al.* Drug interactions of H2-receptor antagonists. *Scand J Gastroenterol Suppl.* 1994;206:14-9.

Bader G, Plohmann B, Hiller K, Franz G. Cytotoxicity of triterpenoid saponins. Part 1: Activities against tumor cells in vitro and hemolytical index. *Pharmazie.* 1996 Jun;51(6):414-7.

Baghdikian B, Lanhers MC, Fleurentin J, Ollivier E, Maillard C, Balansard G, Mortier F. An analytical study, anti-inflammatory and analgesic effects of Harpagophytum procumbens and Harpagophytum zeyheri. *Planta Med.* 1997 Apr;63(2):171-6.

Baghdikian B, Ollivier E, Faure R, Debrauwer L, Rathelot P, Balansard G. Two new pyridine monoterpene alkaloids by chemical conversion of a commercial extract of harpagophytum procumbens. *J Nat Prod.* 1999 Feb;62(2):211-3.

Baharav E, Mor F, Halpern M, Weinberger A. Lactobacillus GG bacteria ameliorate arthritis in Lewis rats. *J Nutr.* 2004 Aug;134(8):1964-9.

Baker DH. Comparative nutrition and metabolism: explication of open questions with emphasis on protein and amino acids. *Proc Natl Acad Sci U S A.* 2005 Dec 13;102(50):17897-902.

Baker DH. Utilization of isomers and analogs of amino acids and other sulfur-contiaining compounds. *Prog. Food Nutr Sci.* 1986.

Baker SM. *Detoxification and Healing.* Chicago: Contemporary Books, 2004.

Balch P, Balch J. *Prescription for Nutritional Healing.* New York: Avery, 2000.

Baldwin CT, Cupples LA, Joost O, Demissie S, Chaisson C, Mcalindon T, Myers RH, Felson D. Absence of linkage or association for osteoarthritis with the vitamin D receptor/type II collagen locus: the Framingham Osteoarthritis Study. *J Rheumatol.* 2002 Jan;29(1):161-5.

Ballentine R. *Diet & Nutrition: A holistic approach.* Honesdale, PA: Himalayan Int., 1978.

Ballentine R. *Radical Healing.* New York: Harmony Books, 1999.

Banno N, Akihisa T, Yasukawa K, Tokuda H, Tabata K, Nakamura Y, Nishimura R, Kimura Y, Suzuki T. Anti-inflammatory activities of the triterpene acids from the resin of Boswellia carteri. *J Ethnopharmacol.* 2006 Sep 19;107(2):249-53.

Barclay TS, Tsourounis C, McCart GM. Glucosamine. *Ann Pharmacother.* 1998 May;32(5):574-9.

Barnaulov OD, Denisenko PP. Anti-ulcer action of a decoction of the flowers of the dropwort, Filipendula ulmaria (L.) Maxim. *Farmakol Toksikol.* 1980 Nov-Dec;43(6):700-5.

Barnaulov OD, Denisenko PP. Anti-ulcer action of a decoction of the flowers of the dropwort, Filipendula ulmaria (L.) Maxim. *Farmakol Toksikol.* 1980 Nov-Dec;43(6):700-5.

Barnhill JG, Fye CL, Williams DW, Reda DJ, Harris CL, Clegg DO. Chondroitin product selection for the glucosamine/chondroitin arthritis intervention trial. *J Am Pharm Assoc* (2003). 2006 Jan-Feb;46(1):14-24.

Basu A, Devaraj S, Jialal I. Dietary factors that promote or retard inflammation. *Arterioscler Thromb Vasc Biol.* 2006 May;26(5):995-1001.

Bateman HE, Kirou KA, Paget SA, Crow MK, Yee AM. Remission of juvenile rheumatoid arthritis after infection with parvovirus B19. *J Rheumatol.* 1999 Nov;26(11):2482-4.

Bates DW, Cullen DJ, Laird N, Petersen LA, Small SD, Servi D, Laffel G, Sweitzer BJ, Shea BF, Hallisey R, *et al.* Incidence of adverse drug events and potential adverse drug events. Implications for prevention. ADE Prevention Study Group. *JAMA.* 1995 Jul 5;274(1):29-34.

Batmanghelidj F. Neurotransmitter histamine: an alternative view point, *Science in Medicine Simplified.* Falls Church, VA: Foundation for the Simple in Medicine, 1990.

Batmanghelidj F. *How to Deal Simply with Back Pain and Rheumatoid Joint Pain.* Vienna, VA: Global Health, 1991.

Batmanghelidj F. *Your Body's Many Cries for Water.* 2nd Ed. Vienna, VA: Global Health, 1997.

Baum J. Infection and rheumatoid arthritis. *Arthritis Rheum.* 1971;14:135–137.

Beasley R, Clayton T, Crane J, von Mutius E, Lai CK, Montefort S, Stewart A; ISAAC Phase Three Study Group. Association between paracetamol use in infancy and childhood, and risk of asthma, rhinoconjunctivitis, and eczema in children aged 6-7 years: analysis from Phase Three of the ISAAC programme. *Lancet.* 2008 Sep. 20;372(9643):1039-48.

Becker KG, Simon RM, Bailey-Wilson JE, *et al.*: Clustering of non-major histocompatibility complex susceptibility candidate loci in human autoimmune diseases. *Proc Natl Acad Sci USA* 1998;95(17):9979-9984.

Beddoe AF. *Biologic Ionization as Applied to Human Nutrition.* Warsaw: Wendell Whitman, 2002.

Beecher GR. Phytonutrients' role in metabolism: effects on resistance to degenerative processes. *Nutr Rev.* 1999 Sep;57(9 Pt 2):S3-6.

Bell IR, Baldwin CM, Schwartz GE, Illness from low levels of environmental chemicals: relevance to chronic fatigue syndrome and fibromyalgia. *Am J Med.* 1998;105 (suppl 3A).:74-82. S.

Bellamy N, Duffy D, Martin N, *et al.* Rheumatoid arthritis in twins: a study of aetiopathogenesis based on the Australian Twin Registry. *Ann Rheum Dis* 1992;51(5): 588-593.

Bengmark S. Curcumin, an atoxic antioxidant and natural NFkappaB, cyclooxygenase-2, lipooxygenase, and inducible nitric oxide synthase inhibitor: a shield against acute and chronic diseases. *JPEN J Parenter Enteral Nutr.* 2006 Jan-Feb;30(1):45-51.

Bennett GJ, Update on the neurophysiology of pain transmission and modulation: focus on the NMDA-receptor. *J Pain Symptom Manage.* 2000;19 (suppl 1):S.:2-6.

Bensky D, Gable A, Kaptchuk T (transl.). *Chinese Herbal Medicine Materia Medica.* Seattle: Eastland Press, 1986.

Bergner P. *The Healing Power of Garlic.* Prima Publishing, Rocklin CA 1996.

Berkow R., (Ed.) *The Merck Manual of Medical Information Home Edition.* New York: Pocket Books, 1997.

Berkow R., (Ed.) *The Merck Manual of Diagnosis and Therapy.* 16th Edition. Rahway, N.J.: Merck Research Labs, 1992.

Berteau O and Mulloy B. 2003. Sulfated fucans, fresh perspectives: structures, functions, and biological properties of sulfated fucans and an overview of enzymes active toward this class of polysaccharide. *Glycobiology.* Jun;13(6):29R-40R.

Bhandari U, Sharma JN, Zafar R. The protective action of ethanolic ginger (Zingiber officinale) extract in cholesterol fed rabbits. *J Ethnopharmacol.* 1998 Jun;61(2):167-71.

Biegert C, Wagner I, Lüdtke R, Kötter I, Lohmüller C, Günaydin I, Taxis K, Heide L. Efficacy and safety of willow bark extract in the treatment of osteoarthritis and rheumatoid arthritis: results of 2 randomized double-blind controlled trials. *J Rheumatol.* 2004 Nov;31(11):2121-30.

Bishop B. Pain: its physiology and rationale for management. Part III. Consequences of current concepts of pain mechanisms related to pain management. *Phys Ther.* 1980 Jan;60(1):24-37.

Blackburn WD, Jr, Dunn TL, Alarcon GS. Infection versus disease activity in rheumatoid arthritis: eight years' experience. *South Med J.* 1986;79:1238–1241.

Bland CM, Thomas S. Micafungin plus fluconazole in an infected knee with retained hardware due to Candida albicans. *Ann Pharmacother.* 2009 Mar;43(3):528-31.

Block AA, Marshall C, Ratcliffe A, Athan E. Staphylococcal pyomyositis in a temperate region: epidemiology and modern management. *Med J Aust.* 2008 Sep 15;189(6):323-5.

Bobel D, Sadkowska-Todys M. Yersiniosis in Poland in 2006. *Przegl Epidemiol.* 2008;62(2):287-93.

Boivin DB, Czeisler CA. Resetting of circadian melatonin and cortisol rhythms in humans by ordinary room light. Neuroreport. 1998 Mar 30;9(5):779-82.

Boje K, Lechtenberg M, Nahrstedt A. New and known iridoid- and phenylethanoid glycosides from Harpagophytum procumbens and their in vitro inhibition of human leukocyte elastase. *Planta Med.* 2003 Sep;69(9):820-5.

Boltin D, Katzir M, Bugoslavsky V, Yalashvili I, Brosh-Nissimov T, Fried M, Elkayam O. Corynebacterium striatum—a classic pathogen eluding diagnosis. *Eur J Intern Med.* 2009 May;20(3):e49-52.

Bombardier C, Laine L, Reicin A, *et al.* Comparison of upper gastrointestinal toxicity of rofecoxib and naproxen in patients with rheumatoid arthritis. VIGOR Study Group. *N. Engl. J. Med.* 2000;343(21):1520–8, 2 p following 1528.

Bombardier C, Laine L, Reicin A, Shapiro D, Burgos-Vargas R, Davis B, Day R, Ferraz MB, Hawkey CJ, Hochberg MC, Kvien TK, Schnitzer TJ; VIGOR Study Group. Comparison of upper gastrointestinal toxicity of rofecoxib and naproxen in patients with rheumatoid arthritis. VIGOR Study Group. *N Engl J Med.* 2000 Nov 23;343(21):1520-8, 2 p following 1528.

Bombardier C. An evidence-based evaluation of the gastrointestinal safety of coxibs. *Am J Cardiol.* 2002 Mar 21;89(6A):3D-9D.

Bongartz D, Hesse A. Selective extraction of quercetrin in vegetable drugs and urine by off-line coupling of boronic acid affinity chromatography and high-performance liquid chromatography. *J Chromatogr B Biomed Appl.* 1995 Nov 17;673(2):223-30.

Borchers AT, Hackman RM, Keen CL, Stern JS, Gershwin ME. Complementary medicine: a review of immunomodulatory effects of Chinese herbal medicines. *Am J Clin Nutr.* 1997 Dec;66(6):1303-12.

Borchert VE, Czyborra P, Fetscher C, Goepel M, Michel MC. Extracts from Rhois aromatica and Solidaginis virgaurea inhibit rat and human bladder contraction. *Naunyn Schmiedebergs Arch Pharmacol.* 2004 Mar;369(3):281-6.

Boston University. Effects Of Vitamin D And Skin's Physiology Examined. *ScienceDaily.* 2008 February 24. Retrieved February 24, 2008, from http://www.sciencedaily.com/releases/ 2008/02/ 080220161707.htm

Boyd B, Zungoli P, Benson E. 2006. *Dust Mites.* HGIC 2551; Clemson University. http://hgic.clemson.edu.

Bradette-Hébert ME, Legault J, Lavoie S, Pichette A. A new labdane diterpene from the flowers of Solidago canadensis. *Chem Pharm Bull.* 2008 Jan;56(1):82-4.

Breedveld FC, LaFeber GJM, Barselaar MT van den, van Dissel JT, Leijh PCJ. Phagocytosis and intracellular killing of Staphylococcus aureus by polymorophonuclear cells from synovial fluid of patients with rheumatoid arthritis. *Arthritis Rheum.* 1986;29:166–173.

Bresalier RS, Sandler RS, Quan H, *et al.* Cardiovascular events associated with rofecoxib in a colorectal adenoma chemoprevention trial. *N. Engl. J. Med.* 2005;352(11):1092–102.

Brighenti F, Valtuena S, Pellegrini N, *et al.* Total Antioxidant Capacity of the Diet Is Inversely and Independently Related to Plasma Concentration of High-Sensitivity C-Reactive Protein in Adult Italian Subjects. *Br J Nutr.* 2005;93(5):619-25.

Brinkhaus B, Witt CM, Jena S, Linde K, Streng A, Hummelsberger J, Irnich D, Hammes M, Pach D, Melchart D, Willich SN. Physician and treatment characteristics in a randomised multicentre trial of acupuncture in patients with osteoarthritis of the knee. *Complement Ther Med.* 2007 Sep;15(3):180-9.

Brody J. *Jane Brody's Nutrition Book.* New York: WW Norton, 1981.

Bronner F, Worrell RV. *Orthopaedics: Principles of Basic and Clinical Science.* London: Informa HealthCare, 1999.

Brown JM, Chung S, Sawyer JK, Degirolamo C, Alger HM, Nguyen T, Zhu X, Duong MN, Wibley AL, Shah R, Davis MA, Kelley K, Wilson MD, Kent C, Parks JS, Rudel LL. Inhibition of stearoyl-coenzyme A desaturase 1 dissociates insulin resistance and obesity from atherosclerosis. *Circulation.* 2008 Sep 30;118(14):1467-75.

Brownstein D. *Salt: Your Way to Health.* West Bloomfield, MI: Medical Alternatives, 2006.

Brzeski M, Madhok R, Capell HA. Evening primrose oil in patients with rheumatoid arthritis and side-effects of non-steroidal anti-inflammatory drugs. *Br J Rheumatol.* 1991 Oct;30(5):370-2.

Budzianowski J. Coumarins, caffeoyltartaric acids and their artifactual methyl esters from Taraxacum officinale leaves. *Planta Med.* 1997 Jun;63(3):288.

Bundy R, Walker AF, Middleton RW, Booth J. Turmeric extract may improve irritable bowel syndrome symptomology in otherwise healthy adults: a pilot study. *J Altern Complement Med.* 2004 Dec;10(6):1015-8.

Burdge GC, Jones AE, Wootton SA. Eicosapentaenoic and docosapentaenoic acids are the principal products of alpha-linolenic acid metabolism in young men. *B J Nutr.* 2002 Oct;88(4):355-63.

Burdge GC, Wootton SA. Conversion of alpha-linolenic acid to eicosapentaenoic, docosapenta-enoic and docosahexaenoic acids in young women. *B J Nutr.* 2002 Oct;88(4):411-20.

Burits M, Asres K, Bucar F. The antioxidant activity of the essential oils of Artemisia afra, Artemisia abyssinica and Juniperus procera. *Phytother Res.* 2001 Mar;15(2):103-8.

Busch A. Hydrotherapy improves pain, knee strength, and quality of life in women with fibromyalgia. *Aust J Physiother.* 2007;53(1):64.

Butani L, Afshinnik A, Johnson J, Javaheri D, Peck S, German JB, Perez RV. Amelioration of tacrolimus-induced nephrotoxicity in rats using juniper oil. *Transplantation.* 2003 Jul 27;76(2):306-11.

Cahn J, Borzeix MG. Administration of procyanidolic oligomers in rats. Observed effects on changes in the permeability of the blood-brain barrier. *Sem Hop.* 1983 Jul 7;59(27-28):2031-4.

Calder PC. Dietary modification of inflammation with lipids. *Proc Nutr Soc.* 2002 Aug;61(3):345-58.

Callender ST, Spray GH. Latent pernicious anemia. *Br J Haematol* 1962;8:230-240.

Calliste CA, Trouillas P, Allais DP, Simon A, Duroux JL. Free radical scavenging activities measured by electron spin resonance spectroscopy and B16 cell antiproliferative behaviors of seven plants. *J Agric Food Chem.* 2001 Jul;49(7):3321-7.

Cameron JS, Moro F, Simmonds HA. Gout, uric acid and purine metabolism in paediatric nephrology. *Pediatr Nephrol.* 1993 Feb;7(1):105-18.

Cao G, Alessio HM, Cutler RG. Oxygen-radical absorbance capacity assay for antioxidants. *Free Radic Biol Med.* 1993 Mar;14(3):303-11.

Cao G, Giovanoni M, Prior RL. Antioxidant capacity in different tissues of young and old rats. *Proc Soc Exp Biol Med.* 1996 Apr;211(4):359-65.

Cao G, Russell RM, Lischner N, Prior RL. Serum antioxidant capacity is increased by consumption of strawberries, spinach, red wine or vitamin C in elderly women. *J Nutr.* 1998 Dec;128(12):2383-90.

Cao G, Shukitt-Hale B, Bickford PC, Joseph JA, McEwen J, Prior RL. Hyperoxia-induced changes in antioxidant capacity and the effect of dietary antioxidants. *J Appl Physiol.* 1999 Jun;86(6):1817-22.

Caramia G. [The essential fatty acids omega-6 and omega-3: from their discovery to their use in therapy]. *Minerva Pediatr.* 2008 Apr;60(2):219-33.

Cardoso ML, Xavier CA, Bezerra MB, Paiva AO, Carvalho MF, Benevides NM, Rocha FA, Leite EL. Assessment of Zymosan-Induced Leukocyte Influx in a Rat Model using Sulfated Polysaccharides. *Planta Med.* 2009 Aug 3.

Carroll D. *The Complete Book of Natural Medicines.* New York: Summit, 1980.

Carron PN, Yerly S, Ksontini R, Calandra T, Meylan P. [Pyoderma gangrenosum: diagnostic and therapeutic challenge]. *Rev Med Suisse.* 2008 Sep 10;4(170):1938-40, 1942-3.

Carson R. *Silent Spring.* Houghton Mifflin: Mariner Books, 1962.

Cavaleiro C, Pinto E, Gonçalves MJ, Salgueiro L. Antifungal activity of Juniperus essential oils against dermatophyte, Aspergillus and Candida strains. *J Appl Microbiol.* 2006 Jun;100(6):1333-8.

Cesarone MR, Belcaro G, Nicolaides AN, Ricci A, Geroulakos G, Ippolito E, Brandolini R, Vinciguerra G, Dugall M, Griffin M, Ruffini I, Acerbi G, Corsi M, Riordan NH, Stuard S, Bavera P, Di Renzo A, Kenyon J, Errichi BM. Prevention of venous thrombosis in long-haul flights with Flite Tabs: the LONFLIT-FLITE randomized, controlled trial. *Angiology.* 2003 Sep-Oct;54(5):531-9.

Chaitow L, Trenev N. *ProBiotics.* New York: Thorsons, 1990.

Chaitow L. *Conquer Pain the Natural Way.* San Francisco: Chronicle Books, 2002.

Chakürski I, Matev M, Koĭchev A, Angelova I, Stefanov G. Treatment of chronic colitis with an herbal combination of Taraxacum officinale, Hipericum perforatum, Melissa officinaliss, Calendula officinalis and Foeniculum vulgare. *Vutr Boles.* 1981;20(6):51-4.

Chaney M, Ross M. *Nutrition.* New York: Houghton Mifflin, 1971.

Chang CI, Chen WC, Shao YY, Yeh GR, Yang NS, Chiang W, Kuo YH. A new labdane-type diterpene from the bark of Juniperus chinensis Linn. *Nat Prod Res.* 2008;22(13):1158-62.

Chantre P, Cappelaere A, Leblan D, Guedon D, Vandermander J, Fournie B. Efficacy and tolerance of Harpagophytum procumbens versus diacerhein in treatment of osteoarthritis. *Phytomedicine.* 2000 Jun;7(3):177-83.

Chapat L, Chemin K, Dubois B, Bourdet-Sicard R, Kaiserlian D. Lactobacillus casei reduces CD8+ T cell-mediated skin inflammation. *Eur J Immunol.* 2004 Sep;34(9):2520-8.

Characterization and quantitation of Antioxidant Constituents of Sweet Pepper (Capsicum annuum - Cayenne). *J Agric Food Chem.* 2004 Jun 16;52(12):3861-9.

Chaudhary R, Jahan S, Goyal PK. Chemopreventive potential of an Indian medicinal plant (Tinospora cordifolia) on skin carcinogenesis in mice. *J Environ Pathol Toxicol Oncol.* 2008;27(3):233-43.

Chavali SR, Weeks CE, Zhong WW, Forse RA. Increased production of TNF-alpha and decreased levels of dienoic eicosanoids, IL-6 and IL-10 in mice fed menhaden oil and juniper oil diets in response to an intraperitoneal lethal dose of LPS. Prostaglandins Leukot Essent Fatty Acids. 1998 Aug;59(2):89-93.

Chen YF, Jobanputra P, Barton P, Bryan S, Fry-Smith A, Harris G, Taylor RS. Cyclooxygenase-2 selective non-steroidal anti-inflammatory drugs (etodolac, meloxicam, celecoxib, rofecoxib, etoricoxib, valdecoxib and lumiracoxib) for osteoarthritis and rheumatoid arthritis: a systematic review and economic evaluation. *Health Technol Assess.* 2008 Apr;12(11):1-278, iii.

Chen Z. Clinical study of 96 cases with chronic hepatitis B treated with jiedu yanggan gao by a double-blind method. *Zhong Xi Yi Jie He Za Zhi.* 1990 Feb;10(2):71-4, 67.

Chevrier MR, Ryan AE, Lee DY, Zhongze M, Wu-Yan Z, Via CS. Boswellia carterii extract inhibits TH1 cytokines and promotes TH2 cytokines in vitro. *Clin Diagn Lab Immunol.* 2005 May;12(5):575-80.

Chilton F, Tucker L. *Win the War Within.* New York: Rodale, 2006.

Chilton FH, Rudel LL, Parks JS, Arm JP, Seeds MC. Mechanisms by which botanical lipids affect inflammatory disorders. *Am J Clin Nutr.* 2008 Feb;87(2):498S-503S.

Chinnadurai SK, Troan BV, Wolf KN, DeVoe RS, Huijsmans CJ, Hermans MH, Wever PC. Septicemia, endocarditis, and cerebral infarction due to Staphylococcus aureus in a harp seal (Phoca groenlandica). *J Zoo Wildl Med.* 2009 Jun;40(2):393-7.

Cho SY, Park JY, Park EM, Choi MS, Lee MK, Jeon SM, Jang MK, Kim MJ, Park YB. Alternation of hepatic antioxidant enzyme activities and lipid profile in streptozotocin-induced diabetic rats by supplementation of dandelion water extract. *Clin Chim Acta.* 2002 Mar;317(1-2):109-17.

Choi HK, De Vera MA, Krishnan E. Gout and the risk of type 2 diabetes among men with a high cardiovascular risk profile. *Rheumatology.* 2008 Oct;47(10):1567-70.

Choi SZ, Choi SU, Lee KR. Phytochemical constituents of the aerial parts from Solidago virga-aurea var. gigantea. *Arch Pharm Res.* 2004 Feb;27(2):164-8.

Chopra A, Lavin P, Patwardhan B, Chitre D. A 32-Week Randomized, Placebo-Controlled Clinical Evaluation of RA-11, an Ayurvedic Drug, on Osteoarthritis of the Knees. *J Clin Rheumatol.* 2004 Oct;10(5):236-245.

Chopra RN, Nayar SL, Chopra IC, eds. *Glossary of Indian Medicinal plants.* New Delhi: CSIR, 1956.

Chorny A, Anderson P, Gonzalez-Rey E, Delgado M. Ghrelin protects against experimental sepsis by inhibiting high-mobility group box 1 release and by killing bacteria. *J Immunol.* 2008 Jun 15;180(12):8369-77.

Christopher J. *School of Natural Healing.* Springville UT: Christopher Publ, 1976.

Chrubasik S, Eisenberg E, Balan E, Weinberger T, Luzzati R, Conradt C. Treatment of low back pain exacerbations with willow bark extract: a randomized double-blind study. *Am J Med.* 2000 Jul;109(1):9-14.

Chrubasik S, Junck H, Breitschwerdt H, Conradt C, Zappe H. Effectiveness of Harpagophytum extract WS 1531 in the treatment of exacerbation of low back pain: a randomized, placebo-controlled, double-blind study. *Eur J Anaesthesiol.* 1999 Feb;16(2):118-29.

Chrubasik S, Künzel O, Black A, Conradt C, Kerschbaumer F. Potential economic impact of using a proprietary willow bark extract in outpatient treatment of low back pain: an open non-randomized study. *Phytomedicine.* 2001 Jul;8(4):241-51.

Chrubasik S, Künzel O, Model A, Conradt C, Black A. Treatment of low back pain with a herbal or synthetic anti-rheumatic: a randomized controlled study. Willow bark extract for low back pain. *Rheumatology.* 2001 Dec;40(12):1388-93.

Chrubasik S, Pollak S. Pain management with herbal antirheumatic drugs. *Wien Med Wochenschr.* 2002;152(7-8):198-203.

Chu YF, Liu RH. Cranberries inhibit LDL oxidation and induce LDL receptor expression in hepatocytes. *Life Sci.* 2005;77(15):1892-1901. 27.

Chun LJ, Tong MJ, Busuttil RW, Hiatt JR. Acetaminophen hepatotoxicity and acute liver failure. *J Clin Gastroenterol.* 2009 Apr;43(4):342-9.Becker R. *The Body Electric.* New York: Morrow, Inc., 1985.

Churin AA, Masnaia NV, Sherstoboev EIu, Shilova IV. Effect of Filipendula ulmaria extract on immune system of CBA/CaLac and C57Bl/6 mice. *Eksp Klin Farmakol.* 2008 Sep-Oct;71(5):32-6.

Churin AA, Masnaia NV, Sherstoboev EIu, Shilova IV. Effect of Filipendula ulmaria extract on immune system of CBA/CaLac and C57Bl/6 mice. *Eksp Klin Farmakol.* 2008 Sep-Oct;71(5):32-6.

Clarkson C, Staerk D, Hansen SH, Smith PJ, Jaroszewski JW. Identification of major and minor constituents of Harpagophytum procumbens (Devil's claw) using HPLC-SPE-NMR and HPLC-ESIMS/APCIMS. *J Nat Prod.* 2006 Sep;69(9):1280-8.

Clegg DO, Reda DJ, Harris CL, Klein MA, O'Dell JR, Hooper MM, Bradley JD, Bingham CO 3rd, Weisman MH, Jackson CG, Lane NE, Cush JJ, Moreland LW, Schumacher HR Jr, Oddis CV, Wolfe F, Molitor JA, Yocum DE, Schnitzer TJ, Furst DE, Sawitzke AD, Shi H, Brandt KD, Moskowitz RW, Williams HJ. Glucosamine, chondroitin sulfate, and the two in combination for painful knee osteoarthritis. *N Engl J Med.* 2006 Feb 23;354(8):795-808.

Clegg DO, Reda DJ, Harris CL, Klein MA, O'Dell JR, Hooper MM, Bradley JD, Bingham CO 3rd, Weisman MH, Jackson CG, Lane NE, Cush JJ, Moreland LW, Schumacher HR Jr, Oddis CV, Wolfe F, Molitor JA, Yocum DE, Schnitzer TJ, Furst DE, Sawitzke AD, Shi H, Brandt KD, Moskowitz RW, Williams HJ. Glucosamine, chondroitin sulfate, and the two in combination for painful knee osteoarthritis. *N Engl J Med.* 2006 Feb 23;354(8):795-808.

Conquer JA, Holub BJ. Dietary docosahexaenoic acid as a source of eicosapentaenoic acid in vegetarians and omnivores. *Lipids.* 1997 Mar;32(3):341-5.

Cooper C, McAlindon T, Coggon D, Egger P, Dieppe P. Occupational activity and osteoarthritis of the knee. *Ann Rheum Dis.* 1994 Feb;53(2):90-3.

Cooper GS, Miller FW, Germolec DR: Occupational exposures and autoimmune diseases. *Int Immunopharm* 2002, 2:303-313.

Cooper K. *The Aerobics Program for Total Well-Being.* New York: Evans, 1980.

Corbe C, Boissin JP, Siou A. Light vision and chorioretinal circulation. Study of the effect of procyanidolic oligomers (Endotelon). *J Fr Ophtalmol.* 1988;11(5):453-60.

Couzy F, Kastenmayer P, Vigo M, Clough J, Munoz-Box R, Barclay DV. Calcium bioavailability from a calcium- and sulfate-rich mineral water, compared with milk, in young adult women. *Am J Clin Nutr.* 1995 Dec;62(6):1239-44.

Crescente M, Jessen G, Momi S, Höltje HD, Gresele P, Cerletti C, de Gaetano G. Interactions of gallic acid, resveratrol, quercetin and aspirin at the platelet cyclooxygenase-1 level. Functional and modelling studies. *Thromb Haemost.* 2009 Aug;102(2):336-46.

Cruccu G, Aziz TZ, Garcia-Larrea L, Hansson P, Jensen TS, Lefaucheur JP, Simpson BA, Taylor RS. EFNS guidelines on neurostimulation therapy for neuropathic pain. *Eur J Neurol.* 2007 Sep;14(9):952-70.

Cummings M. *Human Heredity: Principles and Issues.* St. Paul, MN: West, 1988.

Cunnane G, Doran M, Bresnihan B. Infection and biological therapy in rheumatoid arthritis. *Best Pract Res Clin Rheumatol.* 2003;17:345–363.

Curtis *et al.* and Steel, K. Too Many Elderly Are Taking Dangerous Drugs. *Arch Internal Med.* 2004;164:1621-1625, 1603-1604.

Cwikla C, Schmidt K, Matthias A, Bone KM, Lehmann R, Tiralongo E. Investigations into the antibacterial activities of phytotherapeutics against Helicobacter pylori and Campylobacter jejuni. *Phytother Res.* 2009 Aug 3.

da Costa AC, Luna AS, Pafumé R. Characterization of thermostructural damages observed in a seaweed used for biosorption of cadmium: effects on the kinetics and uptake. *Appl Biochem Biotechnol.* 2007 Apr;137-140(1-12):835-45.

Danko JR, Gilliland WR, Miller RS, Decker CF. Disseminated Mycobacterium marinum infection in a patient with rheumatoid arthritis receiving infliximab therapy. *Scand J Infect Dis.* 2009;41(4):252-5.

Davies G. *Timetables of Medicine.* New York: Black Dog & Leventhal, 2000.

de Almeida AE, Schroeder LF, Caldeira NG, da Silva NM, Batista PR, Gallo MP, de Filippis I. Septic arthritis due to Haemophilus influenzae serotype a in the post-vaccination era in Brazil. *J Med Microbiol.* 2008 Oct;57(Pt 10):1311-2.

de Freitas MV, Netto Rde C, da Costa Huss JC, de Souza TM, Costa JO, Firmino CB, Penha-Silva N. Influence of aqueous crude extracts of medicinal plants on the osmotic stability of human erythrocytes. *Toxicol In Vitro.* 2008 Feb;22(1):219-24.

de Haan J, Vreeling AW, van Hellemondt GG. Reactivation of ancient joint tuberculosis of the knee following total knee arthroplasty after 61 years: a case report. *Knee.* 2008 Aug;15(4):336-8.

de la Torre, J.C., *et al.* Modifications of experimental spinal cord injuries using dimethyl sulfoxide. *Trans Am Neurol Assoc.* 1971;97:230.

De Lucca AJ, Bland JM, Vigo CB, Cushion M, Selitrennikoff CP, Peter J, Walsh TJ. CAY-I, a fungicidal saponin from Capsicum sp. fruit. *Med Mycol.* 2002 Apr;40(2):131-7.

De Smet PA. Herbal remedies. *N Engl J Med.* 2002;347:2046–2056.

Dean C. *Death by Modern Medicine.* Belleville, ON: Matrix Verite-Media, 2005.

Deapen D, Escalante A, Weinrib L. A revised estimate of twin concordance in systemic lupus erythematosus. *Arthritis Rheum.* 1992;35:311-318.

Delcomyn F. *Foundations of Neurobiology.* New York: W.H. Freeman and Co., 1998.

Demos, C.H., Beckloff, G.L., Donin, M.N., Oliver, P.M. Dimethyl sulfoxide in musculoskeletal disorders. *Ann NY Acad Sci.* 1967;141:517-523.

Deutsche Gesellschaft für Ernährung. Drink distilled water? *Med. Mo. Pharm.* 1993;16:146.

Devaraj TL. *Speaking of Ayurvedic Remedies for Common Diseases.* New Delhi: Sterling, 1985.

Devirian TA, Volpe SL. The physiological effects of dietary boron. *Crit Rev Food Sci Nutr.* 2003;43(2):219-31

Di Munno O, Mazzantini M, Delle Sedie A, Mosca M, Bombardieri S. Risk factors for osteoporosis in female patients with systemic lupus erythematosus. *Lupus.* 2004;13(9):724-30.

Dickens E. (Ed.) *The Da Vinci Notebooks.* London: Profile, 2005.

Diğrak M, Ilçim A, Hakki Alma M. Antimicrobial activities of several parts of Pinus brutia, Juniperus oxycedrus, Abies cilicia, Cedrus libani and Pinus nigra. *Phytother Res.* 1999 Nov;13(7):584-7.

Ding X, Staudinger JL. The ratio of constitutive androstane receptor to pregnane X receptor determines the activity of guggulsterone against the Cyp2b10 promoter. *J Pharmacol Exp Ther.* 2005 Jul;314(1):120-7.

Donato F, Monarca S, Premi S., and Gelatti, U. Drinking water hardness and chronic degenerative diseases. Part III. Tumors, urolithiasis, fetal malformations, deterioration of the cognitive function in the aged and atopic eczema. *Ann. Ig.* 2003;15:57-70.

Dooley, M.A. and Hogan S.L. Environmental epidemiology and risk factors for autoimmune disease. *Curr Opin Rheum.* 2003;15(2):99-103.

D'Orazio N, Ficoneri C, Riccioni G, Conti P, Theoharides TC, Bollea MR. Conjugated linoleic acid: a functional food? Int J Immunopathol Pharmacol. 2003 Sep-Dec;16(3):215-20.

Dotolo Institute. *The Study of Colon Hydrotherapy.* Pinellas Park, FL: Dotolo, 2003.

Drubaix I, Maraval M, Robert L, Robert AM. Hyaluronic acid (hyaluronan) levels in pathological human saphenous veins. Effects of procyanidol oligomers, *Pathol Biol.* 1997 Jan;45(1):86-91.

Drubaix I, Robert L, Maraval M, Robert AM. Synthesis of glycoconjugates by human diseased veins: modulation by procyanidolic oligomers. *Int J Exp Pathol.* 1997 Apr;78(2):117-21.

Du Q, Jerz G, Shen L, Xiu L, Winterhalter P. Isolation and structure determination of a lignan from the bark of Salix alba. *Nat Prod Res.* 2007 May;21(5):451-4.

Dubnov-Raz G, Scheuerman O, Chodick G, Finkelstein Y, Samra Z, Garty BZ. Invasive Kingella kingae infections in children: clinical and laboratory characteristics. *Pediatrics.* 2008 Dec;122(6):1305-9.

Dubost JJ, Fis I, Lopitaux R, Soubrier M, Ristori JM, Bussiere JL, Sirot J. Polyarticular Septic Arthritis. *Medicin.* 1993;72:296–310.

Duke J. *The Green Pharmacy.* New York: St. Martins, 1997.

Dumoulin M, Pille F, Van den Abeele AM, Haesebrouck F, Oosterlinck M, Gasthuys F, Martens A. Evaluation of an automated blood culture system for the isolation of bacteria from equine synovial fluid. *Vet J.* 2009 Feb 18.

Dunstan JA, Roper J, Mitoulas L, Hartmann PE, Simmer K, Prescott SL. The effect of supplementation with fish oil during pregnancy on breast milk immunoglobulin A, soluble CD14, cytokine levels and fatty acid composition. *Clin Exp Allergy.* 2004 Aug;34(8):1237-42.

Dupeux S, Pouchot J. Osteomyelitis and septic arthritis. Vertebral osteomyelitis. *Rev Prat.* 2008 Nov 15;58(17):1943-51.

Duwiejua M, Zeitlin IJ, Waterman PG, Chapman J, Mhango GJ, Provan GJ. Anti-inflammatory activity of resins from some species of the plant family Burseraceae. *Planta Med.* 1993 Feb;59(1):12-6.

Ebers GC, Kukay K, Bulman DE, Sadovnick AD, Rice G, Anderson C, Armstrong H, Cousin K, Bell RB, Hader W, Paty DW, Hashimoto S, Oger J, Duquette P, Warren S, Gray T, O'Connor P, Nath A, Auty A, Metz L, Francis G, Paulseth JE, Murray TJ, Pryse-Phillips W, Nelson R, Freedman M, Brunet D, Bouchard JP, Hinds D, Risch N. A full genome search in multiple sclerosis. *Nat Genet.* 1996 Aug;13(4):472-6.

Edris AE. Pharmaceutical and therapeutic potentials of essential oils and their individual volatile constituents: a review. *Phytother Res.* 2007 Apr;21(4):308-23.

el-Ghazaly M, Khayyal MT, Okpanyi SN, Arens-Corell M. Study of the anti-inflammatory activity of Populus tremula, Solidago virgaurea and Fraxinus excelsior. *Arzneimittelforschung.* 1992 Mar;42(3):333-6.

El-Ghorab A, Shaaban HA, El-Massry KF, Shibamoto T. Chemical composition of volatile extract and biological activities of volatile and less-volatile extracts of juniper berry (Juniperus drupacea L.) fruit. *J Agric Food Chem.* 2008 Jul 9;56(13):5021-5.

El-Shemy HA, Aboul-Enein AM, Aboul-Enein MI, Issa SI, Fujita K. The effect of willow leaf extracts on human leukemic cells in vitro. *J Biochem Mol Biol.* 2003; 36 (4): 387-389.

Ellingwood F. *American Materia Medica, Therapeutics and Pharmacognosy.* Portland: Eclectic Medical Publ., 1983.

Elwood PC. Epidemiology and trace elements. *Clin Endocrinol Metab.* 1985 Aug;14(3):617-28.

Engel, M.F., Dimethyl sulfoxide in the treatment of scleroderma. *South Med J.* 1972;65:71.

Engell V, Bach A, Davidsen M, Moller-Madsen B. Purulent coxitis in 8-year-old boy caused by Salmonella enteritidis. *Ugeskr Laeger.* 2009 Apr 27;171(18):1515-6.

Environmental Working Group. *Human Toxome Project.* 2007. http://www.ewg.org/sites/ humantoxome/. Accessed: 2007 Sep.

Environmental Working Group. *Human Toxome Project.* 2007. http://www.ewg.org/sites/humantoxome/. Accessed: 2007 Sep.

EPA. *A Brief Guide to Mold, Moisture and Your Home.* Environmental Protection Agency, Office of Air and Radiation/Indoor Environments Division. EPA 2002;402-K-02-003.

Epstein JH, Zimmerman B, Ho G. Polyarticular septic arthritis. *J Rheumatol.* 1986;13:1105–1107.

Ernst E. Frankincense: systematic review. *BMJ.* 2008 Dec 17;337:a2813.

Evans P, Forte D, Jacobs C, Fredhoi C, Aitchison E, Hucklebridge F, Clow A. Cortisol secretory activity in older people in relation to positive and negative well-being. *Psychoneuroendocrinology.* 2007 Aug 7

Evans, M.S., Reid, K.H., Sharp, J.B. Dimethyl sulfoxide (DMSO) blocks conduction in peripheral nerve C fibers: A possible mechanism of analgesia. *Neurosci Lett.* 1993;150:145-148..

Everhart JE. *Digestive Diseases in the United States.* Darby, PA: Diane Pub, 1994.

Fan AY, Lao L, Zhang RX, Zhou AN, Wang LB, Moudgil KD, Lee DY, Ma ZZ, Zhang WY, Berman BM. Effects of an acetone extract of Boswellia carterii Birdw. (Burseraceae) gum resin on adjuvant-induced arthritis in lewis rats. *J Ethnopharmacol.* 2005 Oct 3;101(1-3):104-9.

Fanella S, Schantz D, Karlowsky J, Rubinstein E. Septic Arthritis Due To Roseomonas gilardii In An Immunocompetent Adolescent. *J Med Microbiol.* 2009 Jul 2.

FAO/WHO Expert Committee. Fats and Oils in Human Nutrition. Food and Nutrition Paper. 1994;(57).

Favero M, Schiavon F, Riato L, Carraro V, Punzi L. Rheumatoid arthritis is the major risk factor for septic arthritis in rheumatological settings. *Autoimmun Rev.* 2008 Oct;8(1):59-61.

Fawell J, Nieuwenhuijsen MJ. Contaminants in drinking water. *Br Med Bull.* 2003;68:199-208.

Fawthrop F, Hornby J, Swan A, Hutton C, Doherty M, Dieppe P. A comparison of normal and pathological synovial fluid. *Br J Rheumatol.* 1985 Feb;24(1):61-9.

Fe Marqués A, Maestre Vera JR, Mateo Maestre M, González Romo F, Castrillo Amores MA. Septic arthritis of the knee due to Prevotella loescheii following tooth extraction. *Med Oral Patol Oral Cir Bucal.* 2008 Aug 1;13(8):E505-7.

Fecka I. Qualitative and quantitative determination of hydrolysable tannins and other polyphenols in herbal products from meadowsweet and dog rose. *Phytochem Anal.* 2009 May;20(3):177-90.

Fernandes G, Bhattacharya A, Rahman M, Zaman K, Banu J. Effects of n-3 fatty acids on autoimmunity and osteoporosis. *Front Biosci.* 2008 May 1;13:4015-20.

Feskanich D, Willett W, Colditz G. Calcium, vitamin D, milk consumption, and hip fractures: a prospective study among postmenopausal women. *Am J Clin Nutr.* 2003 Feb;77(2): 504-511.

Field T, Hernandez-Reif M, Seligman S, Krasnegor J, Sunshine W, Rivas-Chacon R, Schanberg S, Kuhn C. Juvenile rheumatoid arthritis: benefits from massage therapy. *J Pediatr Psychol.* 1997 Oct;22(5):607-17.

Filipowicz N, Kamiński M, Kurlenda J, Asztemborska M, Ochocka JR. Antibacterial and antifungal activity of juniper berry oil and its selected components. *Phytother Res.* 2003 Mar;17(3):227-31.

Fisher P. Homeopathy and The Lancet. *Evid Based Complement Alternat Med.* 2006 March; 3(1):145–147. Folic acid metabolism in human subjects revisited: potential implications for proposed mandatory folic acid fortification in the UK. *Brit J Nutr.* 2007; Oct;98(4).

Flandrin, J, Montanari M(eds.). *Food: A Culinary History from Antiquity to the Present.* New York: Penguin Books, 1999.

Foster S, Hobbs C. *Medicinal Plants and Herbs.* Boston: Houghton Mifflin, 2002.

Fox RD, *Algoculture.* Doctorate Disseration, 1983 Jul.

Franciotta D, Salvetti M, Lolli F, Serafini B, Aloisi F. B cells and multiple sclerosis. *Lancet Neurol.* 2008 Sep;7(9):852-8.

Frawley D, Lad V. *The Yoga of Herbs.* Sante Fe: Lotus Press, 1986.

Frech TM, Clegg DO. The utility of nutraceuticals in the treatment of osteoarthritis. *Curr Rheumatol Rep.* 2007 Apr;9(1):25-30.

French SD, Cameron M, Walker BF, Reggars JW, Esterman AJ. Superficial heat or cold for low back pain. *Cochrane Database Syst Rev.* 2006 Jan 25;(1):CD004750.

Fritioff A, Greger M. Aquatic and terrestrial plant species with potential to remove heavy metals from stormwater. *Int J Phytoremediation.* 2003;5(3):211-24.

Gaby AR. Natural treatments for osteoarthritis. *Altern Med Rev.* 1999 Oct;4(5):330-41.

Gagnier JJ, DeMelo J, Boon H, Rochon P, Bombardier C. Quality of reporting of randomized controlled trials of herbal medicine interventions. *Am J Med.* 2006;119:1–11.

Gagnier JJ, van Tulder M, Berman B, Bombardier C. Herbal medicine for low back pain. *Cochrane Database Syst Rev.* 2006 Apr 19;(2):CD004504

Gagnier JJ, van Tulder MW, Berman B, Bombardier C. Herbal medicine for low back pain: a Cochrane review. *Spine* 2007 Jan 1;32(1):82-92.

Galkin A, Jokela J, Wahlsten M, Tammela P, Sivonen K, Vuorela P. Discovering protein kinase C active plants growing in Finland utilizing automated bioassay combined to LC/MS. *Nat Prod Commun.* 2009 Jan;4(1):139-42.

Gandhi T, Weingart S, Borus J, Seger A, Peterson J, Burdick E, Seger D, Shu K, Federico F, Leape L, Bates D. Adverse drug events in ambulatory care. *N Engl J Med.* 2003 Apr 17;348(16):1556-64.

Gao JX, Issekutz AC, Issekutz TB. Neutrophils migrate to delayed-type hypersensitivity reactions in joints, but not in skin. Mechanism is leukocyte function-associated antigen-1-/Mac-1-independent. *J Immunol.* 1994 Dec 15;153(12):5689-97.

Garcia Gomez LJ, Sanchez-Muniz FJ. Review: cardiovascular effect of garlic (Allium sativum). *Arch Latinoam Nutr.* 2000 Sep;50(3):219-29.

García-Lechuz J, Bouza E. Treatment recommendations and strategies for the management of bone and joint infections. *Expert Opin Pharmacother.* 2009 Jan;10(1):35-55.

Gardner GC, Weisman MH. Pyarthrosis in patients with rheumatoid arthritis: A report of 13 cases and a review on the literature from the past 40 years. *Am J Med.* 1990;88:503–511.

Geller DS, Pope JB, Thornhill BA, Dorfman HD. Cryptococcal pyarthrosis and sarcoidosis. *Skeletal Radiol.* 2009 Jul;38(7):721-7.

Georgian Med News. Phitochemical investigation of juniper rufescens Juniperus oxycedrus L. leaves and fruits. 2009 Mar;(168):107-11.

Gerosa M, De Angelis V, Riboldi P, Meroni PL. Rheumatoid arthritis: a female challenge. *Womens Health* 2008 Mar;4(2):195-201.

Ghadioungui P. (transl.) *The Ebers Papyrus.* Academy of Scientific Research. Cairo, 1987.

Ghayur MN, Gilani AH. Ginger lowers blood pressure through blockade of voltage-dependent calcium Channels acting as a cardiotonic pump activator in mice, rabbit and dogs. *J Cardiovasc Pharmacol.* 2005 Jan;45(1):74-80.

Gibbons E. *Stalking the Healthful Herbs.* New York: David McKay, 1966.

Gibson RA. Docosa-hexaenoic acid (DHA) accumulation is regulated by the polyunsaturated fat content of the diet: Is it synthesis or is it incorporation? *Asia Pac J Clin Nutr.* 2004;13(Suppl):S78.

Giovannucci E. The epidemiology of vitamin D and cancer incidence and mortality: *Cancer Causes Control.* 2005 Mar;16(2):83-95.

Glück U, Gebbers J. Ingested probiotics reduce nasal colonization with pathogenic bacteria (Staphylococcus aureus, Streptococcus pneumoniae, and b-hemolytic streptococci. Am J. Clin. Nutr. 2003;77:517-520.

Göbel H, Heinze A, Ingwersen M, Niederberger U, Gerber D. Effects of Harpagophytum procumbens LI 174 (devil's claw) on sensory, motor und vascular muscle reagibility in the treatment of unspecific back pain. *Schmerz.* 2001 Feb;15(1):10-8.

Gohil K, Packer L. Bioflavonoid-Rich Botanical Extracts Show Antioxidant and Gene Regulatory Activity. *Ann N Y Acad Sci.* 2002:957:70-7.

Goldbach-Mansky R, Wilson M, Fleischmann R, Olsen N, Silverfield J, Kempf P, Kivitz A, Sherrer Y, Pucino F, Csako G, Costello R, Pham TH, Snyder C, van der Heijde D, Tao X, Wesley R, Lipsky PE. Comparison of Tripterygium wilfordii Hook F versus sulfasalazine in the treatment of rheumatoid arthritis: a randomized trial. *Ann Intern Med.* 2009 Aug 18;151(4):229-40, W49-51.

Goldenberg DL, Red JI. Bacterial Arthritis. *N Engl J Med.* 1985;312:764–771.

Goldenberg DL. Infectious arthritis complicating rheumatoid arthritis and other chronic rheumatic disorders. *Arthritis Rheum.* 1989;32:496–502. doi: 10.1002/anr.1780320422.

Golub E. *The Limits of Medicine.* New York: Times Books, 1994.

Gonzales, *et al.* 1987. Polysaccharides as antiviral agents: antiviral activity of carrageenan, *Antimicrobial Agents and Chemotherapy.* 31:1388-1393.

Govindarajan VS, Sathyanarayana MN. Capsicum-production, technology, chemistry, and quality. Part V. Impact on physiology, pharmacology, nutrition, and metabolism; structure, pungency, pain, and desensitization sequences. *Crit Rev Food Sci Nutr.* 1991;29(6):435-74.

Grant WB, Holick MF. Benefits and requirements of vitamin D for optimal health: a review. *Altern Med Rev.* 2005 Jun;10(2):94-111.

Grant WB. Solar ultraviolet irradiance and cancer incidence and mortality. *Adv Exp Med Biol.* 2008;624:16-30.

Grasmuller S, Irnich D. Acupuncture in pain therapy. *MMW Fortschr Med.* 2007 Jun 21;149(25-26):37-9.

Gray H. *Anatomy, Descriptive and Surgical.* 15th Edition. New York: Random House, 1977.

Gray-Davison F. *Ayurvedic Healing.* New York: Keats, 2002.

Griffith HW. *Healing Herbs: The Essential Guide.* Tucson: Fisher Books, 2000.

Grupper M, Potasman I, Rosner I, Slobodin G, Rozenbaum M. Septic arthritis due to Staphylococcus lugdunensis in a native joint. *Rheumatol Int.* 2009 Jul 1.

Grzanna R, Lindmark L, Frondoza CG. Ginger—an herbal medicinal product with broad anti-inflammatory actions. *J Med Food.* 2005 Summer;8(2):125-32.

Guerin M, Huntley ME, Olaizola M. Haematococcus astaxanthin: applications for human health and nutrition. *Trends Biotechnol.* 2003 May;21(5):210-6.

Guillén Fiel G, Gonzalez-Granado LI, Mosqueda R, Negreira S, Giangaspro E. [Arthritis caused by Candida in an immunocompetent infant with a history of systemic candidiasis in the neonatal period.]. *An Pediatr.* 2009 Apr;70(4):383-5.

Gundermann KJ, Müller J. Phytodolor—effects and efficacy of a herbal medicine. *Wien Med Wochenschr.* 2007;157(13-14):343-7.

Guo J. Chronic fatigue syndrome treated by acupuncture and moxibustion in combination with psychological approaches in 310 cases. *J Tradit Chin Med.* 2007 Jun;27(2):92-5.

Gutmanis J. *Hawaiian Herbal Medicine.* Waipahu, HI: Island Heritage, 2001.

Haines JL, Ter-Minassian M, Bazyk A, Gusella JF, Kim DJ, Terwedow H, Pericak-Vance MA, Rimmler JB, Haynes CS, Roses AD, Lee A, Shaner B, Menold M, Seboun E, Fitoussi RP, Gartioux C, Reyes C,

REFERENCES AND BIBLIOGRAPHY

Ribierre F, Gyapay G, Weissenbach J, Hauser SL, Goodkin DE, Lincoln R, Usuku K, Oksenberg JR, *et al.* A complete genomic screen for multiple sclerosis underscores a role for the major histocompatability complex. The Multiple Sclerosis Genetics Group. *Nat Genet.* 1996 Aug;13(4):469-71.

Hambäck PA, Stenberg JA, Ericson L. Asymmetric indirect interactions mediated by a shared parasitoid: connecting species traits and local distribution patterns for two chrysomelid beetles. *Oecologia.* 2006 Jun;148(3):475-81.

Hammond B, Mayhew D, *et al.* Safety assessment of DHA-rich microalgae from Schizochytrium sp. Regul *Toxicol Pharmacol.* 2002;35(2 Pt 1):255-65.

Han Y. Rutin has therapeutic effect on septic arthritis caused by Candida albicans. *Int Immunopharmacol.* 2009 Feb;9(2):207-11.

Hardy CJ, Palmer RP, Muir KR, *et al.* Systemic lupus erythematosus (SLE) and hair treatment: a large community based case-control study. *Lupus.* 1999;8(7): 541-544.

Harkins T, Grissom C. Magnetic Field Effects on B12 Ethanolamine Ammonia Lyase: Evidence for a Radical Mechanism. *Science.* 1994;263:958-960.

Harvald B, Hauge M: Hereditary factors elucidated by twin studies. *In Genetics and the Epidemiology of Chronic Disease.* Edited by Neel JV, Shaw MV, Schull WJ. Washington, DC: Department of Health, Education and Welfare, 1965:64-76.

Hata K, Ishikawa K, Hori K, Konishi T. Differentiation-inducing activity of lupeol, a lupane-type triterpene from Chinese dandelion root (Hokouei-kon), on a mouse melanoma cell line. *Biol Pharm Bull.* 2000 Aug;23(8):962-7.

Haugen MA, Kjeldsen-Kragh J, Skakkebaek N, Landaas S, Sjaastad O, Movinkel P, Førre O. The influence of fast and vegetarian diet on parameters of nutritional status in patients with rheumatoid arthritis. *Clin Rheumatol.* 1993 Mar;12(1):62-9.

Heaney RP, Dowell MS. Absorbability of the calcium in a high-calcium mineral water. *Osteoporos Int.* 1994 Nov;4(6):323-4.

Heck AM, DeWitt BA, Lukes AL. Potential interactions between alternative therapies and warfarin. *Am J Health Syst Pharm.* 2000 Jul 1;57(13):1221-7; quiz 1228-30.

Hedner T, Everts B. The early clinical history o f salicylates in rheumatology and pain. *Clin Rheumatol.* 1998;17(1): 17-25.

Heilpern AJ, Wertheim W, He J, Perides G, Bronson RT, Hu LT. Matrix metalloproteinase 9 plays a key role in lyme arthritis but not in dissemination of Borrelia burgdorferi. *Infect Immun.* 2009 Jul;77(7):2643-9.

Hendel B, Ferreira P. *Water & Salt: The Essence of Life.* Gaithersburg: Natural Resources, 2003.

Henih HIa, Ladna LIa. Phytochemical study of the dropworts, Filipendula ulmaria and F. hexapetala, from the flora of Lvov Province. *Farm Zh.* 1980;(1):50-2.

Herbert V. Vitamin B12: Plant sources, requirements, and assay. *Am J Clin Nutr.* 1988;48:852-858.

Herschler, R., Jacob, S.W. The case of dimethyl sulfoxide. In: Lasagna, L. (Ed.), *Controversies in Therapeutics.* Philadelphia: W.B. Saunders, 1980.

Hess EV: Environmental lupus syndromes. *Br J Rheumatol* 1995, 34(7): 597-599.

Ho YW, Yeung JS, Chiu PK, Tang WM, Lin ZB, Man RY, Lau CS. Ganoderma lucidum polysaccharide peptide reduced the production of proinflammatory cytokines in activated rheumatoid synovial fibroblast. *Mol Cell Biochem.* 2007 Jul;301(1-2):173-9.

Hobbs. C. *Herbal Remedies for Dummies.* New York: Wiley Publ., 1998.

Hobbs C. *Medicinal Mushrooms.* Summertown, TN: Botanica Press, 1986.

Hobbs C. *Stress & Natural Healing.* Loveland, CO: Interweave Press, 1997.

Hoffmann D. *Holistic Herbal.* London: Thorsons, 1983-2002.

Holick MF. Sunlight and vitamin D for bone health and prevention of autoimmune diseases, cancers, and cardiovascular disease. *Am J Clin Nutr.* 2004 Dec;80(6 Suppl):1678S-88S.

Holick MF. The vitamin D deficiency pandemic and consequences for nonskeletal health: mechanisms of action. *Mol Aspects Med.* 2008 Dec;29(6):361-8

Holick MF. Vitamin D for health and in chronic kidney disease. *Semin Dial.* 2005 Jul-Aug;18(4):266-75.

Holick MF. Vitamin D status: measurement, interpretation, and clinical application. *Ann Epidemiol.* 2009 Feb;19(2):73-8.

Holick MF. Vitamin D: importance in the prevention of cancers, type 1 diabetes, heart disease, and osteoporosis. *Am J Clin Nutr.* 2004 Mar;79(3):362-71.

Holladay, S.D. Prenatal Immunotoxicant Exposure and Postnatal Autoimmune Disease. *Environ Health Perspect.* 1999; 107(suppl 5):687-691.

Holmquist G. Susumo Ohno left us January 13, 2000, at the age of 71. *Cytogenet and Cell Genet.* 2000;88:171-172.

Hönscheid A, Rink L, Haase H. T-lymphocytes: a target for stimulatory and inhibitory effects of zinc ions. *Endocr Metab Immune Disord Drug Targets.* 2009 Jun;9(2):132-44.

Horino T, Takao T, Hashimoto K. Invasive Streptococcus agalactiae septic arthritis mimicking polymyalgia rheumatica. *South Med J*. 2009 Jan;102(1):109-10.

Horrobin DF. Effects of evening primrose oil in rheumatoid arthritis. *Ann Rheum Dis*. 1989 Nov;48(11):965-6.

Hoskin M.(ed.). *The Cambridge Illustrated History of Astronomy*. Cambridge: Cambridge Press, 1997.

Hostanska K, Jürgenliemk G, Abel G, Nahrstedt A, Saller R. Willow bark extract (BNO1455) and its fractions suppress growth and induce apoptosis in human colon and lung cancer cells. *Cancer Detect Prev*. 2007;31(2):129-39.

Hu C, Kitts DD. Antioxidant, prooxidant, and cytotoxic activities of solvent-fractionated dandelion (Taraxacum officinale) flower extracts in vitro. *J Agric Food Chem*. 2003 Jan 1;51(1):301-10.

Hu C, Kitts DD. Dandelion (Taraxacum officinale) flower extract suppresses both reactive oxygen species and nitric oxide and prevents lipid oxidation in vitro. *Phytomedicine*. 2005 Aug;12(8):588-97.

Hu C, Kitts DD. Luteolin and luteolin-7-O-glucoside from dandelion flower suppress iNOS and COX-2 in RAW264.7 cells. *Mol Cell Biochem*. 2004 Oct;265(1-2):107-13.

Huang D, Ou B, Prior RL. The chemistry behind antioxidant capacity assays. J Agric Food Chem. 2005 Mar 23;53(6):1841-56.

Huang TH, Tran VH, Duke RK, Tan S, Chrubasik S, Roufogalis BD, Duke CC. Harpagoside suppresses lipopolysaccharide-induced iNOS and COX-2 expression through inhibition of NF-kappa B activation. *J Ethnopharmacol*. 2006 Mar 8;104(1-2):149-55.

Hunt RH, Barkun AN, Baron D, Bombardier C, Bursey FR, Marshall JR, Morgan DG, Paré P, Thomson AB, Whittaker JS. Recommendations for the appropriate use of anti-inflammatory drugs in the era of the coxibs: defining the role of gastroprotective agents. *Can J Gastroenterol*. 2002 Apr;16(4):231-40.

Iida N, Inatomi Y, Murata H, Inada A, Murata J, Lang FA, Matsuura N, Nakanishi T. A new flavone xyloside and two new flavan-3-ol glucosides from Juniperus communis var. depressa. *Chem Biodivers*. 2007 Jan;4(1):32-42.

Innis SM, Hansen JW. Plasma fatty acid responses, metabolic effects, and safety of microalgal and fungal oils rich in arachidonic and docosahexaenoic acids in adults. *Am J Clin Nutr*. 1996 Aug;64(2):159-67.

Innocenti M, Michelozzi M, Giaccherini C, Ieri F, Vincieri FF, Mulinacci N. Flavonoids and biflavonoids in Tuscan berries of Juniperus communis L.: detection and quantitation by HPLC/DAD/ESI/MS. *J Agric Food Chem*. 2007 Aug 8;55(16):6596-602.

Int J Toxicol. Final report on the safety assessment of Juniperus communis Extract, Juniperus oxycedrus Extract, Juniperus oxycedrus Tar, Juniperus phoenicea extract, and Juniperus virginiana Extract. *Int J Toxicol*. 2001;20 Suppl 2:41-56.

Iwami O, Watanabe T, Moon CS, Nakatsuka H, Ikeda M. Motor neuron disease on the Kii Peninsula of Japan: excess manganese intake from food coupled with low magnesium in drinking water as a risk factor. *Sci. Total Environ*. 1994;149:121-135.

Jagetia GC, Aggarwal BB. "Spicing up" of the immune system by curcumin. *J Clin Immunol*. 2007 Jan;27(1):19-35.

Jagetia GC, Nayak V, Vidyasagar MS. Evaluation of the antineoplastic activity of guduchi (Tinospora cordifolia) in cultured HeLa cells. *Cancer Lett*. 1998 May 15;127(1-2):71-82.

Jagetia GC, Rao SK. Evaluation of Cytotoxic Effects of Dichloromethane Extract of Guduchi (Tinospora cordifolia Miers ex Hook F & THOMS) on Cultured HeLa Cells. *Evid Based Complement Alternat Med*. 2006 Jun;3(2):267-72.

Jagetia GC, Rao SK. Evaluation of the antineoplastic activity of guduchi (Tinospora cordifolia) in Ehrlich ascites carcinoma bearing mice. *Biol Pharm Bull*. 2006 Mar;29(3):460-6.

James JA, Kaufman KM, Farris AD, et al. An increased prevalence of Epstein-Barr virus infection in young patients suggests a possible etiology for systemic lupus erythematosus. *J Clin Invest*. 1997, 100:3019-3026.

Jarvis DC. *Folk Medicine*. Greenwich, CN: Fawcett, 1958.

Jawaheer D, Thomson W, MacGregor AJ, et al. Homozygosity for the HLA-DR shared epitope contributes the highest risk for rheumatoid arthritis concordance in identical twins. *Arthritis Rheum*. 1994;37(5):681-686.

Jensen B. *Foods that Heal*. Garden City Park, NY: Avery Publ, 1988, 1993.

Jensen B. *Nature Has a Remedy*. Los Angeles: Keats, 2001.

Jeon HJ, Kang HJ, Jung HJ, Kang YS, Lim CJ, Kim YM, Park EH. Anti-inflammatory activity of Taraxacum officinale. *J Ethnopharmacol* 2008 Jan 4;115(1):82-8.

Jerie P. Milestones of cardivascular pharmacotherapy: salicylates and aspirin. *Cas Lek Cesk*. 2006;145(12):901-4.

Jhon MS. *The Water Puzzle and the Hexagonal Key*. Uplifting, 2004.

Jin ZX, Yang G, Piao YA. Chemical constituents of tannin in Filipendula palmata Pall. *Zhongguo Zhong Yao Za Zhi.* 1994 Jan;19(1):32-3, 62.

Johari H. *Ayurvedic Massage: Traditional Indian Techniques for Balancing Body and Mind.* Rochester, VT: Healing Arts, 1996.

Johnson LM. Gitksan medicinal plants—cultural choice and efficacy. *J Ethnobiol Ethnomed.* 2006 Jun 21;2:29.

Johnston WH, Karchesy JJ, Constantine GH, Craig AM. Antimicrobial activity of some Pacific Northwest woods against anaerobic bacteria and yeast. *Phytother Res.* 2001 Nov;15(7):586-8.

Jones MA, Silman AJ, Whiting S, *et al.* Occurrence of rheumatoid arthritis is not increased in the first degree relatives of a population based inception cohort of inflammatory polyarthritis. *Ann Rheum Dis.* 1996;55(2): 89-93.

Jones R. Nonsteroidal anti-inflammatory drug prescribing: past, present, and future. *Am J Med.* 2001,110 (1A):4S-7S.

Jones SM, Zhong Z, Enomoto N, Schemmer P, Thurman RG. Dietary juniper berry oil minimizes hepatic reperfusion injury in the rat. *Hepatology.* 1998 Oct;28(4):1042-50.

Jürgenliemk G, Petereit F, Nahrstedt A. Flavan-3-ols and procyanidins from the bark of Salix purpurea L. *Pharmazie.* 2007 Mar;62(3):231-4.

Julie G, Julie C, Anne G, Bernard F, Philippe V, Madeleine C, Jolivet-Gougeon A. Childhood delayed septic arthritis of the knee caused by Serratia fonticola. *Knee.* 2009 Apr 27.

Julkunen-Tiitto R, Meier B. Variation in growth and secondary phenolics among field-cultivated clones of Salix myrsinifolia. *Planta Med.* 1992; 58 (1): 77-80.

Julkunen-Tiitto R. A chemotaxonomic survey of phenolics in leaves of northern Salicaceae species. *Phytochemistry.* 1986;25(3):663-667.

Jurenka JS. Anti-inflammatory properties of curcumin, a major constituent of Curcuma longa: a review of preclinical and clinical research. *Altern Med Rev.* 2009 Feb;14(2):141-153.

Kaandorp CJE, van Schaardenburg D, Krijnen P, Habbema JDF, Laar MAFJ ven de. Risk factor for septic arthritis in patients with joint disease. *Arthritis Rheum.* 1995;38:1819–1825.

Kähkönen MP, Hopia AI, Vuorela HJ, Rauha JP, Pihlaja K, Kujala TS, Heinonen M. Antioxidant activity of plant extracts containing phenolic compounds. *J Agric Food Chem.* 1999 Oct;47(10):3954-62.

Kammerer B, Kahlich R, Biegert C, Gleiter CH, Heide L. HPLC-MS/MS analysis of willow bark extracts contained in pharmaceutical preparations. *Phytochem Anal.* 2005 Nov-Dec;16(6):470-8.

Kandel E, Siegelbaum S, Schwartz J. Synaptic transmission. *Principles of Neural Science.* New York: Elsevier, 1991.

Kaptchuk TJ. The placebo effect in alternative medicine: can the performance of a healing ritual have clinical significance? *Ann Intern Med.* 2002 Jun 4;136(11):817-25.

Karaman I, Sahin F, Güllüce M, Ogütçü H, Sengül M, Adigüzel A. Antimicrobial activity of aqueous and methanol extracts of Juniperus oxycedrus L. *J Ethnopharmacol.* 2003 Apr;85(2-3):231-5.

Kashiwada Y, Takanaka K, Tsukada H, Miwa Y, Taga T, Tanaka S, Ikeshiro Y. Sesquiterpene glucosides from anti-leukotriene B4 release fraction of Taraxacum officinale. *J Asian Nat Prod Res.* 2001;3(3):191-7.

Katina ZF, Silant'eva KN. Filipendula hexapetala Bilib., its distribution and possibilities of use. *Farm Zh.* 1968;23(4):72-5.

Kazansky DB. MHC restriction and allogeneic immune responses. *J Immunotoxicol.* 2008 Oct;5(4):369-84.

Kearney PM, Baigent C, Godwin J, Halls H, Emberson JR, Patrono C. Do selective cyclo-oxygenase-2 inhibitors and traditional non-steroidal anti-inflammatory drugs increase the risk of atherothrombosis? Meta-analysis of randomised trials. *BMJ* 2006;332 (7553): 1302–8.

Kelder P. *Ancient Secret of the Fountain of Youth: Book 1.* New York: Doubleday, 1998.

Kelley GA, Kelley KS, Tran ZV. Aerobic exercise and lipids and lipoproteins in women: a meta-analysis of randomized controlled trials. *J Womens Health.* 2004 Dec;13(10):1148-64.

Kellgren JH, Ball J, Fairbrother RW, Barnes KL. Suppurative arthritis complicating rheumatoid arthritis. *Br Med J.* 1958;1:1193–1199.

Keogh JB, Grieger JA, Noakes M, Clifton PM. Flow-Mediated Dilatation Is Impaired by a High-Saturated Fat Diet but Not by a High-Carbohydrate Diet. *Arterioscler Thromb Vasc Biol.* 2005 Mar 17

Kerckhoffs DA, Brouns F, Hornstra G, Mensink RP. Effects on the human serum lipoprotein profile of beta-glucan, soy protein and isoflavones, plant sterols and stanols, garlic and tocotrienols. *J Nutr.* 2002 Sep;132(9):2494-505.

Kessel S, Wittenberg CE. Joint infection in a young patient caused by Streptococcus uberis, a pathogen of bovine mastitis—a case report. *Z Orthop Unfall.* 2008 Jul-Aug;146(4):507-9.

Kesson AM, Bellemore MC, O'Mara TJ, Ellis DH, Sorrell TC. Scedosporium prolificans osteomyelitis in an immunocompetent child treated with a novel agent, hexadecylphospocholine (miltefosine), in combination with terbinafine and voriconazole: a case report. *Clin Infect Dis.* 2009 May 1;48(9):1257-61.

Keville K, Green M. *Aromatherapy: A Complete Guide to the Healing Art.* Freedom, CA: Crossing Press, 1995.

Key T, Appleby P, Davey G, Allen N, Spencer E, Travis R. Mortality in British vegetarians: review and preliminary results from EPIC-Oxford. *Amer. Jour. Clin. Nutr. Suppl.* 2003;78(3): 533S-538S.

Keynes SA, Due SL, Paul B. Pseudomonas arthropathy in an older patient. *Age Ageing.* 2009 Mar;38(2):245-6.

Khayyal MT, El-Ghazaly MA, Abdallah DM, Okpanyi SN, Kelber O, Weiser D. Mechanisms involved in the anti-inflammatory effect of a standardized willow bark extract. *Arzneimittelforschung.* 2005; 55 (11): 677-687.

Kim HM, Shin HY, Lim KH, Ryu ST, Shin TY, Chae HJ, Kim HR, Lyu YS, An NH, Lim KS. Taraxacum officinale inhibits tumor necrosis factor-alpha production from rat astrocytes. *Immunopharmacol Immunotoxicol.* 2000 Aug;22(3):519-30.

Kim JT, Ren CJ, Fielding GA, Pitti A, Kasumi T, Wajda M, Lebovits A, Bekker A. Treatment with lavender aromatherapy in the post-anesthesia care unit reduces opioid requirements of morbidly obese patients undergoing laparoscopic adjustable gastric banding. *Obes Surg.* 2007 Jul;17(7):920-5.

Kim LS, Axelrod LJ, Howard P, Buratovich N, Waters RF. Efficacy of methylsulfonylmethane (MSM) in osteoarthritis pain of the knee: a pilot clinical trial. *Osteoarthritis Cartilage.* 2006 Mar;14(3):286-94.

Kim SJ, Jung JY, Kim HW, Park T. Anti-obesity effects of Juniperus chinensis extract are associated with increased AMP-activated protein kinase expression and phosphorylation in the visceral adipose tissue of rats. *Biol Pharm Bull.* 2008 Jul;31(7):1415-21.

Kim YH, Kim KS, Han CS, Yang HC, Park SH, Ko KI, Lee SH, Kim KH, Lee NH, Kim JM, Son K. Inhibitory effects of natural plants of Jeju Island on elastase and MMP-1 expression. *Int J Cosmet Sci.* 2007 Dec;29(6):487-8.

Kimmatkar N, Thawani V, Hingorani L, Khiyani R. Efficacy and tolerability of Boswellia serrata extract in treatment of osteoarthritis of knee—a randomized double blind placebo controlled trial. *Phytomedicine.* 2003 Jan;10(1):3-7.

Kimmitt PT, Kirby A, Perera N, Nicholson KG, Schober PC, Rajakumar K, Chapman CA. Identification of Neisseria gonorrhoeae as the causative agent in a case of culture-negative dermatitis-arthritis syndrome using real-time PCR. *J Travel Med.* 2008 Sep-Oct;15(5):369-71.

Kisiel W, Barszcz B. Further sesquiterpenoids and phenolics from Taraxacum officinale. *Fitoterapia.* 2000 Jun;71(3):269-73.

Kisiel W, Michalska K. Sesquiterpenoids and phenolics from Taraxacum hondoense. *Fitoterapia.* 2005 Sep;76(6):520-4.

Kjeldsen-Kragh J, Haugen M, Borchgrevink CF, Forre O. Vegetarian diet for patients with rheumatoid arthritis—status: two years after introduction of the diet. Clin Rheumatol. 1994 Sep;13(3):475-82. Erratum in: *Clin Rheumatol.* 1994 Dec;13(4):649.

Kjeldsen-Kragh J, Haugen M, Borchgrevink CF, Laerum E, Eek M, Mowinkel P, Hovi K, Forre O. Controlled trial of fasting and one-year vegetarian diet in rheumatoid arthritis. *Lancet.* 1991 Oct 12;338(8772):899-902.

Kjeldsen-Kragh J, Haugen M, Forre O, Laache H, Malt UF. Vegetarian diet for patients with rheumatoid arthritis: can the clinical effects be explained by the psychological characteristics of the patients? *Br J Rheumatol.* 1994 Jun;33(6):569-75.

Kjeldsen-Kragh J. Rheumatoid arthritis treated with vegetarian diets. *Am J Clin Nutr.* 1999 Sep;70(3 Suppl):594S-600S.

Klarica J, Jajić I. The frequency of gout and other disorders of uric acid metabolism in Dalmatia in comparison with these disorders in Croatia. *Reumatizam.* 1993;40(2):1-5.

Klatz RM, Goldman RM, Cebula C. *Infection Protection.* New York: HarperResource, 2002.

Klein R, Landau MG. *Healing: The Body Betrayed.* Minneapolis: DCI:Chronimed, 1992.

Klein-Galczinsky C. Pharmacological and clinical effectiveness of a fixed phytogenic combination trembling poplar (Populus tremula), true goldenrod (Solidago virgaurea) and ash (Fraxinus excelsior) in mild to moderate rheumatic complaints. *Wien Med Wochenschr.* 1999;149(8-10):248-53.

Klickstein LB, Shapleigh C, Goetzl EJ. Lipoxygenation of arachidonic acid as a source of polymorphonuclear leukocyte chemotactic factors in synovial fluid and tissue in rheumatoid arthritis and spondyloarthritis. *J Clin Invest.* 1980 Nov;66(5):1166-70.

Kloss J. *Back to Eden.* Twin Oaks, WI: Lotus Press, 1939-1999.

Kneer W, Kühnau S, Bias P, Haag RF. Dimethylsulfoxide (DMSO) gel in treatment of acute tendopathies. A multicenter, placebo-controlled, randomized study. *Fortschr Med.* 1994 Apr 10;112(10):142-6.

Knudsen JF, Sokol GH. Potential glucosamine-warfarin interaction resulting in increased international normalized ratio: case report and review of the literature and MedWatch database. *Pharmacotherapy.* 2008 Apr;28(4):540-8.

Kobayashi H, Hall GS, Tuohy MJ, Knothe U, Procop GW, Bauer TW. Bilateral periprosthetic joint infection caused by Salmonella enterica serotype Enteritidis, and identification of Salmonella sp using molecular techniques. *Int J Infect Dis.* 2009 Mar 6.

Kobayashi S, Momohara S, Kamatani N, Okamoto H. Molecular aspects of rheumatoid arthritis: role of environmental factors. *FEBS J.* 2008 Sep;275(18):4456-62.

Kolb, K.H., Jaenicke, G., Kramer, M., Schulze, P.E. Absorption, distribution, and elimination of labeled dimethyl sulfoxide in man and animals. *Ann NY Acad Sci.* 1967;141:85-95, 1967.

Kolodziej H. Olimeric flavan-3-ols from medicinal willow bark. Phytochemistry. 1990; 29 (3): 955-960.

Komano Y, Harigai M, Koike R, Sugiyama H, Ogawa J, Saito K, Sekiguchi N, Inoo M, Onishi I, Ohashi H, Amamoto F, Miyata M, Ohtsubo H, Hiramatsu K, Iwamoto M, Minota S, Matsuoka N, Kageyama G, Imaizumi K, Tokuda H, Okoehi Y, Kudo K, Tanaka Y, Takeuchi T, Miyasaka N. Pneumocystis jiroveci pneumonia in patients with rheumatoid arthritis treated with infliximab: a retrospective review and case-control study of 21 patients. *Arthritis Rheum.* 2009 Mar 15;61(3):305-12.

Konrad L, Muller HH, Lenz C, Laubinger H, Aumüller G, Lichius JJ. Antiproliferative effect on human prostate cancer cells by a stinging nettle root (Urtica dioica) extract. *Planta Med.* 2000;66:44–47.

Koo HN, Hong SH, Song BK, Kim CH, Yoo YH, Kim HM. Taraxacum officinale induces cytotoxicity through TNF-alpha and IL-1alpha secretion in Hep G2 cells. *Life Sci.* 2004 Jan 16;74(9):1149-57.

Kowalchik C, Hylton W (eds). *Rodale's Illustrated Encyclopedia of Herbs.* Emmaus, PA: 1987.

Kowalczyk E, Krzesiński P, Kura M, Niedworok J, Kowalski J, Blaszczyk J. Pharmacological effects of flavonoids from Scutellaria baicalensis. *Przgl Lek.* 2006;63(2):95-6.

Kozan E, Küpeli E, Yesilada E. Evaluation of some plants used in Turkish folk medicine against parasitic infections for their in vivo anthelmintic activity. *J Ethnopharmacol.* 2006 Nov 24;108(2):211-6.

Kozlowski LT, Mehta NY, Sweeney CT, *et al.* Filter ventilation and nicotine content of tobacco in cigarettes from Canada, the United Kingdom, and the United States. *Tob Control.* 1998;7(4): 369-375.

Kreig M. *Black Market Medicine.* New York: Bantam, 1968.

Kris-Etherton, PM *et al.* High-monounsaturated Fatty Acid Diets Lower Both Plasma Cholesterol and Triacylglycerol Concentrations. *Am J Clin Nutr.* 1999;70:1009-15

Krivoy N, Pavlotzky E, Chrubasik S, Eisenberg E, Brook G. Effect of salicis cortex extract on human platelet aggregation. *Planta Medica.* 2001; 67 (3): 209-212.

Krsnich-Shriwise S. Fibromyalgia syndrome: an overview. *Phys Ther.* 1997;77:68-75.

Kruger K, Kamilli I, Schattenkirchner M. Blastocystis hominis as a rare arthritogenic pathogen. *Z Rheumatol.* 1994 Mar-Apr;53(2):83-5.

Krüger P, Kanzer J, Hummel J, Fricker G, Schubert-Zsilavecz M, Abdel-Tawab M. Permeation of Boswellia extract in the Caco-2 model and possible interactions of its constituents KBA and AKBA with OATP1B3 and MRP2. *Eur J Pharm Sci.* 2009 Feb 15;36(2-3):275-84.

Kubo I, Fujita K, Kubo A, Nihei K, Ogura T. Antibacterial activity of coriander volatile compounds against Salmonella choleraesuis. *J Agric Food Chem.* 2004 Jun 2;52(11):3329-32.

Kudriashov BA, Ammosova IaM, Liapina LA, Osipova NN, Azieva LD, Liapin GIu, Basanova AV. Heparin from the meadowsweet (Filipendula ulmaria) and its properties. *Izv Akad Nauk SSSR Biol.* 1991 Nov-Dec;(6):939-43.

Kudriashov BA, Liapina LA, Azieva LD. The content of a heparin-like anticoagulant in the flowers of the meadowsweet (Filipendula ulmaria). *Farmakol Toksikol.* 1990 Jul-Aug;53(4):39-41.

Kuipers JG, Sibilia J, Bas S, Gaston H, Granfors K, Vischer TL, Hajjaj-Hassouni N, Ladjouze-Rezig A, Sellami S, Wollenhaupt J, Zeidler H, Schumacher HR, Dougados M. Reactive and undifferentiated arthritis in North Africa: use of PCR for detection of Chlamydia trachomatis. *Clin Rheumatol.* 2009 Jan;28(1):11-6.

Kulkarni RR, Patki PS, Jog VP, Gandage SG, Patwardhan B. Treatment of osteoarthritis with a herbomineral formulation: a double-blind, placebo-controlled, cross-over study. *J Ethnopharmacol.* 1991 May-Jun;33(1-2):91-5.

Kung HC, Hoyert DL, Xu J, Murphy SL. Deaths: Final Data for 2005. *National Vital Statistics Reports.* 2008;56(10). http://www.cdc.gov/nchs/data/ nvsr/nvsr56/nvsr56_10.pdf. Accessed: 2008 Jun.

Kuo CH, Dai ZK, Wu JR, Hsieh TJ, Hung CH, Hsu JH. Septic arthritis as the initial manifestation of fatal Vibrio vulnificus septicemia in a patient with thalassemia and iron overload. *Pediatr Blood Cancer.* 2009 Jul 9.

Kuo IC, Lu PL, Lin WR, Lin CY, Chang YW, Chen TC, Chen YH. Sphingomonas paucimobilis bacteremia and septic arthritis in a diabetic patient presenting with septic pulmonary emboli. *J Med Microbiol.* 2009 Jun 15.

Kurowska M, Rudnicka W, Kontny E, Janicka I, Chorazy M, Kowalczewski J, Ziółkowska M, Ferrari-Lacraz S, Strom TB, Maśliński W. Fibroblast-like synoviocytes from rheumatoid arthritis patients express functional IL-15 receptor complex: endogenous IL-15 in autocrine fashion enhances cell proliferation and expression of Bcl-x(L) and Bcl-2. *J Immunol.* 2002 Aug 15;169(4):1760-7.

Kuznetsova TA, *et al.* Biological activity of fucoidans from brown algae and the prospects of their use in medicine. *Antibiot Khimioter.* 2004;49(5):24-30.

Lad V. Ayurveda: *The Science of Self-Healing.* Twin Lakes, WI: Lotus Press.

Laine L, Bombardier C, Hawkey CJ, Davis B, Shapiro D, Brett C, Reicin A. Stratifying the risk of NSAID-related upper gastrointestinal clinical events: results of a double-blind outcomes study in patients with rheumatoid arthritis. *Gastroenterology.* 2002 Oct;123(4):1006-12.

Laine L, Connors LG, Reicin A, Hawkey CJ, Burgos-Vargas R, Schnitzer TJ, Yu Q, Bombardier C. Serious lower gastrointestinal clinical events with nonselective NSAID or coxib use. *Gastroenterology.* 2003 Feb;124(2):288-92.

Lamaison JL, Carnat A, Petitjean-Freytet C. Tannin content and inhibiting activity of elastase in Rosaceae. *Ann Pharm Fr.* 1990;48(6):335-40.

Lamblin F, Hano C, Fliniaux O, Mesnard F, Fliniaux MA, Lainé E. Interest of lignans in prevention and treatment of cancers. *Med Sci.* 2008 May;24(5):511-9.

Lanhers MC, Fleurentin J, Mortier F, Vinche A, Younos C. Anti-inflammatory and analgesic effects of an aqueous extract of Harpagophytum procumbens. *Planta Med.* 1992 Apr;58(2):117-23.

Lappe FM. *Diet for a Small Planet.* New York: Ballantine, 1971.

Laudahn D, Walper A. Efficacy and tolerance of Harpagophytum extract LI 174 in patients with chronic non-radicular back pain. *Phytother Res.* 2001 Nov;15(7):621-4.

Lauder RM. Chondroitin sulphate: a complex molecule with potential impacts on a wide range of biological systems. *Complement Ther Med.* 2009 Jan;17(1):56-62.

LaValle JB. *The Cox-2 Connection.* Rochester, VT: Healing Arts, 2001.

Lazarou J, Pomeranz BH, Corey PN. Incidence of adverse drug reactions in hospitalized patients: a meta-analysis of prospective studies. *JAMA.* 1998 Apr 15;279(15):1200-5.

Lean G. US study links more than 200 diseases to pollution. London Independent. 2004 Nov 14.

Leape L. Lucian Leape on patient safety in U.S. hospitals. Interview by Peter I Buerhaus. *J Nurs Scholarsh.* 2004;36(4):366-70.

Leblan D, Chantre P, Fournié B. Harpagophytum procumbens in the treatment of knee and hip osteoarthritis. Four-month results of a prospective, multicenter, double-blind trial versus diacerhein. *Joint Bone Spine.* 2000;67(5):462-7.

Lee CK, Cheng YS. Diterpenoids from the leaves of Juniperus chinensis var. kaizuka. *J Nat Prod.* 2001 Apr;64(4):511-4.

Lee HS, Lee CS, Yang CJ, Su SL, Salter DM. Candida albicans induces cyclo-oxygenase 2 expression and prostaglandin E2 production in synovial fibroblasts through an extracellular-regulated kinase 1/2 dependent pathway. *Arthritis Res Ther.* 2009;11(2):R48.

Lee JH, Lee JH, Lee NY, Ha CW, Chung DR, Peck KR. [Two Cases of Septic Arthritis by Mycoplasma hominis after Total Knee Replacement Arthroplasty.]. *Korean J Lab Med.* 2009 Apr;29(2):135-9.

Lehmann B. The vitamin D3 pathway in human skin and its role for regulation of biological processes. *Photochem Photobiol.* 2005 Nov-Dec;81(6):1246-51.

Leitzmann C. Vegetarian diets: what are the advantages? *Forum Nutr.* 2005;(57):147-56.

Lenaers C, Brunet D, Ladegaillerie K, Pinel M, Closs B. Presented at the 16(th) DGK Symposium, March 2-4, 2005, Leipzig, Germany - Received the Award for the Best Poster Presentation 1 Influencing the equilibrium of the cutaneous ecosystem to improve the properties of skin prone to acne. *Int J Cosmet Sci.* 2007 Apr;29(2):143-4.

Leu YL, Shi LS, Damu AG. Chemical constituents of Taraxacum formosanum. Chem *Pharm Bull* . 2003 May;51(5):599-601.

Leu YL, Wang YL, Huang SC, Shi LS. Chemical constituents from roots of Taraxacum formosanum. *Chem Pharm Bull.* 2005 Jul;53(7):853-5.

Leventhal LJ, Boyce EG, Zurier RB. Treatment of rheumatoid arthritis with gammalinolenic acid. *Ann Intern Med.* 1993 Nov 1;119(9):867-73.

Lévesque H, Lafont O. [Aspirin throughout the ages: a historical review]. *Rev Med Intern.* 2000 Mar;21 Suppl 1:8s-17s.

Lewis WH, Elvin-Lewis MPF. *Medical Botany: Plants Affecting Man's Health.* New York: Wiley, 1977.

Lewontin R. *The Genetic Basis of Evolutionary Change.* New York: Columbia Univ Press, 1974.

Leyel CF. *Culpeper's English Physician & Complete Herbal.* Hollywood, CA: Wilshire, 1971.

Li X, Liu Z, Zhang XF, Wang LJ, Zheng YN, Yuan CC, Sun GZ. Isolation and characterization of phenolic compounds from the leaves of Salix matsudana. *Molecules.* 2008 Aug 3;13(8):1530-7.

Liapina LA, Koval'chuk GA. A comparative study of the action on the hemostatic system of extracts from the flowers and seeds of the meadowsweet (Filipendula ulmaria (L.) Maxim.). *Izv Akad Nauk Ser Biol.* 1993 Jul-Aug;(4):625-8.

Libby DB, Bearman G. Bacteremia due to Clostridium difficile-review of the literature. *Int J Infect Dis.* 2009 Apr 25.

Lim JP, Song YC, Kim JW, Ku CH, Eun JS, Leem KH, Kim DK. Free radical scavengers from the heartwood of Juniperus chinensis. *Arch Pharm Res.* 2002 Aug;25(4):449-52.

Lininger S, Gaby A, Austin S, Brown D, Wright J, Duncan A. *The Natural Pharmacy.* New York: Three Rivers, 1999.

Lipski E. *Digestive Wellness.* Los Angeles, CA: Keats, 2000.

Lloyd JU. *American Materia Medica, Therapeutics and Pharmacognosy.* Portland, OR: Eclectic Medical Publications, 1989-1983.

Lloyd-Still JD, Powers CA, Hoffman DR, Boyd-Trull K, Lester LA, Benisek DC, Arterburn LM. Bioavailability and safety of a high dose of docosahexaenoic acid triacylglycerol of algal origin in cystic fibrosis patients: a randomized, controlled study. *Nutrition.* 2006 Jan;22(1):36-46.

Lo GH, et al. (2003). Intra-articular hyaluronic acid in treatment of knee osteoarthritis. *JAMA,* 290(23): 3115-3121.

Lo GH, Niu J, McLennan CE, Kiel DP, McLean RR, Guermazi A, Genant HK, McAlindon TE, Hunter DJ. Meniscal damage associated with increased local subchondral bone mineral density: a Framingham study. *Osteoarthritis Cartilage.* 2008 Feb;16(2):261-7.

Lockie, L.M., Norcross, B. A clinical study on the effects of dimethyl sulfoxide in 103 patients with acute and chronic musculoskeletal injures and inflammation. *Ann NY Acad Sci.* 1967;141:599-602.

Loew D, Möllerfeld J, Schrödter A, Puttkammer S, Kaszkin M. Investigations on the pharmacokinetic properties of Harpagophytum extracts and their effects on eicosanoid biosynthesis in vitro and ex vivo. *Clin Pharmacol Ther.* 2001 May;69(5):356-64.

Loizzo MR, Saab AM, Tundis R, Statti GA, Menichini F, Lampronti I, Gambari R, Cinatl J, Doerr HW. Phytochemical analysis and in vitro antiviral activities of the essential oils of seven Lebanon species. *Chem Biodivers.* 2008 Mar;5(3):461-70.

Lomax AR, Calder PC. Probiotics, immune function, infection and inflammation: a review of the evidence from studies conducted in humans. *Curr Pharm Des.* 2009;15(13):1428-518.

Lopez-Garcia E, Schulze MB, Meigs JB, Manson JE, Rifai N, Stampfer MJ, Willett WC, Hu FB. Consumption of trans fatty acids is related to plasma biomarkers of inflammation and endothelial dysfunction. *J Nutr.* 2005 Mar;135(3):562-6.

Lovchik MA, Fráter G, Goeke A, Hug W. Total synthesis of junionone, a natural monoterpenoid from Juniperus communis L., and determination of the absolute configuration of the naturally occurring enantiomer by ROA spectroscopy. *Chem Biodivers.* 2008 Jan;5(1):126-39.

Luo W, Yu H, Cao Z, Schoeb TR, Marron M, Dybvig K. Association of Mycoplasma arthritidis mitogen with lethal toxicity but not with arthritis in mice. *Infect Immun.* 2008 Nov;76(11):4989-98.

Lykken DT, Tellegen A, DeRubeis R: Volunteer bias in twin research: the rule of two-thirds. *Soc Biol* 1978, 25(1): 1-9. Phillips DI: Twin studies in medical research: can they tell us whether diseases are genetically determined? *Lancet* 1993;341(8851): 1008-1009.

Mabey R, ed. *The New Age Herbalist.* New York: Simon & Schuster, 1941.

Maes HH, Silberg JL, Neale MC, Eaves LJ. Genetic and cultural transmission of antisocial behavior: an extended twin parent model. *Twin Res Hum Genet.* 2007 Feb;10(1):136-50.

Mahady GB, Pendland SL, Stoia A, Hamill FA, Fabricant D, Dietz BM, Chadwick LR. In vitro susceptibility of Helicobacter pylori to botanical extracts used traditionally for the treatment of gastrointestinal disorders. *Phytother Res.* 2005 Nov;19(11):988-91.

Mahdi JG, Mahdi AJ, Mahdi AJ, Bowen ID. The historical analysis of aspirin discovery, its relation to the willow tree and antiproliferative and anticancer potential. *Cell Prolif.* 2006;39(2):147-155.

Makrides M, Neumann M, Gibson R. Effect of maternal docosahexaenoic acid (DHA) supplementation on breast milk composition. *Europ Jrnl of Clin Nutr.* 1996;50:352-357.

Maksimović Z, Petrović S, Pavlović M, Kovacević N, Kukić J. Antioxidant activity of Filipendula hexapetala flowers. *Fitoterapia.* 2007 Apr;78(3):265-7.

Maliakal PP, Wanwimolruk S. Effect of herbal teas on hepatic drug metabolizing enzymes in rats. *J Pharm Pharmacol.* 2001 Oct;53(10):1323-9.

Mamalis IP, Panagopoulos MI, Papanastasiou DA, Bricteux G. [Sacroiliitis and osteomyelitis of the humeral bone du to Brucella melitensis in an adolescent]. *Rev Med Liege.* 2008 Dec;63(12):742-5.

Manso-Silván L, Vilei EM, Sachse K, Djordjevic SP, Thiaucourt F, Frey J. Mycoplasma leachii sp. nov. as a new species designation for Mycoplasma sp. bovine group 7 of Leach, and reclassification of Mycoplasma mycoides subsp. mycoides LC as a serovar of Mycoplasma mycoides subsp. capri. *Int J Syst Evol Microbiol.* 2009 Jun;59(Pt 6):1353-8.

Manz F. Hydration and disease. *J Am Coll Nutr.* 2007 Oct;26(5 Suppl):535S-541S.

Margioris AN. Fatty acids and postprandial inflammation. *Curr Opin Clin Nutr Metab Care.* 2009 Mar;12(2):129-37.

Martí-Bonmatí L, Sanz-Requena R, Rodrigo JL, Alberich-Bayarri A, Carot JM. Glucosamine sulfate effect on the degenerated patellar cartilage: preliminary findings by pharmacokinetic magnetic resonance modeling. *Eur Radiol.* 2009 Jun;19(6):1512-8.

Martinez M. Docosahexaenoic acid therapy in docosahexaenoic acid-deficient patients with disorders of peroxisomal biogenesis. Versicherungsmedizin. 1996;31 Suppl:145-152

Matsumoto AK, Bathon J, Bingham CO. Rheumatoid Arthritis Treatment. Johns Hopkins Medical Center. http://www.hopkins-arthritis.org/arthritis-info/rheumatoid-arthritis/rheum_treat.html. Accessed July, 2009.

Matsumoto, J. Clinical trials of dimethyl sulfoxide in rheumatoid arthritis patients in Japan. *Ann NY Acad Sci.* 1967;141:560-568.

Mattoli L, Cangi F, Maidecchi A, Ghiara C, Ragazzi E, Tubaro M, Stella L, Tisato F, Traldi P. Metabolomic fingerprinting of plant extracts. *J Mass Spectrom.* 2006 Dec;41(12):1534-45.

Mayes MD. Epidemiologic studies of environmental agents and systemic autoimmune diseases. *Environ Health Perspect.* 1999 Oct;107 Suppl 5:743-8.

Mazzio EA, Soliman KF. In vitro screening for the tumoricidal properties of international medicinal herbs. *Phytother Res.* 2009 Mar;23(3):385-98.

McAlindon T, Formica M, Schmid CH, Fletcher J. Changes in barometric pressure and ambient temperature influence osteoarthritis pain. *Am J Med.* 2007 May;120(5):429-34.

McAlindon T, Giannotta L, Taub N, *et al.* Environmental factors predicting nephritis in systemic lupus erythematosus. *Ann Rheum Dis.* 1993;52(10): 720-724.

McAlindon TE, Biggee BA. Nutritional factors and osteoarthritis: recent developments. *Curr Opin Rheumatol.* 2005 Sep;17(5):647-52.

McAlindon TE, Jacques P, Zhang Y, Hannan MT, Aliabadi P, Weissman B, Rush D, Levy D, Felson DT. Do antioxidant micronutrients protect against the development and progression of knee osteoarthritis? *Arthritis Rheum.* 1996 Apr;39(4):648-56.

McAlindon TE, Teale JD, Dieppe PA. Levels of insulin related growth factor 1 in osteoarthritis of the knee. *Ann Rheum Dis.* 1993 Mar;52(3):229-31.

McAlindon TE. Nutraceuticals: do they work and when should we use them? *Best Pract Res Clin Rheumatol.* 2006 Feb;20(1):99-115.

McConnaughey E. *Sea Vegetables.* Happy Camp, CA: Naturegraph, 1985.

McCune LM, Johns T. Antioxidant activity in medicinal plants associated with the symptoms of diabetes mellitus used by the indigenous peoples of the North American boreal forest. *J Ethnopharmacol.* 2002 Oct;82(2-3):197-205.

McDougall J, McDougall M. *The McDougal Plan.* Clinton, NJ: New Win, 1983.

McNally ME, Atkinson SA, Cole DE. Contribution of sulfate and sulfoesters to total sulfur intake in infants fed human milk. *J Nutr.* 1991 Aug;121(8):1250-4.

Medina JM, Thomas A, Denegar CR. Knee osteoarthritis: should your patient opt for hyaluronic acid injection? *J Fam Pract.* 2006 Aug;55(8):669-75.

Mehra PN, Puri HS. Studies on Gaduchi satwa. *Indian J Pharm.* 1969;31:180-2.

Meier B, Shao Y, Julkunen-Tiitto R, Bettschart A, Sticher O. A chemotaxonomic survey of phenolic compounds in Swiss willow species. Planta Med. 1992;58:A698.

Meier B, Sticher O, Julkunen-Tiitto R. Pharmaceutical aspects of the use of willows in herbal remedies. *Planta Med.* 1988;54(6):559-560.

Meini S, Maggi CA. Knee osteoarthritis: a role for bradykinin? *Inflamm Res.* 2008 Aug;57(8):351-61.

Melcion C, Verroust P, Baud L, Ardaillou N, Morel-Maroger L, Ardaillou R. Protective effect of procyanidolic oligomers on the heterologous phase of glomerulonephritis induced by anti-glomerular basement membrane antibodies. *C R Seances Acad Sci III.* 1982 Dec 6;295(12):721-6.

Melzig MF. Goldenrod—a classical exponent in the urological phytotherapy. *Wien Med Wochenschr.* 2004 Nov;154(21-22):523-7.

Menkes CJ, Renoux M, Laoussadi S, Mauborgne A, Bruxelle J, Cesselin F. Substance P levels in the synovium and synovial fluid from patients with rheumatoid arthritis and osteoarthritis. *J Rheumatol.* 1993 Apr;20(4):714-7.

Merchant RE and Andre CA. 2001. A review of recent clinical trials of the nutritional supplement Chlorella pyrenoidosa in the treatment of fibromyalgia, hypertension, and ulcerative colitis. *Altern Ther Health Med.* May-Jun;7(3):79-91.

Meyer A, Kirsch H, Domergue F, Abbadi A, Sperling P, Bauer J, Cirpus P, Zank TK, Moreau H, Roscoe TJ, Zahringer U, Heinz E. Novel fatty acid elongases and their use for the reconstitution of docosahex-aenoic acid biosynthesis. *J Lipid Res.* 2004 Oct;45(10):1899-909.

Miceli N, Trovato A, Dugo P, Cacciola F, Donato P, Marino A, Bellinghieri V, La Barbera TM, Güvenç A, Taviano MF. Comparative Analysis of Flavonoid Profile, Antioxidant and Antimicrobial Activity of the Berries of Juniperus communis L. var. communis and Juniperus communis L. var. saxatilis Pall. *J Agric Food Chem.* 2009 Jul 6.

Michalska K, Kisiel W. Sesquiterpene lactones from Taraxacum obovatum. *Planta Med.* 2003 Feb;69(2):181-3.

Miller GT. *Living in the Environment.* Belmont, CA: Wadsworth, 1996.

Miller K. Cholesterol and In-Hospital Mortality in Elderly Patients. Am Family Phys. 2004 May.

Mills SY, Jacoby RK, Chacksfield M, Willoughby M. Effect of a proprietary herbal medicine on the relief of chronic arthritis pain: a double-blind study. *Br J Rheumatol.* 1996; 35 (9): 874-878.

Milne BW, Arnold MH, Hudson B, Coolican MR. Infectious arthritis of the knee caused by Mycobacterium terrae: a case report. *J Orthop Surg.* 2009 Apr;17(1):103-8.

Mindell E, Hopkins V. *Prescription Alternatives.* New Canaan, CT: Keats, 1998.

Mindikoglu AL, Magder LS, Regev A. Outcome of liver transplantation for drug-induced acute liver failure in the United States: analysis of the united network for organ sharing database. *Liver Transpl.* 2009 Jul;15(7):719-29.

Mitchell AE, Hong YJ, Koh E, Barrett DM, Bryant DE, Denison RF, Kaffka S. Ten-year comparison of the influence of organic and conventional crop management practices on the content of flavonoids in to-matoes. *J Agric Food Chem.* 2007 Jul 25;55(15):6154-9.

Mohowald ML. Animal models of infectious arthritis. *Clin Rheum Dis.* 1986;12:403–421.

Monarca S, Donato F, Zerbini I, Calderon RL, Craun GF. Review of epidemiological studies on drinking water hardness and cardiovascular diseases. Eur J Cardiovasc Prev Rehabil. 2006 Aug;13(4):495-506.

Monarca S. Zerbini I, Simonati C, Gelatti U. Drinking water hardness and chronic degenerative diseases. Part II. Cardiovascular diseases. *Ann. Ig.* 2003;15:41-56.

Montero M, Horcajada JP, Sorlí L, Alvarez-Lerma F, Grau S, Riu M, Sala M, Knobel H. Effectiveness and Safety of Colistin for the Treatment of Multidrug-Resistant Pseudomonas aeruginosa Infections. *Infection.* 2009 Jun 4.

Moorhead KJ, Morgan HC. *Spirulina: Nature's Superfood.* Kailua-Kona, HI: Nutrex, 1995.

Mor A, Mitnick HJ, Greene JB, Azar N, Budnah R, Fetto J. Relapsing oligoarticular septic arthritis during etanercept treatment of rheumatoid arthritis. *J Clin Rheumatol.* 2006;12:87–9.

Morel AF, Dias GO, Porto C, Simionatto E, Stuker CZ, Dalcol II. Antimicrobial activity of extractives of Solidago microglossa. *Fitoterapia.* 2006 Sep;77(6):453-5.

Mortensen NP, Kuijf ML, Wim Ang C, Schiellerup P, Krogfelt KA, Jacobs BC, van Belkum A, Endtz HP, Bergman MP. Sialylation of Campylobacter jejuni lipo-oligosaccharides is associated with severe gas-tro-enteritis and reactive arthritis. *Microbes Infect.* 2009 Jul 21.

Mortia M, Nakamura H, Kitano T. Comparison of clinical outcome after treatment of hip arthritis caused by MRSA with that caused by non-MRSA in infants. *J Pediatr Orthop B.* 2009 Jan;18(1):1-5.

Moujir L, Seca AM, Silva AM, Barreto MC. Cytotoxic activity of diterpenes and extracts of Juniperus brevi-folia. *Planta Med.* 2008 Jun;74(7):751-3.

Moussaieff A, Shein NA, Tsenter J, Grigoriadis S, Simeonidou C, Alexandrovich AG, Trembovler V, Ben-Neriah Y, Schmitz ML, Fiebich BL, Munoz E, Mechoulam R, Shohami E. Incensole acetate: a novel neuroprotective agent isolated from Boswellia carterii. *J Cereb Blood Flow Metab.* 2008 Jul;28(7):1341-52.

Moussard C, Alber D, Toubin MM, Thevenon N, Henry JC. A drug used in traditional medicine, harpago-phytum procumbens: no evidence for NSAID-like effect on whole blood eicosanoid production in human. *Prostaglandins Leukot Essent Fatty Acids.* 1992 Aug;46(4):283-6.

Mozaffarian D, Aro A, Willett WC. Health effects of trans-fatty acids: experimental and observational evidence. *Eur J Clin Nutr.* 2009 May;63 Suppl 2:S5-21.

Muangchan C, Nilganuwong S. The study of clinical manifestation of osteoarticular tuberculosis in Siriraj Hospital, Thailand. *J Med Assoc Thai.* 2009 Mar;92 Suppl 2:S101-9.

Mühlbauer RC, Lozano A, Palacio S, Reinli A, Felix R. Common herbs, essential oils, and monoterpenes potently modulate bone metabolism. *Bone.* 2003 Apr;32(4):372-80.

Mundy GR. Osteoporosis and inflammation. *Nutr Rev.* 2007 Dec;65(12 Pt 2):S147-51.

Munkombwe NM. Acetylated phenolic glycosides from Harpagophytum procumbens. *Phytochemistry.* 2003 Apr;62(8):1231-4.

Muñoz-Mahamud E, Casanova L, Font L, Fernández-Valencia JA, Bori G. Septic arthritis of the hip caused by nontyphi Salmonella after urinary tract infection. *Am J Emerg Med.* 2009 Mar;27(3):373.e5-373.e8.

Murphy WA Jr, Nedden Dz D, Gostner P, Knapp R, Recheis W, Seidler H. The iceman: discovery and imaging. *Radiology.* 2003 Mar;226(3):614-29.

235

Murray M and Pizzorno J. *Encyclopedia of Natural Medicine.* 2nd Edition. Roseville, CA: Prima Publishing, 1998.

Na HJ, Koo HN, Lee GG, Yoo SJ, Park JH, Lyu YS, Kim HM. Juniper oil inhibits the heat shock-induced apoptosis via preventing the caspase-3 activation in human astrocytes CCF-STTG1 cells. *Clin Chim Acta.* 2001 Dec;314(1-2):215-20.

Nadkarni AK, Nadkarni KM. *Indian Materia Medica.* (Vols 1 and 2). Bombay, India: Popular Pradashan, 1908, 1976.

Nag HL, Neogi DS, Nataraj AR, Kumar VA, Yadav CS, Singh U. Tubercular infection after arthroscopic anterior cruciate ligament reconstruction. *Arthroscopy.* 2009 Feb;25(2):131-6.

Naghii MR, Samman S. The role of boron in nutrition and metabolism. *Prog Food Nutr Sci.* 1993 Oct-Dec;17(4):331-49.

Nahrstedt A, Schmidt M, Jäggi R, Metz J, Khayyal MT. Willow bark extract: the contribution of polyphenols to the overall effect. *Wien Med Wochenschr.* 2007;157(13-14):348-51.

Naqvi G, Malik S, Jan W. Necrotizing Fasciitis of the lower extremity: a case report and current concept of diagnosis and management. *Scand J Trauma Resusc Emerg Med.* 2009 Jun 15;17(1):28.

Nau R, Christen HJ, Eiffert H. Lyme disease—current state of knowledge. *Dtsch Arztebl Int.* 2009 Jan;106(5):72-81; quiz 82, I.

NDL, BHNRC, ARS, USDA. *Oxygen Radical Absorbance Capacity (ORAC) of Selected Foods - 2007.* Beltsville, MD: USDA-ARS. 2007.

Newall CA, Anderson LA, Philpson JD. *Herbal Medicine: A Guide for Healthcare Professionals.* London: Pharmaceutical Press, 1996.

Newmark T, Schulick P. *Beyond Aspirin.* Prescott, AZ: Holm, 2000.

Newnham RE. Essentiality of boron for healthy bones and joints. *Environ Health Perspect.* 1994 Nov;102 Suppl 7:83-5.

Nicholls SJ, Lundman P, Harmer JA, Cutri B, Griffiths KA, Rye KA, Barter PJ, Celermajer DS. Consumption of saturated fat impairs the anti-inflammatory properties of high-density lipoproteins and endothelial function. *J Am Coll Cardiol.* 2006 Aug 15;48(4):715-20.

Niederau C, Göpfert E. The effect of chelidonium- and turmeric root extract on upper abdominal pain due to functional disorders of the biliary system. Results from a placebo-controlled double-blind study. *Med Klin.* 1999 Aug 15;94(8):425-30.

Nielsen JD, Lind JW, Bruun B. Two cases of invasive Haemophilus influenzae type f infection. *Ugeskr Laeger.* 2009 Jan 19;171(4):247.

Nolla JM, Gomez-Vaquero C, Fiter J, Mateo L, Juanola X, Rodriguez-Moreno J. Pyarthrosis in patients with rheumatoid arthritis: A detailed analysis of 10 cases and literature review. *Semin Arthritis Rheum.* 2000;30:121–126.

Norton WL, Meisinger MA. An overview of nonsteroidal antiinflammatory agents (NSAIA). *Inflammation.* 1977 Mar;2(1):37-46.

NPSF. One Hundred Million Americans See Medical Mistakes Directly Touching Them as Patients, Friends, Relatives. *National Patient Safety Foundation.* Press Release. 1997 Oct 9. http://npsf.org/pr/pressrel/final-sur.htm. Acc. 2007 Mar.

Nuñez YO, Salabarria IS, Collado IG, Hernández-Galán R. Sesquiterpenes from the wood of Juniperus lucayana. *Phytochemistry.* 2007 Oct;68(19):2409-14.

Nyman T, Julkunen-Tiitto R. Chemical variation within and among six northern willow species. *Phytochemistry.* 2005; 66 (24): 2836-2843.

O'Connor A. The Claim: Raisins Soaked in Gin Can Ease Arthritis Pain. *NY Times.* 2006 Oct 3.

O'Connor J., Bensky D. (ed). *Shanghai College of Traditional Chinese Medicine: Acupuncture: A Comprehensive Text.* Seattle: Eastland Press, 1981.

O'Connor MI. Warming strengthens an herbivore-plant interaction. *Ecology.* 2009 Feb;90(2):388-98.

Oehme FW (ed.). *Toxicity of heavy metals in the environment. Part 1.* New York: M.Dekker, 1979.

Ogrendik M. Rheumatoid arthritis is linked to oral bacteria: etiological association. *Mod Rheumatol.* 2009 Jun 24.

Oh CK, Lücker PW, Wetzelsberger N, Kuhlmann F. The determination of magnesium, calcium, sodium and potassium in assorted foods with special attention to the loss of electrolytes after various forms of food preparations. *Mag.-Bull.* 1986;8:297-302.

Oh R. Practical applications of fish oil (Omega-3 fatty acids) in primary care. *J Am Board Fam Pract.* 2005 Jan-Feb;18(1):28-36.

Okasaka M, Takaishi Y, Kashiwada Y, Kodzhimatov OK, Ashurmetov O, Lin AJ, Consentino LM, Lee KH.Terpenoids from Juniperus polycarpus var. seravschanica. *Phytochemistry.* 2006 Dec;67(24):2635-40.

Olsson AR, Skogh T, Wingren G: Comorbidity and lifestyle, reproductive factors, and environmental exposures associated with rheumatoid arthritis. *Ann Rheum Dis.* 2001;60:934-939.

Ostensson A, Geborek P. Septic arthritis as a non-surgical complication in rheumatoid arthritis: Relation to disease severity and therapy. *Br J Rheumatol.* 1991;30:35–38.

Ottaviani S, Kemiche F, Thibault M, Cerf-Payrastre I, Pertuiset E. Polyarticular septic arthritis due to Moraxella canis revealing multiple myeloma. *Joint Bone Spine.* 2009 May;76(3):319-20.

Otto SJ, van Houwelingen AC, Hornstra G. The effect of supplementation with docosahexaenoic and arachidonic acid derived from single cell oils on plasma and erythrocyte fatty acids of pregnant women in the second trimester. *Prostaglandins Leukot Essent Fatty Acids.* 2000 Nov;63(5):323-8.

Ou CC, Tsao SM, Lin MC, Yin MC. Protective action on human LDL against oxidation and glycation by four organosulfur compounds derived from garlic. *Lipids.* 2003 Mar;38(3):219-24.

Pak CH, Oleneva VA, Agadzhanov SA. Dietetic aspects of preventing urolithiasis in patients with gout and uric acid diathesis. *Vopr Pitan.* 1985 Jan-Feb;(1).21-4.

Palazzi C, D'Angelo S, Olivieri I. Hepatitis C virus-related arthritis. *Autoimmun Rev.* 2008 Oct;8(1):48-51.

Parcell S. Sulfur in human nutrition and applications in medicine. *Altern Med Rev.* 2002 Feb;7(1):22-44.

Patberg WR, Rasker JJ. Weather effects in rheumatoid arthritis: from controversy to consensus. A review. *J Rheumatol.* 2004 Jul;31(7):1327-34.

Patwardhan B, Gautam M. Botanical immunodrugs: scope and opportunities. *Drug Discov Today.* 2005 Apr 1;10(7):495-502.

Payment P, Franco E, Richardson L, Siemiatyck, J. Gastrointestinal health effects associated with the consumption of drinking water produced by point-of-use domestic reverse-osmosis filtration units. *Appl Environ. Microbiol.* 1991;57:945-948.

Payment, P. (1989) Bacterial colonization of reverse-osmosis water filtration units. *Can. J. Microbiol.* 1989;35:1065-1067.

Pehowich DJ, Gomes AV, Barnes JA. Fatty acid composition and possible health effects of coconut constituents. *West Indian Med J.* 2000 Jun;49(2):128-33.

Peña-Sagredo JL, Hernández MV, Fernandez-Llanio N, Giménez-Ubeda E, Muñoz-Fernandez S, Ortiz A, Gonzalez-Gay MA, Fariñas MC; Biobadaser group. Listeria monocytogenes infection in patients with rheumatic diseases on TNF-alpha antagonist therapy: the Spanish Study Group experience. *Clin Exp Rheumatol.* 2008 Sep-Oct;26(5):854-9.

Pendell D. *Plant Powers, Poisons, and Herbcraft.* San Francisco: Mercury House, 1995.

Pepeljnjak S, Kosalec I, Kalodera Z, Blazević N. Antimicrobial activity of juniper berry essential oil (Juniperus communis L., Cupressaceae). *Acta Pharm.* 2005 Dec;55(4):417-22.

Percy, E.C., Carson, J.D. The use of DMSO in tennis elbow and rotator cuff tendinitis: A double-blind study. *Med Sci Sports Exercise.* 1981;13:215-219.

Pereira HL, Ribeiro SL, Pennini SN, Sato EI. Leprosy-related joint involvement. *Clin Rheumatol.* 2009 Jan;28(1):79-84.

Peresun'ko AP, Bespalov VG, Limarenko AI, Aleksandrov VA. Clinico-experimental study of using plant preparations from the flowers of Filipendula ulmaria (L.) Maxim for the treatment of precancerous changes and prevention of uterine cervical cancer. *Vopr Onkol.* 1993;39(7-12):291-5.

Pérez A, Herranz M, Padilla E, Ferres F. [Usefulness of synovial fluid inoculation in blood culture bottles for diagnosing Kingella kingae septic arthritis: State of the question.]. *Enferm Infecc Microbiol Clin.* 2009 Apr 29.

Perez-Galvez A, Martin HD, Sies H, Stahl W. Incorporation of carotenoids from paprika oleoresin into human chylomicrons. *Br J Nutr.* 2003 Jun;89(6):787-93.

Perez-Pena R. Secrets of the Mummy's Medicine Chest. *NY Times.* 2005 Sept 10.

Petlevski R, Hadzija M, Slijepcević M, Juretić D, Petrik J. Glutathione S-transferases and malondialdehyde in the liver of NOD mice on short-term treatment with plant mixture extract P-9801091. *Phytother Res.* 2003 Apr;17(4):311-4.

Petlevski R, Hadzija M, Slijepcević M, Juretić D. Toxicological assessment of P-9801091 plant mixture extract after chronic administration in CBA/HZg mice—a biochemical and histological study. *Coll Antropol.* 2008 Jun;32(2):577-81.

Petrek J, Havel L, Petrlova J, *et al.* Analysis of salicylic acid in willow barks and branches by en electrochemical method. *Russ J Plant Physiol.* 2007; 54 (4): 553-558.

Petri M, Allbritton J: Hair product use in systemic lupus erythematosus: a case-control study. *Arthritis Rheum.* 1992;35(6):625-629.

Petri M, Yadla N: Predictors of new development of proteinuria in SLE (suppl). *Arthritis Rheum.* 1995;S314.

Physicians' Desk Reference. Montvale, NJ: Thomson, 2003-2008

Picardo MC, de Melo Ferreira AC, Augusto da Costa AC. Biosorption of radioactive thorium by Sargassum filipendula. *Appl Biochem Biotechnol.* 2006 Sep;134(3):193-206.

Picardo MC, Ferreira AC, da Costa AC. Continuous thorium biosorption—dynamic study for critical bed depth determination in a fixed-bed reactor. *Bioresour Technol.* 2009 Jan;100(1):208-10.

Pintado-García V. Infectious spondylitis. *Enferm Infecc Microbiol Clin.* 2008 Oct;26(8):510-7.

Pitt-Rivers R, Trotter WR. *The Thyroid Gland.* London: Butterworth Publ, 1954.

Plohmann B, Bader G, Hiller K, Franz G. Immunomodulatory and antitumoral effects of triterpenoid saponins. *Pharmazie.* 1997 Dec;52(12):953-7.

Poblocka-Olech L, Krauze-Baranowska M. SPE-HPTLC of procyanidins from the barks of different species and clones of Salix. *J Pharm Biomed Anal.* 2008 Nov 4;48(3):965-8.

Poblocka-Olech L, van Nederkassel AM, Vander Heyden Y, Krauze-Baranowska M, Glód D, Baczek T. Chromatographic analysis of salicylic compounds in different species of the genus Salix. *J Sep Sci.* 2007 Nov;30(17):2958-66.

Pohl D. Epstein-Barr virus and multiple sclerosis. *J Neurol Sci.* 2009 Apr 9.

Ponsonby AL, McMichael A, van der Mei I. Ultraviolet radiation and autoimmune disease: insights from epidemiological research. *Toxicology.* 2002 Dec 27;181-182:71-8.

Postlethwait EM. Scavenger receptors clear the air. *J Clin Invest.* 2007 Mar;117(3):601-4.

Potterton D. (Ed.) *Culpeper's Color Herbal.* New York: Sterling, 1983.

Poukens-Renwart P, Tits M, Wauters JN, Angenot L. Densitometric evaluation of spiraeoside after derivatization in flowers of Filipendula ulmaria (L.) Maxim. *J Pharm Biomed Anal.* 1992 Oct-Dec;10(10-12):1085-8.

Preisinger E, Quittan M. Thermo- and hydrotherapy. *Wien Med Wochenschr.* 1994;144(20-21):520-6.

Prete PE, Gurakar-Osborne A, Kashyap ML. Synovial fluid lipoproteins: review of current concepts and new directions. *Semin Arthritis Rheum.* 1993 Oct;23(2):79-89.

Prucksunand C, Indrasukhsri B, Leethochawalit M, Hungspreugs K. Phase II clinical trial on effect of the long turmeric (Curcuma longa Linn) on healing of peptic ulcer. *Southeast Asian J Trop Med Public Health.* 2001 Mar;32(1):208-15.

Pruthi S, Thapa MM. Infectious and inflammatory disorders. *Magn Reson Imaging Clin N Am.* 2009 Aug;17(3):423-38, v.

Qi G, Hua H, Gao Y, Lin Q, Yu GY. Effects of Ganoderma lucidum spores on sialoadenitis of nonobese diabetic mice. *Chin Med J.* 2009 Mar 5;122(5):556-60.

Qi J, Chen JJ, Cheng ZH, Zhou JH, Yu BY, Qiu SX. Iridoid glycosides from Harpagophytum procumbens D.C. (devil's claw). *Phytochemistry.* 2006 Jul;67(13):1372-7.

Radulović N, Misić M, Aleksić J, Doković D, Palić R, Stojanović G. Antimicrobial synergism and antagonism of salicylaldehyde in Filipendula vulgaris essential oil. *Fitoterapia.* 2007 Dec;78(7-8):565-70.

Rahman MM, Bhattacharya A, Fernandes G. Docosahexaenoic acid is more potent inhibitor of osteoclast differentiation in RAW 264.7 cells than eicosapentaenoic acid. *J Cell Physiol.* 2008 Jan;214(1):201-9.

Raloff J. Ill Winds. *Science News:* 2001;160(14):218.

Randall CF. Stinging nettles for osteoarthritis pain of the hip. *Br J Gen Pract.* 1994 Nov;44(388):533-4.

Rao SK, Rao PS, Rao BN. Preliminary investigation of the radiosensitizing activity of guduchi (Tinospora cordifolia) in tumor-bearing mice. *Phytother Res.* 2008 Nov;22(11):1482-9.

Rappoport J. Both sides of the pharmaceutical death coin. *Townsend Letter for Doctors and Patients.* 2006 Oct.

Rauha JP, Remes S, Heinonen M, Hopia A, Kähkönen M, Kujala T, Pihlaja K, Vuorela H, Vuorela P. Antimicrobial effects of Finnish plant extracts containing flavonoids and other phenolic compounds. *Int J Food Microbiol.* 2000 May 25;56(1):3-12.

Rauma A. Antioxidant status in vegetarians versus omnivores. *Nutrition.* 2003;16(2): 111-119.

Raut AA, Sunder S, Sarkar S, Pandita NS, Vaidya AD. Preliminary study on crystal dissolution activity of Rotula aquatica, Commiphora wightii and Boerhaavia diffusa extracts. *Fitoterapia.* 2008 Dec;79(7-8):544-7.

Reger D, Goode S, Mercer E. *Chemistry: Principles & Practice.* Fort Worth, TX: Harcourt Brace, 1993.

Regis E. *Virus Ground Zero.* New York: Pocket, 1996.

Reichenbach S, Sterchi R, Scherer M, Trelle S, Bürgi E, Bürgi U, Dieppe PA, Jüni P. Meta-analysis: chondroitin for osteoarthritis of the knee or hip. *Ann Intern Med.* 2007 Apr 17;146(8):580-90.

Reichling J, Schmökel H, Fitzi J, Bucher S, Saller R. Dietary support with Boswellia resin in canine inflammatory joint and spinal disease. *Schweiz Arch Tierheilkd.* 2004 Feb;146(2):71-9.

Reiffenberger DH, Amundson LH. Fibromyalgia syndrome: a review. *Am Fam Physician.* 1996;53:1698-704.

Renoux M, Hilliquin P, Galoppin L, Florentin I, Menkes CJ. Release of mast cell mediators and nitrites into knee joint fluid in osteoarthritis—comparison with articular chondrocalcinosis and rheumatoid arthritis. *Osteoarthritis Cartilage.* 1996 Sep;4(3):175-9.

Renoux M, Hilliquin P, Galoppin L, Florentin J, Menkes CJ. Cellular activation products in osteoarthritis synovial fluid. *Int J Clin Pharmacol Res.* 1995;15(4):135-8.

Robert AM, Groult N, Six C, Robert L. The effect of procyanidolic oligomers on mesenchymal cells in culture II—Attachment of elastic fibers to the cells. *Pathol Biol.* 1990 Jun;38(6):601-7.

Robert AM, Robert L, Renard G. Protection of cornea against proteolytic damage. Experimental study of procyanidolic oligomers (PCO) on bovine cornea. *J Fr Ophtalmol.* 2002 Apr;25(4):351-5.

Robert AM, Tixier JM, Robert L, Legeais JM, Renard G. Effect of procyanidolic oligomers on the permeability of the blood-brain barrier. *Pathol Biol.* 2001 May;49(4):298-304.

Rodale R. *Our Next Frontier.* Emmaus, PA: Rodale, 1981.

Rodgers JT, Puigserver P. Fasting-dependent glucose and lipid metabolic response through hepatic sirtuin 1. Proc Natl Acad Sci USA. 2007 Jul 31;104(31):12861-6.

Rodriguez-Fragoso L, Reyes-Esparza J, Burchiel SW, Herrera-Ruiz D, Torres E. Risks and benefits of commonly used herbal medicines in Mexico. *Toxicol Appl Pharmacol.* 2008 Feb 15;227(1):125-35.

Rohekar S, Tsui FW, Tsui HW, Xi N, Riarh R, Bilotta R, Inman RD. Symptomatic acute reactive arthritis after an outbreak of salmonella. *J Rheumatol.* 2008 Aug;35(8):1599 602.

Rohner Mächler M, Glaus TM, Reusch CE. Life threatening intestinal bleeding in a Bearded Collie associated with a food supplement for horses. *Schweiz Arch Tierheilkd.* 2004 Oct;146(10):479-82.

Rooney PJ. Tuberculosis and secondary reactive arthritis. *J Rheumatol.* 2009 Jan;36(1):200; author reply 200.

Ros E, Mataix J. Fatty acid composition of nuts—implications for cardiovascular health. *Br J Nutr.* 2006 Nov;96 Suppl 2:S29-35. Erratum in: Br J Nutr. 2008 Feb;99(2):447-8.

Rosenau BJ, Schur PH. Association of measles virus with rheumatoid arthritis. *J Rheumatol.* 2009 May;36(5):893-7.

Rostom S, Bahiri R, Srifi N, Hajjaj-Hassouni N. [Multifocal septic arthritis and spondylitis due to salmonella complicating drepanocytosis]. *Presse Med.* 2009 Jul-Aug;38(7-8):1189-91.

Routasalo P, Isola A. The right to touch and be touched. *Nurs Ethics.* 1996 Jun;3(2):165-76.

Rozycki VR, Baigorria CM, Freyre MR, Bernard CM, Zannier MS, Charpentier M. Nutrient content in vegetable species from the Argentine Chaco. *Arch Latinoam Nutr.* 1997 Sep;47(3):265-70.

Rubin E., Farber JL. *Pathology.* 3rd Ed. Philadelphia: Lippincott-Raven, 1999.

Russell IJ. Advances in fibromyalgia: possible role for central neurochemicals. *Am J Med Sci.* 1998;315:377-84.

Ryman D. *Aromatherapy: The Complete Guide to Plant and Flower Essences for Health and Beauty.* New York: Bantam, 1993.

Ryzhikov MA, Ryzhikova VO. Application of chemiluminescent methods for analysis of the antioxidant activity of herbal extracts. *Vopr Pitan.* 2006;75(2):22-6.

Salem N, Wegher B, Mena P, Uauy R. Arachidonic and docosahexaenoic acids are biosynthesized from their 18-carbon precursors in human infants. Proc Natl Acad Sci. 1996;93:49-54.

Salido S, Altarejos J, Nogueras M, Sánchez A, Pannecouque C, Witvrouw M, De Clercq E. Chemical studies of essential oils of Juniperus oxycedrus ssp. badia. *J Ethnopharmacol.* 2002 Jun;81(1):129-34.

Salim, A.S., Role of oxygen-derived free radical scavengers in the management of recurrent attacks of ulcerative colitis: A new approach. *J. Lab Clin Med.* 1992;119:740-747.

Salman SA, Baharoon SA. Septic arthritis of the knee joint secondary to prevotella bivia. *Saudi Med J.* 2009 Mar;30(3):426-8.

Salom IL, Silvis SE, Doscherholmen A. Effect of cimetidine on the absorption of vitamin B12. *Scand J Gastroenterol.* 1982;17:129-31.

Samoylenko V, Dunbar DC, Gafur MA, Khan SI, Ross SA, Mossa JS, El-Feraly FS, Tekwani BL, Bosselaers J, Muhammad I. Antiparasitic, nematicidal and antifouling constituents from Juniperus berries. *Phytother Res.* 2008 Dec;22(12):1570-6.

Sanchez-Guerrero J, Karlson EW, Colditz GA, *et al.* Hair dye use and the risk of developing systemic lupus erythematosus. *Arthritis Rheum.* 1996;39(4):657-662.

Santos, L., Tipping, P.G. Attenuation of adjuvant arthritis in rats by treatment with oxygen radical scavengers. *Immunol Cell Biol.* 1994;72:406-414.

Santos-García Cuéllar MT, Negreira Cepeda S, Barrios López M. Listeria monocytogenes induced-chronic arthritis in an immunoincompetent child. *An Pediatr.* 2008 Nov;69(5):493-4.

Sassi AB, Harzallah-Skhiri F, Bourgougnon N, Aouni M. Antiviral activity of some Tunisian medicinal plants against Herpes simplex virus type 1. *Nat Prod Res.* 2008 Jan 10;22(1):53-65.

Satyanarayana S, Sushruta K, Sarma GS, Srinivas N, Subba Raju GV. Antioxidant activity of the aqueous extracts of spicy food additives—evaluation and comparison with ascorbic acid in in-vitro systems. *J Herb Pharmacother.* 2004;4(2):1-10.

Saur M, Distler O, Müller N. Septic arthritis? Gonococcal infection despite negative bacterial cultures. *Praxis.* 2008 Sep 10;97(18):977-83.

Sawitzke AD, Shi H, Finco MF, Dunlop DD, Bingham CO 3rd, Harris CL, Singer NG, Bradley JD, Silver D, Jackson CG, Lane NE, Oddis CV, Wolfe F, Lisse J, Furst DE, Reda DJ, Moskowitz RW, Williams HJ, Clegg DO. The effect of glucosamine and/or chondroitin sulfate on the progression of knee osteoarthritis: a report from the glucosamine/chondroitin arthritis intervention trial. *Arthritis Rheum.* 2008 Oct;58(10):3183-91.

Schauenberg P, Paris F. *Guide to Medicinal Plants.* New Canaan, CT: Keats Publ, 1977.

Schauss AG, Wu X, Prior RL, Ou B, Huang D, Owens J, Agarwal A, Jensen GS, Hart AN, Shanbrom E. Antioxidant capacity and other bioactivities of the freeze-dried Amazonian palm berry, Euterpe oleraceae mart. (acai). *J Agric Food Chem.* 2006 Nov 1;54(22):8604-10.

Scheer T, Wichtl M. On the Occurrence of Kaempferol-4'-O-beta-D-glucopyranoside in Filipendula ulmaria and Allium cepa. *Planta Med.* 1987 Dec;53(6):573-574.

Schempp H, Weiser D, Elstner EF. Biochemical model reactions indicative of inflammatory processes. Activities of extracts from Fraxinus excelsior and Populus tremula. *Arzneimittelforschung.* 2000 Apr;50(4):362-72.

Schepetkin IA, Faulkner CL, Nelson-Overton LK, Wiley JA, Quinn MT. Macrophage immunomodulatory activity of polysaccharides isolated from Juniperus scopolorum. *Int Immunopharmacol.* 2005 Dec;5(13-14):1783-99.

Scherbel, A.L., McCormack, L.J., Layle, J.K. Further observations on the effect of dimethyl sulfoxide in patients with generalized scleroderma (progressive systemic sclerosis). *Ann NY Acad Sci.* 1967;141:613-629.

Schilcher H, Leuschner F. The potential nephrotoxic effects of essential juniper oil. *Arzneimittelforschung.* 1997 Jul;47(7):855-8.

Schillaci D, Arizza V, Dayton T, Camarda L, Di Stefano V. In vitro anti-biofilm activity of Boswellia spp. oleogum resin essential oils. *Lett Appl Microbiol.* 2008 Nov;47(5):433-8.

Schmid B, Kötter I, Heide L. Pharmacokinetics of salicin after oral administration of a standardised willow bark extract. *Eur J Clin Pharmacol.* 2001 Aug;57(5):387-91.

Schmid B, Lüdtke R, Selbmann HK, Kötter I, Tschirdewahn B, Schaffner W, Heide L. Efficacy and tolerability of a standardized willow bark extract in patients with osteoarthritis: randomized placebo-controlled, double blind clinical trial. *Phytother Res.* 2001 Jun;15(4):344-50.

Schmid B, Lüdtke R, Selbmann HK, Kötter I, Tschirdewahn B, Schaffner W, Heide L. Effectiveness and tolerance of standardized willow bark extract in arthrosis patients. Randomized, placebo controlled double-blind study. *Z Rheumatol.* 2000 Oct;59(5):314-20.

Schneider I, Gibbons S, Bucar F. Inhibitory activity of Juniperus communis on 12(S)-HETE production in human platelets. *Planta Med.* 2004 May;70(5):471-4.

Schneider L, Ehlinger M, Stanchina C, Giacomelli MC, Gicquel P, Karger C, Clavert JM. Salmonella enterica subsp. arizonae bone and joints sepsis. A case report and literature review. *Orthop Traumatol Surg Res.* 2009 May;95(3):237-42.

Schottner M, Gansser D, Spiteller G. Lignans from the roots of Urtica dioica and their metabolites bind to human sex hormone binding globulin (SHBG). *Planta Med.* 1997;63:529–532.

Schulick P. *Ginger: Common Spice & Wonder Drug.* Brattleboro, VT: Herbal Free Perss, 1996.

Schumacher P. *Biophysical Therapy Of Allergies.* Stuttgart: Thieme, 2005.

Schütz K, Carle R, Schieber A. Taraxacum—a review on its phytochemical and pharmacological profile. *J Ethnopharmacol.* 2006 Oct 11;107(3):313-23.

Schwaninger M, Sallmann S, Petersen N, Schneider A, Prinz S, Libermann TA, Spranger M. Bradykinin induces interleukin-6 expression in astrocytes through activation of nuclear factor-kappaB. *J Neurochem.* 1999 Oct;73(4):1461-6.

Schwellenbach LJ, Olson KL, McConnell KJ, Stolepart RS, Nash JD, Merenich JA. The triglyceride-lowering effects of a modest dose of docosahexaenoic acid alone versus in combination with low dose eicosapentaenoic acid in patients with coronary artery disease and elevated triglycerides. *J Am Coll Nutr.* 2006;25(6):480-485.

Scott GN. Interaction of warfarin with glucosamine—chondroitin. *Am J Health Syst Pharm.* 2004 Jun 1;61(11):1186; author reply 1186.

Scott JT. New knowledge of the pathogenesis of gout. *J Clin Pathol Suppl.* 1978;12:205-13.

Seca AM, Silva AM, Bazzocchi IL, Jimenez IA. Diterpene constituents of leaves from Juniperus brevifolia. *Phytochemistry.* 2008 Jan;69(2):498-505.

Seca AM, Silva AM. The chemical composition of hexane extract from bark of Juniperus brevifolia. *Nat Prod Res.* 2008;22(11):975-83.

Selby A. *Aromatherapy.* New York: Macmillan, 1996.

Sengupta K, Alluri KV, Satish AR, Mishra S, Golakoti T, Sarma KV, Dey D, Raychaudhuri SP. A double blind, randomized, placebo controlled study of the efficacy and safety of 5-Loxin for treatment of osteoarthritis of the knee. *Arthritis Res Ther.* 2008;10(4):R85.

Seo K, Jung S, Park M, Song Y, Choung S. Effects of leucocyanidines on activities of metabolizing enzymes and antioxidant enzymes. *Biol Pharm Bull.* 2001 May;24(5):592-3.

REFERENCES AND BIBLIOGRAPHY

Seo SW, Koo HN, An HJ, Kwon KB, Lim BC, Seo EA, *et al*. Taraxacum officinale protects against chole-cystokinin-induced acute pancreatitis in rats. *World J Gastroenterol*. 2005;11:597–599.

Shams F, Asnis D, Lombardi C, Segal-Maurer S. A report of two cases of tuberculous arthritis of the ankle. *J Foot Ankle Surg*. 2009 Jul-Aug;48(4):452-6.

Sharma JN, Sharma JN. Comparison of the anti-inflammatory activity of Commiphora mukul (an indigenous drug) with those of phenylbutazone and ibuprofen in experimental arthritis induced by mycobacterial adjuvant. *Arzneimittelforschung*. 1977 Jul;27(7):1455-7.

Sherman G, Zeller L, Avriel A, Friger M, Harari M, Sukenik S. Intermittent balneotherapy at the Dead Sea area for patients with knee osteoarthritis. *Isr Med Assoc J*. 2009 Feb;11(2):88-93.

Shi S, Zhao Y, Zhou H, Zhang Y, Jiang X, Huang K. Identification of antioxidants from Taraxacum mongo-licum by high-performance liquid chromatography-diode array detection-radical scavenging detection electrospray ionization mass spectrometry and nuclear magnetic resonance experiments. *J Chromatogr A*. 2008 Oct 31;1209(1-2):145-52

Shi S, Zhou H, Zhang Y, Huang K, Liu S. Chemical constituents from Neo-Taraxacum siphonathum. *Zhongguo Zhong Yao Za Zhi*. 2009 Apr;34(8):1002-4.

Shi SY, Zhou CX, Xu Y, Tao QF, Bai H, Lu FS, Lin WY, Chen HY, Zheng W, Wang LW, Wu YH, Zeng S, Huang KX, Zhao Y, Li XK, Qu J. Studies on chemical constituents from herbs of Taraxacum mongo-licum. *Zhongguo Zhong Yao Za Zhi*. 2008 May;33(10):1147-57.

Shilova IV, Zhavoronok TV, Souslov NI, Novozheeva TP, Mustafin RN, Losseva AM. Hepatoprotective properties of fractions from meadowsweet extract during experimental toxic hepatitis. *Bull Exp Biol Med*. 2008 Jul;146(1):49-51.

Shilova IV, Zhavoronok TV, Suslov NI, Krasnov EA, Novozheeva TP, Veremeev AV, Nagaev MG, Petina GV. Hepatoprotective and antioxidant activity of meadowsweet extract during experimental toxic hepatitis. *Bull Exp Biol Med*. 2006 Aug;142(2):216-8.

Shirley, S.W., Stewart, B.H., Mirelman, S. Dimethyl sulfoxide in treatment of inflammatory genitourinary disorders. *Urology*. 1978;11:215-220.

Shishodia S, Harikumar KB, Dass S, Ramawat KG, Aggarwal BB. The guggul for chronic diseases: ancient medicine, modern targets. *Anticancer Res*. 2008 Nov-Dec;28(6A):3647-64.

Siala M, Gdoura R, Younes M, Fourati H, Cheour I, Meddeb N, Bargaoui N, Baklouti S, Sellami S, Rihl M, Hammami A. Detection and frequency of Chlamydia trachomatis DNA in synovial samples from Tu-nisian patients with reactive arthritis and undifferentiated oligoarthritis. *FEMS Immunol Med Microbiol*. 2009 Mar;55(2):178-86.

Sigstedt SC, Hooten CJ, Callewaert MC, Jenkins AR, Romero AE, Pullin MJ, Kornienko A, Lowrey TK, Slambrouck SV, Steelant WF. Evaluation of aqueous extracts of Taraxacum officinale on growth and invasion of breast and prostate cancer cells. *Int J Oncol*. 2008 May;32(5):1085-90.

Sigurdsson S, Gudbjarnason S. Inhibition of acetylcholinesterase by extracts and constituents from Angelica archangelica and Geranium sylvaticum. *Z Naturforsch C*. 2007 Sep-Oct;62(9-10):689-93.

Silman AJ, MacGregor AJ, Thomson W, *et al*. Twin concordance rates for rheumatoid arthritis: results from a nationwide study. *Br J Rheumatol*. 1993;32(10): 903-907.

Simopoulos AP. Essential fatty acids in health and chronic disease. *Am J Clin Nutr*. 1999 Sep;70(3 Suppl):560S-569S.

Singer P, Shapiro H, Theilla M, Anbar R, Singer J, Cohen J. Anti-inflammatory properties of omega-3 fatty acids in critical illness: novel mechanisms and an integrative perspective. *Intensive Care Med*. 2008 Sep;34(9):1580-92.

Singh BB, Mishra LC, Vinjamury SP, Aquilina N, Singh VJ, Shepard N. The effectiveness of Commiphora mukul for osteoarthritis of the knee: an outcomes study. *Altern Ther Health Med*. 2003 May-Jun;9(3):74-9.

Singh S, Khajuria A, Taneja SC, Johri RK, Singh J, Qazi GN. Boswellic acids: A leukotriene inhibitor also effective through topical application in inflammatory disorders. *Phytomedicine*. 2008 Jun;15(6-7):400-7.

Sipahi OR, Ozkören Calik S, Pullukçu H, Işikgöz Taşbakan M, Arda B, Tünger A, Ulusoy S. [Streptococcus equisimilis associated septic arthritis/prosthetic joint infection]. *Mikrobiyol Bul*. 2008 Jul;42(3):515-8.

Sivadon-Tardy V, Roux AL, Piriou P, Herrmann JL, Gaillard JL, Rottman M. Gardnerella vaginalis acute hip arthritis in a renal transplant recipient. *J Clin Microbiol*. 2009 Jan;47(1):264-5.

Sneader W. The discovery of aspirin: a reappraisal. *BMJ*. 2000 Dec 23;321;1591-1594.

Snowden N. Immunisation of Immunosuppressed Patients with Rheumatic Diseases. *Rep Rheumatic Dis*. 2007 Jun (5):12.

Sobel, D., Klein, A.C. *Arthritis: What Works*. New York: St. Martins Press, 1989.

Sofic E, Denisova N, Youdim K, Vatrenjak-Velagic V, De Filippo C, Mehmedagic A, Causevic A, Cao G, Joseph JA, Prior RL. Antioxidant and pro-oxidant capacity of catecholamines and related compounds.

Effects of hydrogen peroxide on glutathione and sphingomyelinase activity in pheochromocytoma PC12 cells: potential relevance to age-related diseases. *J Neural Transm.* 2001;108(5):541-57.

Sofic E, Rustembegovic A, Kroyer G, Cao G. Serum antioxidant capacity in neurological, psychiatric, renal diseases and cardiomyopathy. *J Neural Transm.* 2002 May;109(5-6):711-9.

Sompamit K, Kukongviriyapan U, Nakmareong S, Pannangpetch P, Kukongviriyapan V. Curcumin improves vascular function and alleviates oxidative stress in non-lethal lipopolysaccharide-induced endotoxaemia in mice. *Eur J Pharmacol.* 2009 Aug 15;616(1-3):192-9.

Spence A. *Basic Human Anatomy.* Menlo Park, CA: Benjamin/Commings, 1986.

Spiller G. *The Super Pyramid.* New York: HRS Press, 1993.

Spiridonov NA, Konovalov DA, Arkhipov VV. Cytotoxicity of some Russian ethnomedicinal plants and plant compounds. *Phytother Res.* 2005 May;19(5):428-32.

Sroka Z, Cisowski W, Seredyńska M, Luczkiewicz M. Phenolic extracts from meadowsweet and hawthorn flowers have antioxidative properties. *Z Naturforsch C.* 2001 Sep-Oct;56(9-10):739-44.

Stachowska E, Dolegowska B, Chlubek D, Wesolowska T, Ciechanowski K, Gutowski P, Szumilowicz H, Turowski R. Dietary trans fatty acids and composition of human atheromatous plaques. *Eur J Nutr.* 2004 Oct;43(5):313-8.

Steele JW, Ronald W. Phytochemistry of the Salicaceae. VI. The use of a gas-liquid chromatographic screening test for the chemotaxonomy of Populus species. *J Chromatogr.* 1973;84(2):315-318.

Stenberg JA, Hambäck PA, Ericson L. Herbivore-induced "rent rise" in the host plant may drive a diet breadth enlargement in the tenant. *Ecology.* 2008 Jan;89(1):126-33.

Stenberg JA, Witzell J, Ericson L. Tall herb herbivory resistance reflects historic exposure to leaf beetles in a boreal archipelago age-gradient. *Oecologia.* 2006 Jun;148(3):414-25.

Stengler M. *The Natural Physician's Healing Therapies.* Stamford, CT: Bottom Line Books, 2008.

Strle F, Stanek G. Clinical manifestations and diagnosis of lyme borreliosis. *Curr Probl Dermatol.* 2009;37:51-110.

Strom BL, Reidenberg MM, West S, *et al.* Shingles, allergies, family medical history, oral contraceptives, and other potential risk factors for systemic lupus erythematosus. *Am J Epidemiol* 1994, 140:632-642.

Strusberg I, Mendelberg RC, Serra HA, Strusberg AM. Influence of weather conditions on rheumatic pain. *J Rheumatol.* 2002 Feb;29(2):335-8.

Sulman FG, Levy D, Lunkan L, Pfeifer Y, Tal E. New methods in the treatment of weather sensitivity. *Fortschr Med.* 1977 Mar 17;95(11):746-52.

Sulman FG. Migraine and headache due to weather and allied causes and its specific treatment. *Ups J Med Sci Suppl.* 1980;31:41-4.

Sumantran VN, Kulkarni AA, Harsulkar A, Wele A, Koppikar SJ, Chandwaskar R, Gaire V, Dalvi M, Wagh UV. Hyaluronidase and collagenase inhibitory activities of the herbal formulation Triphala guggulu. *J Biosci.* 2007 Jun;32(4):755-61.

Sung JH, Lee JO, Son JK, Park NS, Kim MR, Kim JG, Moon DC. Cytotoxic constituents from Solidago virga-aurea var. gigantea MIQ. *Arch Pharm Res.* 1999 Dec;22(6):633-7.

Svendsen AJ, Holm NV, Kyvik K, *et al.* Relative importance of genetic effects in rheumatoid arthritis: historical cohort study of Danish nationwide twin population. *BMJ* 2002;324(7332): 264-266.

Sweeney B, Vora M, Ulbricht C, Basch E. Evidence-based systematic review of dandelion (Taraxacum officinale) by natural standard research collaboration. *J Herb Pharmacother.* 2005;5(1):79-93.

Takada Y, Ichikawa H, Badmaev V, Aggarwal BB. Acetyl-11-keto-beta-boswellic acid potentiates apoptosis, inhibits invasion, and abolishes osteoclastogenesis by suppressing NF-kappa B and NF-kappa B-regulated gene expression. *J Immunol.* 2006 Mar 1;176(5):3127-40.

Takasaki M, Konoshima T, Tokuda H, Masuda K, Arai Y, Shiojima K, Ageta H. Anti-carcinogenic activity of Taraxacum plant. I. *Biol Pharm Bull.* 1999 Jun;22(6):602-5.

Tan DX, Manchester LC, Reiter RJ, Qi WB, Karbownik M, Calvo JR. Significance of melatonin in antioxidative defense system: reactions and products. *Biol Signals Recept.* 2000 May-Aug;9(3-4):137-59.

Tapiero, H., G. N. Ba, *et al.* (2002). Polyunsaturated fatty acids (PUFA) and eicosanoids in human health and pathologies. Biomed Pharmacother. 56(5): 215-22.

Tapsell LC, Hemphill I, Cobiac L, Patch CS, Sullivan DR, Fenech M, Roodenrys S, Keogh JB, Clifton PM, Williams PG, Fazio VA, Inge KE. Health benefits of herbs and spices: the past, the present, the future. *Med J Aust.* 2006 Aug 21;185(4 Suppl):S4-24.

Taussig SJ, Batkin S. Bromelain, the enzyme complex of pineapple (Ananas comosus) and its clinical application. An update. *J Ethnopharmacol.* 1988 Feb-Mar;22(2):191-203.

Taylor RB, Lindquist N, Kubanek J, Hay ME. Intraspecific variation in palatability and defensive chemistry of brown seaweeds: effects on herbivore fitness. *Oecologia.* 2003 Aug;136(3):412-23.

Teitelbaum J. *From Fatigue to Fantastic.* New York: Avery, 2001.

REFERENCES AND BIBLIOGRAPHY

Thampithak A, Jaisin Y, Meesarapee B, Chongthammakun S, Piyachaturawat P, Govitrapong P, Supavilai P, Sanvarinda Y. Transcriptional regulation of iNOS and COX-2 by a novel compound from Curcuma comosa in lipopolysaccharide-induced microglial activation. *Neurosci Lett.* 2009 Sep 22;462(2):171-5.

Theofilopoulos AN, Kono DH: The genes of systemic autoimmunity. *Proc Assoc Am Physicians.* 1999;111(3): 228-240.

Thie J. *Touch for Health.* Marina del Rey, CA: Devorss Publications, 1973-1994.

Thieme H. Isolation of a new phenolic glycoside from the blossoms of Filipendula ulmaria (L.) Maxim. *Pharmazie.* 1966 Feb;21(2):123.

Thomas, R.G., Gebhardt, S.E. 2008. Nutritive value of pomegranate fruit and juice. *Maryland Dietetic Association Annual Meeting, USDA-ARS.* 2008 April 11.

Tierra L. *The Herbs of Life.* Freedom, CA: Crossing Press, 1992.

Tierra M. *The Way of Herbs.* New York: Pocket Books, 1990.

Tisserand R. *The Art of Aromatherapy.* New York: Inner Traditions, 1979.

Tissi L, Bistoni F, Puliti M. IL-4 deficiency decreases mortality but increases severity of arthritis in experimental group B Streptococcus infection. *Mediators Inflamm.* 2009;2009:394021.

Tiwari M. *Ayurveda: A Life of Balance.* Rochester, VT: Healing Arts, 1995.

Tlaskalová-Hogenová H, Stepánková R, Hudcovic T, Tucková L, Cukrowska B, Lodinová-Zádníková R, Kozáková H, Rossmann P, Bártová J, Sokol D, Funda DP, Borovská D, Reháková Z, Sinkora J, Hofman J, Drastich P, Kokesová A. Commensal bacteria (normal microflora), mucosal immunity and chronic inflammatory and autoimmune diseases. *Immunol Lett.* 2004 May 15;93(2-3):97-108.

Todd GR, Acerini CL, Ross-Russell R, Zahra S, Warner JT, McCance D. Survey of adrenal crisis associated with inhaled corticosteroids in the United Kingdom. *Arch Dis Child.* 2002 Dec;87(6):457-61.

Tonkal AM, Morsy TA. An update review on Commiphora molmol and related species. *J Egypt Soc Parasitol.* 2008 Dec;38(3):763-96.

Topçu G, Erenler R, Cakmak O, Johansson CB, Celik C, Chai HB, Pezzuto JM. Diterpenes from the berries of Juniperus excelsa. *Phytochemistry.* 1999 Apr;50(7):1195-9.

Towle A. *Modern Biology.* Austin: Harcourt Brace, 1993.

Travers V, Norotte G, Roger B, Apoil A. Traitement des arthrites aigues a pyogenes des grosses articulations des membres. A propos de 79 cas. *Rev Rhum.* 1988;55:655–660.

Trojanová I, Rada V, Kokoska L, Vlková E. The bifidogenic effect of Taraxacum officinale root. *Fitoterapia.* 2004 Dec;75(7-8):760-3.

Tsong T. Deciphering the language of cells. *Trends in Biochem Sci.* 1989;14:89-92.

Tulk HM, Robinson LE. Modifying the n-6/n-3 polyunsaturated fatty acid ratio of a high-saturated fat challenge does not acutely attenuate postprandial changes in inflammatory markers in men with metabolic syndrome. *Metabolism.* 2009 Jul 20.

Tupin E, Benhnia MR, Kinjo Y, Patsey R, Lena CJ, Haller MC, Caimano MJ, Imamura M, Wong CH, Crotty S, Radolf JD, Sellati TJ, Kronenberg M. NKT cells prevent chronic joint inflammation after infection with Borrelia burgdorferi. *Proc Natl Acad Sci U S A.* 2008 Dec 16;105(50):19863-8.

Turkulov V, Madle-Samardzija N, Canak G, Gavrancić C, Vukadinov J, Doder R. Various clinical manifestations of brucellosis infection. *Med Pregl.* 2008 Sep-Oct;61(9-10):517-20.

Turner RA, Schumacher HR, Myers AR. Phagocytic function of polymorphonuclear leukocytes in rheumatic disease. *J Clin Invest.* 1973;52:1632–1635.

Valle MG, Nano GM, Tira S. The Essential Oil of Filipendula ulmaria. *Planta Med.* 1988 Apr;54(2):181-182.

Van Albada-Kuipers GA, Linthorst J, Peeters EAJ, Breeveld FC, Dijkmans BAC, Hermans J, vanden-broucke JP, Cats A. Frequency of infection among patients with rheumatoid arthritis versus patients with osteoarthritis or soft tissue rheumatism. *Arthritis Rheum.* 1988;31:667–671.

van Beelen VA, Roeleveld J, Mooibroek H, Sijtsma L, Bino RJ, Bosch D, Rietjens IM, Alink GM. A comparative study on the effect of algal and fish oil on viability and cell proliferation of Caco-2 cells. *Food Chem Toxicol.* 2007 May;45(5):716-24.

Van Cauter E, Leproult R, Plat L. Age-related changes in slow wave sleep and REM sleep and relationship with growth hormone and cortisol levels in healthy men. *JAMA.* 2000 Aug 16;284(7):861-8.

Van Slambrouck S, Daniels AL, Hooten CJ, Brock SL, Jenkins AR, Ogasawara MA, Baker JM, Adkins G, Elias EM, Agustin VJ, Constantine SR, Pullin MJ, Shors ST, Kornienko A, Steelant WF. Effects of crude aqueous medicinal plant extracts on growth and invasion of breast cancer cells. *Oncol Rep.* 2007 Jun;17(6):1487-92.

Vanderbroucke JP, Kaaks R, Valkenburg HA, Boersma JW, Cats A, Festen JJM, Hartman AP, Huber-Bruning O, Rasker JJ, Weber J. Frequency of infections among rheumatoid arthritis patients, before and after disease onset. *Arthritis Rheum.* 1987;30:810–813.

Vane JR, Botting RM. The mechanism of action of aspirin. *Thromb Res.* 2003 Jun 15;110(5-6):255-8.

243

Vane JR. The fight against rheumatism: from willow bark to COX-1 sparing drugs. *J Physiol Pharmacol.* 2000 Dec;51(4 Pt 1):573-86.

Vassilopoulos D, Calabrese LH. Virally associated arthritis 2008: clinical, epidemiologic, and pathophysiologic considerations. *Arthritis Res Ther.* 2008;10(5):215.

Venkatachalam KV. Human 3'-phosphoadenosine 5'-phosphosulfate (PAPS) synthase: biochemistry, molecular biology and genetic deficiency. *IUBMB Life.* 2003 Jan;55(1):1-11.

Vidgren HM, Agren JJ, Schwab U, Rissanen T, Hanninen O, Uusitupa MI. Incorporation of n-3 fatty acids into plasma lipid fractions, and erythrocyte membranes and platelets during dietary supplementation with fish, fish oil, and docosahexaenoic acid-rich oil among healthy young men. *Lipids.* 1997 Jul;32(7):697-705.

Vila R, Mundina M, Tomi F, Furlán R, Zacchino S, Casanova J, Cañigueral S. Composition and antifungal activity of the essential oil of Solidago chilensis. *Planta Med.* 2002 Feb;68(2):164-7.

Vílchez Aparicio V, Toledano Martínez E, Narrarro Laredo JL, García Vadillo JA. Septic arthritis and osteomyelitis caused by Pasteurella multocida: a new case. *Rev Clin Esp.* 2009 Apr;209(4):205-6.

Vinson JA, Proch J, Bose P. MegaNatural((R)) Gold Grapeseed Extract: In Vitro Antioxidant and In Vivo Human Supplementation Studies. *J Med Food.* 2001 Spring;4(1):17-26.

Visser S, Tupper J. Septic until proven otherwise: approach to and treatment of the septic joint in adult patients. *Can Fam Physician.* 2009 Apr;55(4):374-5.

Vlachojannis J, Roufogalis BD, Chrubasik S. Systematic review on the safety of Harpagophytum preparations for osteoarthritic and low back pain. *Phytother Res.* 2008 Feb;22(2):149-52.

Vlachojannis JE, Cameron M, Chrubasik S. A systematic review on the effectiveness of willow bark for musculoskeletal pain. *Phytother Res.* 2009 Jul;23(7):897-900.

Vlad SC, LaValley MP, McAlindon TE, Felson DT. Glucosamine for pain in osteoarthritis: why do trial results differ? *Arthritis Rheum.* 2007 Jul;56(7):2267-77.

Vojdani A. Antibodies as predictors of complex autoimmune diseases. *Int J Immunopathol Pharmacol.* 2008 Apr-Jun;21(2):267-78.

Volesky B, Weber J, Park JM. Continuous-flow metal biosorption in a regenerable Sargassum column. *Water Res.* 2003 Jan;37(2):297-306.

von Kruedener S, Schneider W, Elstner EF. A combination of Populus tremula, Solidago virgaurea and Fraxinus excelsior as an anti-inflammatory and antirheumatic drug. A short review. *Arzneimittelforschung.* 1995 Feb;45(2):169-71.

Wagner I, Greim C, Laufer S, Heide L, Gleiter CH. Influence of willow bark extract on cyclooxygenase activity and on tumor necrosis factor alpha or interleukin 1 beta release in vitro and ex vivo. *Clin Pharmacol Ther.* 2003; 73 (3): 272-274.

Wahler D, Gronover CS, Richter C, Foucu F, Twyman RM, Moerschbacher BM, Fischer R, Muth J, Prufer D. Polyphenoloxidase silencing affects latex coagulation in Taraxacum spp. *Plant Physiol.* 2009 Jul 15.

Walsh SJ, Rau LM: Autoimmune diseases: a leading cause of death among young and middle-aged women in the United States. *Am J Public Health* 2000, 90(9): 1463-1466.

Wang C, Ao Y, Wang J, Hu Y, Cui G, Yu J. Septic arthritis after arthroscopic anterior cruciate ligament reconstruction: a retrospective analysis of incidence, presentation, treatment, and cause. *Arthroscopy.* 2009 Mar;25(3):243-9.

Wang CT, et al. Therapeutic effects of hyaluronic acid on osteoarthritis of the knee: A meta-analysis of randomized controlled trials. *J of Bone and Jnt Surg.* 2004;86-A(3): 538–545.

Wang WS, Li EW, Jia ZJ. Terpenes from Juniperus przewalskii and their antitumor activities. *Pharmazie.* 2002 May;57(5):343-5.

Wangsomboonsiri W, Luksananun T, Saksornchai S, Ketwong K, Sungkanuparph S. Streptococcus suis infection and risk factors for mortality. *J Infect.* 2008 Nov;57(5):392-6.

Wanjari K, Baradkar VP, Mathur M, Kumar S. Tuberculous synovitis in a HIV positive patient. *Indian J Med Microbiol.* 2009 Jan-Mar;27(1):72-5.

Warnock M, McBean D, Suter A, Tan J, Whittaker P. Effectiveness and safety of Devil's Claw tablets in patients with general rheumatic disorders. *Phytother Res.* 2007 Dec;21(12):1228-33.

Watkins BA, Hannon K, Ferruzzi M, Li Y. Dietary PUFA and flavonoids as deterrents for environmental pollutants. *J Nutr Biochem.* 2007 Mar;18(3):196-205.

Webster D, Taschereau P, Belland RJ, Sand C, Rennie RP. Antifungal activity of medicinal plant extracts; preliminary screening studies. *J Ethnopharmacol.* 2008 Jan 4;115(1):140-6.

Wedge DE, Tabanca N, Sampson BJ, Werle C, Demirci B, Baser KH, Nan P, Duan J, Liu Z. Antifungal and insecticidal activity of two Juniperus essential oils. *Nat Prod Commun.* 2009 Jan;4(1):123-7.

Wegener T, Lüpke NP. Treatment of patients with arthrosis of hip or knee with an aqueous extract of devil's claw (Harpagophytum procumbens DC.). *Phytother Res.* 2003 Dec;17(10):1165-72.

Wegrowski J, Robert AM, Moczar M. The effect of procyanidolic oligomers on the composition of normal and hypercholesterolemic rabbit aortas. *Biochem Pharmacol.* 1984 Nov 1;33(21):3491-7.

Wei A, Shibamoto T. Antioxidant activities and volatile constituents of various essential oils. *J Agric Food Chem.* 2007 Mar 7;55(5):1737-42.

Weidema IR, Magnussen LS, Philipp M. Gene flow and mode of pollination in a dry-grassland species, Filipendula vulgaris (Rosaceae). *Heredity.* 2000 Mar;84 (Pt 3):311-20.

Weiner MA. *Secrets of Fijian Medicine.* Berkeley, CA: Univ. of Calif., 1969.

Weiss RF. *Herbal Medicine.* Gothenburg, Sweden: Beaconsfield, 1988.

Weissmann G. Aspirin. *Sci Am.* 1991;264 (1): 84-90.

Whitfield KE, Wiggins SA, Belue R, Brandon DT. Genetic and environmental influences on forced expiratory volume in African Americans: the Carolina African-American Twin Study of Aging. *Ethn Dis.* 2004 Spring;14(2):206-11.

Werbach M. *Nutritional Influences on Illness.* Tarzana, CA: Third Line Press, 1996.

West R. Risk of death in meat and non-meat eaters. *BMJ.* 1994 Oct 8;309(6959):955.

White A. Stinging nettles for osteoarthritis pain of the hip. *Br J Gen Pract.* 1995 Mar;45(392):162.

WHO. *Guidelines for Drinking-water Quality.* 2nd ed, vol. 2. Geneva: World Health Organization, 1996.

WHO. *Guidelines on health aspects of water desalination.* ETS/80.4. Geneva: World Health Organization, 1980.

WHO. Health effects of the removal of substances occurring naturally in drinking water, with special reference to demineralized and desalinated water. Report on a working group (Brussels, 20-23 March 1978). *EURO Reports and Studies.* 1979;16.

WHO. How trace elements in water contribute to health. *WHO Chronicle.* 1978;32:382-385.

Wigler I, Grotto I, Caspi D, Yaron M. The effects of Zintona EC (a ginger extract) on symptomatic gonarthritis. *Osteoarthritis Cartilage.* 2003 Nov;11(11):783-9.

Wilson L. *Nutritional Balancing and Hair Mineral Analysis.* Prescott, AZ: LD Wilson, 1998.

Wilson PC, Rinker B. The incidence of methicillin-resistant staphylococcus aureus in community-acquired hand infections. *Ann Plast Surg.* 2009 May;62(5):513-6.

Wilton JMA, Gibson T, Chuck CM. Defective phagocytosis by synovial fluid and blood polymorphonuclear leukocytes in patients with rheumatoid arthritis. *Rheumatol Rehabil.* 1978;17:25-35.

Winchester AM. *Biology and its Relation to Mankind.* New York: Van Nostrand Reinhold, 1969.

Winstein KJ, Armstrong D. Top Pain Scientist Fabricated Data in Studies, Hospital Says. *Wall Street J.* 2009 March 11. http://online.wsj.com/article/SB123672510903888207.html?mod=loomia&loomia_si=t0:a16:g2:r1:c0 .0270612:b22894832. Accessed July, 2009.

Wittenberg JS. *The Rebellious Body.* New York: Insight, 1996.

Wong SL, Anthony EY, Shetty AK. Pyomyositis due to Streptococcus pneumoniae. *Am J Emerg Med.* 2009 Jun;27(5):633.e1-3.

Woo KJ, Kwon TK. Sulforaphane suppresses lipopolysaccharide-induced cyclooxygenase-2 (COX-2) expression through the modulation of multiple targets in COX-2 gene promoter. *Int Immunopharmacol.* 2007 Dec 15;7(13):1776-83.

Wood M. *The Book of Herbal Wisdom.* Berkeley, CA: North Atlantic, 1997.

Worwood VA. *The Complete Book of Essential Oils & Aromatherapy.* San Rafael, CA: New World, 1991.

Wu S, Yang L, Gao Y, Liu X, Liu F. Multi-channel counter-current chromatography for high-throughput fractionation of natural products for drug discovery. *J Chromatogr A.* 2008 Feb 8;1180(1-2):99-107.

Yadav VS, Mishra KP, Singh DP, Mehrotra S, Singh VK. Immunomodulatory effects of curcumin. *Immunopharmacol Immunotoxicol.* 2005;27(3):485-97.

Yamamoto H, Teramoto S, Matsui H, Matsuse T, Toba K, Ouchi Y. [An elderly case with pseudogout exacerbated by the administration of granulocyte-colony stimulating factor during drug-induced granulocytopenia]. *Nippon Ronen Igakkai Zasshi.* 1999 Aug;36(8):572-5.

Yang WC, Huang YC, Tsai MH, Chiu CH, Jaing TH. Salmonella septic arthritis involving multiple joints in a girl with acute lymphoblastic leukemia at diagnosis. *Pediatr Neonatol.* 2009 Feb;50(1):33-5.

Yao Q, Frank M, Glynn M, Altman RD. Rheumatic manifestations in HIV-1 infected in-patients and literature review. *Clin Exp Rheumatol.* 2008 Sep-Oct;26(5):799-806.

Yarnell E. Botanical medicines for the urinary tract. *World J Urol.* 2002 Nov;20(5):285-93.

Yeager S. *The Doctor's Book of Food Remedies.* Emmaus, PA: Rodale Press, 1998.

Yip YB, Tam AC. An experimental study on the effectiveness of massage with aromatic ginger and orange essential oil for moderate-to-severe knee pain among the elderly in Hong Kong. *Complement Ther Med.* 2008 Jun;16(3):131-8.

Youn YN, Lim E, Lee N, Kim YS, Koo MS, Choi SY. Screening of Korean medicinal plants for possible osteoclastogenesis effects in vitro. *Genes Nutr.* 2008 Feb;2(4):375-80.

Zaki SA, Phulsunder A, Shanbag P. Arthritis as the presenting feature of HIV infection in a child. *J Infect.* 2009 May;58(5):391-2.

Zhang J, Zhang X, Lei G, Li B, Chen J, Zhou T. A new phenolic glycoside from the aerial parts of Solidago canadensis. *Fitoterapia.* 2007 Jan;78(1):69-71.

Zhang Y, Hannan MT, Chaisson CE, McAlindon TE, Evans SR, Aliabadi P, Levy D, Felson DT. Bone mineral density and risk of incident and progressive radiographic knee osteoarthritis in women: the Framingham Study. *J Rheumatol.* 2000 Apr;27(4):1032-7.

Zhang Y, McAlindon TE, Hannan MT, Chaisson CE, Klein R, Wilson PW, Felson DT. Estrogen replacement therapy and worsening of radiographic knee osteoarthritis: the Framingham Study. *Arthritis Rheum.* 1998 Oct;41(10):1867-73.

Zheng M. Experimental study of 472 herbs with antiviral action against the herpes simplex virus. *Zhong Xi Yi Jie He Za Zhi.* 1990 Jan;10(1):39-41, 6.

Zizza, C. The nutrient content of the Italian food supply 1961-1992. *Euro J Clin Nutr.* 1997;51: 259-265.

Index